AF770964

Pleasure in the Middle Ages

INTERNATIONAL MEDIEVAL RESEARCH

Editorial Board

Axel E. W. Müller, *University of Leeds* — Executive Editor
John B. Dillon, *University of Wisconsin, Madison*
Richard K. Emmerson, *Manhattan College, New York*
Christian Krötzl, *University of Tampere*
Chris P. Lewis, *University of London*
Pauline Stafford, *University of Leeds / University of Liverpool*

with the assistance of the IMC Programming Committee

Previously published volumes in this series are listed at the back of the book.

VOLUME 24

Pleasure in the Middle Ages

Edited by

Naama Cohen-Hanegbi
and Piroska Nagy

BREPOLS

British Library Cataloguing in Publication Data

A catalogue record for this book is available from the British Library.

© 2018, Brepols Publishers n.v., Turnhout, Belgium

All rights reserved. No part of this publication may be reproduced, stored in a retrieval system, or transmitted, in any form or by any means, electronic, mechanical, photocopying, recording, or otherwise, without the prior permission of the publisher.

D/2018/0095/48
ISBN: 978-2-503-57520-9
e-ISBN: 978-2-503-57521-6
DOI: 10.1484/M.IMR-EB.5.112956
Printed in the EU on acid-free paper

Contents

List of Illustrations viii

Acknowledgements ix

Abbreviations x

Pleasure in the Middle Ages: An Introduction
NAAMA COHEN-HANEGBI and PIROSKA NAGY xi

Pleasured Bodies

Reflections on High Medieval Monastic Pleasures
ESTHER COHEN 3

'It Is Full Merry in Heaven': The Pleasurable Connotations of 'Merriment' in Late Medieval England
PHILIPPA C. MADDERN 21

The Pleasures and Joys of the Humoral Body in Medieval Medicine
FERNANDO SALMÓN 39

Bodily Pleasures: Late Medieval Medical Counsel in Context
NAAMA COHEN-HANEGBI 59

Visual Pleasure and the Illuminated Prayer Book
MAEVE DOYLE 77

Abbasid Concubines and Slave Courtesans in *Adab* Discourse:
Cultural Mediators for an Ethical Appreciation of Pleasure
KAREN MOUKHEIBER 113

Courts and Pleasures: The Neuroscience of Pleasure and
the Pursuit of Favour in Twelfth-Century Courts
WILLIAM M. REDDY 131

Didactic Pleasures

Taking Pleasure in Virtues and Vices:
Alcuin's Manual for Count Wido
BARBARA H. ROSENWEIN 167

Sin, the Business of Pleasure, and the Pleasure of Reading:
Exemplary Narratives and Other Forms of Sinful Pleasure
in William Peraldus's *Summa de vitiis*
RICHARD NEWHAUSER 181

The Role of Pleasure in the Acquisition of Good Virtues:
Giles of Rome's Idea of Education in his
De regimine principum (*c.* 1279)
NOËLLE-LAETITIA PERRET 203

Pleasure as an Affective Tool in Pastoral Care:
The Cases of Simone Fidati and Richard Rolle
in Fourteenth-Century Italy and England
XAVIER BIRON-OUELLET 225

Hell: The Pleasure of the Suffering of Others from Visions
of the Afterlife to Religious Theatre
ÉLYSE DUPRAS 249

Pleasures in God

Holy Gluttons: Bede and the Carolingians
on the Pleasures of Reading
ZACHARY GIULIANO 281

On Leeks and Onions: Pope Gregory VII
and the Rejection of Pleasure
KEN A. GRANT 309

Intoxication and the Song of Songs: Bernard of Clairvaux
and the Rediscovery of Origen in the Twelfth Century
CONSTANT J. MEWS 329

Pleasure in Medieval Christian Mystical Literature:
The Analysis of John of Ruusbroec (1281–1381)
and Hadewijch (Thirteenth Century)
ROB FAESEN 353

Index 379

List of Illustrations

Figure 1, p. 79. 'Cambrai Hours. Hours of the Virgin, Lauds: Temptation of Bed', Cambrai, Bibliothèque municipale, MS 87, fol. 29^{r}. Before 1297.

Figure 2, p. 83. 'Cambrai Hours. Initial with quartered heraldry', Cambrai, Bibliothèque municipale, MS 87, fol. 211^{r} (detail). Before 1297.

Figure 3, p. 88. 'Cambrai Hours. Hours of the Virgin, Sext: Temptation of Food and Drink', Cambrai, Bibliothèque municipale, MS 87, fol. 47^{r} (detail). Before 1297.

Figure 4, p. 89. 'Cambrai Hours. Hours of the Virgin, Vespers: Temptation of Music', Cambrai, Bibliothèque municipale, MS 87, fol. 53^{v} (detail). Before 1297.

Figure 5, p. 93. 'Cambrai Hours. Five Joys of the Virgin: Mary adored by book owner and husband', Cambrai, Bibliothèque municipale, MS 87, fol. 71^{r} (detail). Before 1297.

Figure 6, p. 94. 'Cambrai Hours. Nine Joys of the Virgin', Cambrai, Bibliothèque municipale, MS 87, fols 200^{v}–201^{r}. Before 1297.

Figure 7, p. 97. 'Cambrai Hours. Nine Joys of the Virgin: Book owner in heraldic garments', Cambrai, Bibliothèque municipale, MS 87, fol. 200^{v} (detail). Before 1297.

Figure 8, p. 99. 'Cambrai Hours. Nine Joys of the Virgin: Incarnation', Cambrai, Bibliothèque municipale, MS 87, fol. 201^{r} (detail). Before 1297.

Figure 9, p. 102. 'Cambrai Hours. Nine Joys of the Virgin: Book owner with a rosary', Cambrai, Bibliothèque municipale, MS 87, fol. 203^{r} (detail). Before 1297.

Figure 10, p. 106. 'Cambrai Hours. Hours of the Virgin, Matins: Annunciation', Cambrai, Bibliothèque municipale, MS 87, fol. 19^{r} (detail). Before 1297.

Acknowledgements

The editors would like to extend their deepest thanks to Axel Muller, the editor of the IMR series, and to Guy Carney, our publishing manager, for assisting us throughout the process of assembling this volume. We also thank Deborah A. Oosterhouse for her careful copyediting of the volume and Carle-Gabriel Mérineau for her help in putting together the index for the book.

Abbreviations

CCCM	Corpus Christianorum Continuatio Mediaevalis
CCSL	Corpus Christianorum Series Latina
CSEL	Corpus Scriptorum Ecclesiasticorum Latinorum
GCS	Die Griechischen Christlichen Schriftsteller
PL	*Patrologia cursus completus, Series latina*, ed. by Jacques-Paul Migne, 221 vols (Paris: Migne, 1844–64)

Pleasure in the Middle Ages: An Introduction

Naama Cohen-Hanegbi and Piroska Nagy

L'animo, ch'è creato ad amar presto,
ad ogne cosa è mobile che piace,
tosto che dal piacere in atto è desto.

The mind, disposed to love at its creation,
is readily moved toward anything that pleases
as soon as by that pleasure it is roused to act.[1]

In these condensed lines, Dante's Virgil explains the mechanism by which pleasure is the source of action. Pleasure is defined as an orienting signal, directing one towards one's natural disposition; in other words, pleasure tells us what we love. Dante was clearly standing on the shoulders of giants when recounting this theory, for the association of pleasure with nature and 'the natural' — here, represented by 'disposition', which exists right from a person's creation — runs deep throughout the ages. Plato and Aristotle understood

[1] Dante Alighieri, *Purgatorio*, XVIII.19–21, ed. and trans. by Hollander and Hollander, pp. 288–89.

Naama Cohen-Hanegbi (naamaco@post.tau.ac.il) is a senior lecturer in the History Department of Tel Aviv University. She has published articles on the medical and religious treatment of emotions and on medicine within inter-religious encounter. She is the author of *Caring for the Living Soul: Emotions, Medicine and Penance in the Late Medieval Mediterranean* (Leiden: Brill, 2017).

Piroska Nagy (nagy.piroska@uqam.ca) is professor of Medieval History at the Université du Québec à Montréal (UQAM). She is the author of *Le Don des larmes au Moyen Age: Un instrument spirituel en quête d'institution, v^e^–XIIIe siècle* (Paris: Albin Michel, 2000) and co-author, with Damien Boquet, of *Sensible Moyen Âge: Une histoire des émotions dans l'Occident médiéval* (Paris: Seuil, 2015), forthcoming in English as *Medieval Sensibilities: A History of Emotions in the Middle Ages*. With D. Boquet she launched in 2006 the project EMMA, 'Emotions in the Middle Ages' (http://emma.hypotheses.org) in France; they co-edited a series of volumes on medieval emotions.

Pleasure in the Middle Ages, ed. by Naama Cohen-Hanegbi and Piroska Nagy, IMR 24 (Turnhout: Brepols, 2018), pp. xi–xxiii BREPOLS PUBLISHERS 10.1484/M.IMR-EB.5.113458

pleasure as the restoration of one's nature: the return of the spirit or soul to its natural goal.[2] Later theorists of the classical age would identify the pursuit of pleasure as a natural drive, some ascribing greater moral worth to those who could master these natural inclinations.[3] In addition, we find copious discourse about unnatural pleasures derived from misdirected and unbalanced dispositions.[4] Pleasure stands, therefore, at the very core of the many ways in which the order of being was articulated over centuries. Medieval Christian thought — to which we shall return — inherited these ancient views and reconfigured them to align with the narrative of the Fall and Redemption through Christ and the ethics these imply. Shifting notions of nature and of the natural would thus produce new modes of thinking about pleasure and the pleasurable. For this reason, the deep-seated association between pleasure and nature challenges historians to consider what pleasure was in past societies, the ways in which it was understood, and the ways in which it was propagated. For medieval history, such an investigation offers a further incentive: that of dispelling the popular stigma of a joyless era[5] in which only violence, plague, and suffering took place, revealing instead that pleasure was recognized in medieval times as an important motivating element at the source (or aim) of all movement, as well as, often, a desirable feeling in one's daily life.

Historicizing pleasure requires us, then, both to understand the anthropological framework of the period we study and to rethink our own conventions and connotations concerning pleasure, in order to avoid misunderstanding and anachronism. Western Christian anthropology is built on a series of complementary opposites involving pleasure, which could be rearticulated and emphasized in several ways in different cultural settings through the centuries. As a basic scriptural reference, Christ's Sermon on the Mount concerning the Beatitudes (Matthew 5. 3–12) maintains that to deserve otherworldly salvation and eternal beatitude one must endure sadness, pain, and suffering in this life — an idea understood as an 'entry fee' to pay for eternal pleasure. Conversely, indulging in worldly pleasures leads to eternal death and suffering. According to Saint Augustine, the most influential of Western Church Fathers, the very nature of man, since the Fall, has been vitiated so that his will inclines towards earthly pleasures, which create eternal pain and suffering.[6] Restoring human

[2] Wolfsdorf, *Pleasure in Ancient Greek Philosophy*, pp. 40–50, 106–07.

[3] Van Riel, *Pleasure and the Good Life*, pp. 79–93.

[4] For example, see Cadden, 'Trouble in the Earthly Paradise'.

[5] See for instance Le Goff, 'Le Refus du plaisir'.

[6] See Augustine, *De civitate Dei*, XIV, ed. by Dombart and Kalb.

nature by belonging to the Church thus means restoring the inclination of man towards the ultimate good and pleasure in God, even if this happens through sacrifice and suffering 'in this valley of tears'.

And yet, people of the early Middle Ages did not banish pleasures from their vocabulary. Games, tales, festivities, and music lent pleasure to their daily life; various pleasures — of love, aesthetic beauty, victory in warfare, or foods — were celebrated in poetry, romance, and visual arts. Moderate pleasure was also regarded as necessary to health, whether by invigorating the movement of humours in the body and producing necessary warmth or by inducing positive feelings (joy, delight, hope) and happy thoughts. In addition, any reader of medieval texts must be aware of the ongoing use of similes and metaphors by which authors envisioned pleasure. These literary devices often both conflate and unravel clear distinctions between the physical and the spiritual as well as the categories of good and evil. Whatever the image used, the transmutation of pleasure and its direction towards the 'ultimate good' was an essential theme within medieval thought.

The link between pleasure and pain, on the one hand, and the issues of soteriology and eschatology, on the other, is the landscape behind all medieval discourse on pleasure — a landscape that differs radically from our contemporary Western anthropology of pleasure and pain. Within medieval culture, pleasure, enjoyment, and joy were often construed as interdependent with and complementary to sadness, pain, and suffering.[7] Later medieval religious writing, for instance, is saturated with emotions and sensations of suffering and pain alongside those of love and joy. This is especially true with reference to the Passion of Christ, a common path of devotion in the later Middle Ages. The Passion was imitated in prayers, meditations, and rituals because it was conceived as a prerequisite for eternal peace and beatitude.

Today, predominant post-Freudian conceptions conceive pleasure in terms of a bodily, sensorial, or sensual experience. In this volume, most studies bear witness to the fact that medieval pleasure operated through diverse understandings of the relationship between body, mind, and soul. For religious authors, pleasure could be discussed as a purely spiritual and/or intellectual sensation that emanates from the supreme. At the same time, carnal pleasure and other sensual pleasures were condemned as vices and could represent demonic intervention. These two extreme positions were negotiated throughout the medieval centuries, but it was especially transformed by the new discourse on nature in the twelfth and thirteenth centuries. Here pleasure took a central place in

[7] Cf. Casagrande and Vecchio, *Piacere e dolore*.

the new learned mentalities and the growing legitimization of the body as a natural divine creation. This approach to pleasure encompassing body-mind-spirit receives even greater expressions outside the realm of theology, be it medicine or literature, and it is further visible in social and cultural practices. Nevertheless, as a number of essays in the book suggest, the divide between theology, religious life, and the more 'secular' domains should be cautiously set in the study of medieval pleasure, and perhaps in the study of medieval emotions more generally.

Indicating a major turn in the medieval worldview and what we call medieval anthropology — a term by which we mean the vision and study of man — this new discourse was strongly linked to the renewed investment in the idea of incarnation in theology, and to the growing desire to apply Christian theology to the everyday life of clergy and laity during the central Middle Ages (eleventh to thirteenth centuries). In turn, these innovations were part of the great 'descent of values from heaven to earth', as Jacques Le Goff put it,[8] or in other words, a new attitude which ascribed value to this world and to worldly things. In this context, new questions (from Anselm's *Cur Deus homo?* to Abelard's *Sic et non*) arose and new texts (especially those discovered through translations from Greek and Arabic) opened new pathways for the investigation of creation. New viewpoints were developed for appreciating the meaning of *corpus Christi*, or Christ's humanity, from and around which emanated a new study of earthly life. The human body, and thus human emotions, were reconsidered in this new light. The result was a more positive valuation of the body and its pleasures than that of previous periods dominated by Augustinian theology with its denial of worldly things, seen as pale and imperfect reflections of heavenly reality.

Defining Medieval Pleasure: Vocabulary, Contexts, and Concepts

In such a complex and changing cultural landscape, we cannot escape the question: What do we understand by 'pleasure', a modern term which has no exact equivalent in medieval vocabularies? In other words, how do we *translate* pleasure when explaining medieval *realia* to contemporary readers?

Translation constitutes a vital primary step for making sense of medieval pleasure: it is a mission that requires more than a good dictionary. For while medieval Latin and vernacular languages of the period employ several words that denote pleasure and pleasurable feelings, replacing the medieval word with a twenty-first-century term does not account for the conceptual and cultural considerations

[8] Le Goff, 'Du ciel sur la terre'.

of the word in its original setting. In Latin, *gaudium*, *fruitio*, *delectatio*, *delicia*, *laetitia*, and *voluptas* can all be translated as 'pleasure' in a general sense, just like the Old and Middle French terms of *joy/joi*, *delitacion/delicion*, *delice*, *laece/liece* or *soulas*, *plaisir*, *deduit*, *esbatements*, *gogue*, and *aise*. Yet all these terms — Latin and Old or Middle French — have specific uses and contexts and take on specific meanings conditioned by circumstance. Thus, a specific cultural situation — and in this respect, ours is not so different from that of the medieval West — might define the pleasure in question as either an emotion or a sensation, either spiritual or sexual, as pleasure experienced through the senses or in the rational mind, and it may be either lauded or derided. Such particular meanings, which were often obvious to medieval authors and audiences without necessitating any clarification, may be profoundly alien to the modern connotations of the word. Therefore, the cultural environment and the surrounding text constitute together a pair of essential keys for understanding the precise meaning of a word for pleasure and assessing the exact intention behind that word's usage. Since medieval culture itself was not unified, but rather a mosaic of several cultures, contexts should be examined with particular care. First, cultural and social groups could belong to different 'emotional communities' within the same society and employ divergent notions and evaluations of pleasure, making up slightly (or significantly) distinct affective anthropologies. Second, as we have noted above, some major changes in the later Middle Ages affecting long-term attitudes to pleasure and more generally to emotions also complicate the picture. The reflections on pleasure discussed in this volume — in medieval theological and devotional literature or in secular texts such as poetry and medical treatises — demonstrate the diversified shapes and values pleasure had in medieval societies.

Medieval sources deal with pleasure as it relates to a range of subjects, including divinity, food, the body and the soul, the will, friendship and communal experience, knowledge and discovery, morality, health, aesthetics, and sex. Thus, historicizing pleasure yields many and various types of inquiries and questions. Indeed, the many possibilities of thinking about pleasure in the medieval context was vividly apparent in the 2013 International Medieval Congress at Leeds which was the springboard for this volume as well as other publications. Ian Wood, in keeping with the atmosphere of the conference from which the papers originated, brought together in the digital journal *Mirabilia* an assortment of discussions of diverse pleasures from Late Antiquity to 1500.[9] In a sense, this book follows suit in showcasing a range of methodolo-

[9] Wood and others, *Pleasure in the Middle Ages*.

gies and approaches and in covering a long period — between the ninth and fifteenth centuries. The contributions in this volume reflect on the number of ways in which pleasure was understood and used by a variety of authors and sources, and they examine how pleasure was transformed within specific disciplinary and cultural settings. Nevertheless, one common issue that appears to be quintessential to medieval discourse is the dynamic between body and soul (or mind, sometimes conceived as a further, third entity) in the experience of pleasure. This dynamic shapes attitudes and practices and determines the values that were attributed to pleasure. In medieval contexts, pleasure could be a bodily sensation, as in the case of tasting a delicious meal, or an intellectual and spiritual experience, as in the contemplation of holy texts, or it could be a spiritual feeling, as when experiencing the divine. Or it could be a combination of any and all of these. In any case, pleasure is an *experience*, sometimes difficult to classify within our categories of 'emotion', 'feeling', or 'sensation'. Our categories, in effect, do not have the same boundaries as those employed in medieval times. While bodily pleasure may be considered involuntary and sometimes even opposed to the will, medieval theories of the soul often regarded cognition or mental activity as intimately linked to the body. For example, listening to music, speaking with friends, seeing beautiful images, or imagining delightful affairs were all voluntary actions that were deemed to produce physical joy. Furthermore, pleasure was construed as the implementation of desire, itself understood as both a material urge and a cognitive reaction. Spiritual pleasures, being perhaps the most difficult to attain and describe, further demand intricate examination. Some such pleasures would only be enjoyed in the afterlife, while others could be obtained and even cultivated by the living as well. The ineffability of sublime joy was therefore frequently met by the use of analogous terms for sensual delights, surpassing its unworldly nature by imagination and vision, or by apophatic discourse.

Methods for cultivating some kinds of pleasures, and alternately for encouraging abstinence from others, also constitute a substantial issue when historicizing pleasure. These methods reveal what was deemed pleasant or delightful within specific social and religious cultures. Such practices capture not only the values attributed to particular pleasures but also how they served to construct social, cultural, and religious norms. In addition, while pleasure is often considered a personal emotion or feeling, medieval examples shed light on the ways it functioned as an interpersonal, relational, and communal experience. Whether fostering cohesion in monastic friendships and devotional communities, or serving to show off chivalric prowess, pleasure could function not only to restore one's personal nature, to use Platonic terminology, but also to restore the nature of one's community. Thus, while the essays of this collection present and reflect on specific manifestations of pleasure in medieval culture, they also demonstrate how pleasure captured and constructed medieval ideals and norms.

The research presented here was conducted by scholars belonging to different disciplines of medieval studies: historians, theologians, philosophers, art historians, and literary specialists. Most are based on papers delivered in the above-mentioned 2013 IMC conference that was devoted to the theme of 'Pleasure'. Their approaches are manifold, and they bear witness to the importance of pleasure — and more widely, to the significance of the 'affective turn' — in medieval studies today. Interestingly, however, few of them refer to the works, the epistemological framework, or the methodological questions raised by the new field commonly termed the 'history of emotions' or 'emotion research'.[10] This, we find, is indicative of the current state of the history of emotions as researchers are divided on the necessity for, and even the utility of, a specific theoretical framework for studying emotions in medieval societies. Despite the vibrant 'emotion talk' of contemporary social sciences which highlights the idiosyncratic nature of emotions and emotions' equally unique and powerful contribution to daily life, medievalists often prefer to consider emotions no differently from other cultural practices. Thus, a predominant approach in historical study of emotions is to apply the prism of cultural and intellectual history. A possible explanation for this disengagement with contemporary theories of emotions may be either a hesitance to apply contemporary ideas or, in other cases, the certainty that it would lead us to anachronistic considerations. For instance, the association between emotional and irrational, deriving from post-Cartesian theories of the mind, is irrelevant in most medieval anthropologies.

Nevertheless, several historians proposed innovative methodologies for investigating the roles and actions of emotions in a society, which assist in integrating emotions in our vision of past societies. Some scholars do so by invoking ideas from the social sciences and modifying them to the topic of emotions. Such an approach can be seen in the work of Robert Kaster or Nira Pancer, in their analysis of Roman and early medieval societies, where they suggest view-

[10] For an overview of these questions, see now Plamper, *The History of Emotions*; one can get a good idea of the field of interdisciplinary research on emotions at the page of the International Society for Research on Emotion, <https://isre.org/>, and in the review of the society hosted there.

ing emotional sequences as culturally prefabricated *scripts*.[11] Monique Scheer, as well, proposed considering emotions as social practices, in a Bourdieuian fashion.[12] A more radical position argues that emotions are a key for defining communities. William Reddy proposed that expressions of emotions through language influence the course of history in a manner that is unlike any other syntactic utterance. This specific power of emotions as Reddy proposed in the concept '*emotives*' is to produce a statement which is at once both declarative and performative.[13] Emotions are then inherently formative. Emotions are also an analytical tool for Barbara Rosenwein. Rosenwein's 'emotional communities' are primarily a way of explaining the affective dimension of social and cultural groups, linked by common aims and values. Yet her concept further suggests that analysis of emotion words, and of norms and theories of emotions, can in turn be employed to reveal communal norms and societal boundaries.[14]

The multiple avenues of research can be seen in the light of another divide in the discipline between studies taking emotions as a topic, interested in the histories of emotions and affects themselves, and studies which consider emotions as a gateway or a tool for analysing other issues. It often appears that while scholars of the first branch engage with the research on emotions accomplished outside the discipline of history, the second branch of scholars write primarily within their discipline, in our case on the medieval era. This is nevertheless an implicit and subtle debate. As seen in the essays included in this book, both routes of inquiry can yield studies that do well to inform both interests if they are based on a common assumption that pleasure is culturally constructed. Our knowledge of medieval culture and social conventions is greatly enriched by looking at how pleasure was conceived, taught, and performed. Yet inevitably these studies also ask questions that are fundamental to the 'history of emotions'. Quite naturally, almost all of them discuss questions concerning vocabulary and the issues of cultural meaning around the expressions of pleasure. Many of the studies, analysing theories and norms of emotions, discuss what have been coined in the field as *emotionologies*, smaller *emotional communities*

[11] Rosenwein, *Emotional Communities in the Early Middle Ages*; Kaster, *Emotion, Restraint and Community in Ancient Rome*; Pancer, 'Les Hontes mérovingiennes'.

[12] Scheer, 'Are Emotions a Kind of Practice and Is That What Makes Them Have a History?'.

[13] Reddy, *The Navigation of Feeling*.

[14] See especially Rosenwein, *Emotional Communities in the Early Middle Ages*; Pancer, 'Les Hontes mérovingiennes'.

in a given context or larger *emotional regimes* which define the main *emotional style* of a whole society.[15] For instance, emotional education is a topic discussed at length by the authors in this volume, since dictates against certain kinds of pleasure were a major theme in Christian societies. Medieval theoretical frameworks (i.e. medieval *emotionologies*) for analysing emotions in theology, philosophy, and medicine help us understand the nature and functions of pleasure in the medieval worldview, even if pleasure is not always described as an emotion in medieval sources. Finally, practices of emotions are identified and explored through the multifold representations of pleasures in narrative, spiritual, and iconographic sources.

The Shape of this Book

The volume is divided into three parts, which call attention to distinct realms of pleasure: pleasured bodies, didactic pleasures, and pleasure in God. In these three categories we sought to capture a broad picture of the varieties of pleasure, revealing them in a bottom-up order — from the human to the divine, from the material to the metaphysical, and from the secular to the holy — though in the medieval world (and in the sources we examine), the divine is often mingled with the earthly. In choosing this order (that inverts the 'normal' medieval intellectual structure) we were guided by the recognition that the conceptualization of personal pleasure and the identification of how pleasure is experienced by individuals were often the building blocks of didactic literature and of devotional aids helping to explicate religious and mystical thought. This order challenges earlier views of a Middle Ages devoid of pleasure, which mainly derived from normative and theological sources. Instead we draw attention to the formulation of pleasure, throughout the Middle Ages, as an affect sustained by the interaction between physical and sensory knowledge, between cultural and social mores, and between religious thought and ethics. Medieval pleasures lie within the nexus of all three categories.

The first part opens with an essay by Esther Cohen which discusses the variety of pleasures that monasteries offered to their inhabitants. While the setting was devout, the pleasures recounted in letters and autobiographies were not only of a spiritual nature; they included various worldly experiences, such as singing, listening to music, and friendship. The late (and greatly missed)

[15] For these notions, see in order, Stearns and Stearns, 'Emotionology'; Rosenwein, *Emotional Communities in the Early Middle Ages*; Reddy, *The Navigation of Feeling*.

Philippa C. Maddern (†2014) explores the association between good health and joy in late medieval society by tracing the uses of 'merriment' in a range of textual evidence. Fernando Salmón studies elaborations of the Latin medical understanding of *delicia* and its stimulation within the humoral body, offering examples of the sources of bodily pleasure. Naama Cohen-Hanegbi looks at how fifteenth-century Italian physicians negotiated medical theory and cultural and religious norms in providing advice on the pleasures of the body. Maeve Doyle considers the aesthetic pleasures an illustrated prayer book might have offered its reader. Alongside the pleasure of devotion, she argues, the images invoke processes of mirroring and identification that instill the reader with a sense of pleasure. Turning from Europe to the Middle East, Karen Moukheiber explores the discourse of love and its delights within *adab* literature. Focusing on courtesans and slaves, the author questions the boundaries this culture set between licit and illicit, between respectable and disreputable pleasures. Remaining in the realm of love and desire, William M. Reddy returns our study to a European context in his examination of courtly love and its cultural context. A number of bodily pleasures are discussed in this section: aural, visual, and sexual, and the joys of feeling 'well' generally. While these are examined in their own contexts, several of the essays included here also contribute to a broader understanding of medieval perceptions of the phenomenon of pleasure. Thus, Esther Cohen argues that medieval monastic culture reified pleasure, regarding it as an affect external to the self. Fernando Salmón proposes that the humoral perception of pleasure (and emotions more generally) operated as a cross-cultural system in the premodern world. William M. Reddy engages with the science of the twenty-first century, arguing that its tools for defining emotions are inadequate and should be supplemented by historical contextualization. Social and cultural information, he claims, feed the learning processes which neuroscientists recognize to be requisite for shaping emotional states.

Good and bad pleasures are the focus of the second section, which treats various versions of didactic literature produced between the ninth and fifteenth centuries. A common thread in these sources is the notion of 'good' pleasure achieved by following a moral or virtuous path leading to salvation. Barbara H. Rosenwein studies Alcuin's manual for Count Wido, one of the earliest of medieval manuals of moral self-help written for a lay reader. Her analysis highlights Alcuin's instruction as a path for achieving the pleasure of mastering one's emotional conduct. Within this framework, she suggests considering the moral teaching of vice and virtue as a psychological tool that guides a person towards approved pleasures: worldly peace of mind and otherworldly beatitude. Examining the thirteenth-century work on vices and virtues by

William Peraldus, Richard Newhauser shows, in a similar vein, that the issue of pleasures constituted a vital part of the teaching of vice and virtue, instruction seen as a necessary vehicle for transmitting Christian values. The instructions of Giles of Rome in his *De regimine principum* further accentuate this association between pleasure and ethical behaviour in didactic literature. In her account of Giles's discussion of children's education, Noëlle-Laetitia Perret underlines the calculated measure of exposure to pleasurable habits. While pleasure is essential for successful education, its restraint is reputed to foster modesty and obedience, traits which will in turn secure rational upbringing.

Giles's Aristotelian-influenced pedagogy was primarily written for rulers and the elites of society. A wider audience is envisioned in the pastoral teaching discussed in the essay by Xavier Biron-Ouellet. His examination of pastoral theology traces how pleasure was employed by Simone Fidati and Richard Rolle to advocate adherence to the Church and to the Christian community. Despite their common aim, their paths to salvation involve distinct attitudes towards pleasure: Fidati acknowledges its necessity and advocates using it sensibly, Rolle calls on people to avoid it as much as possible. According to Biron-Ouellet, it is the culture of the community addressed that determines the message. Finally, arriving at the topic from a different angle, Elyse Dupras's study of theatrical texts reminds us that pleasure could be utilized to teach virtues in a less direct manner, through the diverse joys procured by attending morality plays. Thus, the humorous performances incite the rather dubious pleasure of glee in the damnation of sinners guiding their audience to the righteous path to salvation. As these contributions suggest, Christian morality did not merely understand pleasure as something to be suspected for its sinfulness or as an occasion of sin, but also knew how to exploit it as a rhetorical or educational tool. The essays in this second section showcase well Richard Newhauser's important observation that pleasure was often considered a positive, God-given sensation that could direct people to virtue.

The last section turns to delight in God, largely exploring the mystical pleasures of experiencing and uniting with the divine. Interestingly, three of the papers illustrate the centrality of food and drink within the imagery used for the portrayal of spiritual pleasures, either through its rejection or through its metaphorical enjoyment. Zachary Guiliano discusses Bede's notion of 'holy gluttony', by which the holy word is imbibed without satiation. Bede's pleasure in the Word is twofold, Guiliano proposes: it is found both in the commentary and in the aesthetics of the text's composition for the readers' pleasure. Ken A. Grant describes the austerity of Pope Gregory VII from his habit of denying himself foods he loved. Desire for intoxication is a metaphor for pleasure and for love of the divine in Bernard of Clairvaux's commentary on the Song of Songs. Constant J. Mews identifies Bernard's indebtedness to the commentaries of Origen and Gregory the Great in this concept of pleasure, but further shows Bernard's innovation in speaking of a much more personal experience of the soul in its encounter with the divine. Delight in the divine is also the ideal form of mystical union expressed in the writings of the two Flemish mystics, John of Ruusbroec and Hadewijch. Rob Faesen's account of the definition of divine love and mystical enjoyment elucidates their nature according to the formulations of the two mystics.

By opening with friendship in Esther Cohen's essay and concluding with love in Rob Faesen's, this book makes it clear that pleasure must be discussed alongside the feelings and sensations that relate to it. How should particular sensations, feelings, and experiences be studied? By choosing to isolate pleasure or instead to consider it within a cluster of other emotional or sensory states, the contributors to this book implicitly give different answers to this question; but one common method that unites the authors throughout the collection is their attempt to define and analyze pleasures, joys, enjoyments, and delights through the language and mindset of the source material. As the contributions to this volume show, this methodology reinforces the impression that generalizations about 'medieval society', in this field as in any others, tend to gloss over the intricacies of complex and variegated culture. The book of medieval pleasures starts here; by raising new questions and topics, it implicitly hopes for many new studies to follow.

Works Cited

Primary Sources

Augustine, *De civitate Dei*, ed. by Bernhard Dombart and Alfons Kalb, CCSL, 47–48 (Turnhout: Brepols, 1955)

Dante Alighieri, *Purgatorio*, ed. and trans. by Jean Hollander and Robert Hollander (New York: Anchor Books, 2004)

Secondary Works

Cadden, Joan, 'Trouble in the Earthly Paradise: The Regime of Nature in Late Medieval Christian Culture', in *The Moral Authority of Nature*, ed. by Lorraine Daston and Fernando Vidal (Chicago: Chicago University Press, 2003), pp. 207–31

Casagrande, Carla, and Silvana Vecchio, eds, *Piacere e dolore: Materiali per una storia delle passioni nel Medioevo*, Micrologus' Library, 29 (Firenze: SISMEL – Galluzzo, 2009)

Kaster, Robert A., *Emotion, Restraint and Community in Ancient Rome* (Oxford: Oxford University Press, 2005)

Le Goff, Jacques, 'Du ciel sur la terre: La Mutation des valeurs du XIIe siècle au XIIIe siècle dans l'Occident chrétien', in Jacques Le Goff, *Héros du Moyen Âge: Le roi, le saint au Moyen Âge* (Paris: Gallimard, 2004), pp. 1263–87

——, 'Le Refus du plaisir', in Jacques Le Goff, *L'Imaginaire médiéval: Essais*, Bibliothèque des Histoires (Paris: Gallimard, 1985), pp. 136–48

Pancer, Nira, 'Les Hontes mérovingiennes: Essai de méthodologie et cas de figure', *Rives nord-méditerranéennes*, 31 (2008), 41–56

Plamper, Jan, *The History of Emotions: An Introduction* (Oxford: Oxford University Press, 2015)

Reddy, William M., *The Navigation of Feeling: A Framework for the History of Emotions* (Cambridge: Cambridge University Press, 2001)

Rosenwein, Barbara H., *Emotional Communities in the Early Middle Ages* (Ithaca, NY: Cornell University Press, 2006)

Scheer, Monique, 'Are Emotions a Kind of Practice and Is That What Makes Them Have a History? A Bourdieuian Approach to Understanding Emotion', *History and Theory*, 51 (2012), 193–220

Stearns, Peter N., and Carol Z. Stearns, 'Emotionology: Clarifying the History of Emotions and Emotional Standards', *American Historical Review*, 90 (1985), 813–36

Van Riel, Gerd, *Pleasure and the Good Life: Plato, Aristotle, and the Neoplatonists*, Philosophia Antiqua, 85 (Leiden: Brill, 2000)

Wolfsdorf, David, *Pleasure in Ancient Greek Philosophy* (Cambridge: Cambridge University Press, 2013)

Wood, Ian, and others, eds, *Pleasure in the Middle Ages: Collected Papers 2013 Leeds IMC*, special issue, *Mirabilia*, 18 (2014), <http://www.revistamirabilia.com/issues/mirabilia-18-2014-1> [accessed 12 September 2017]

Pleasured Bodies

Reflections on High Medieval Monastic Pleasures

Esther Cohen

Sed longe sunt te omnes inferiores et minores quantum ad singularem hanc, in qua tu exsultas et tripudias suauitatem; sed iucunditatem, sed dulcedinem, sed hilaritatem, sed alacritatem, sed amoenitatem, sed serenitatem, sed sinceritatem, sed delectationem, sed omnis denique (ut breui multa sermone concludam) boni plenitudinem et quamdam illius ad quam suspiramus beatitudinis coelestis imaginem, et similitudinem. O quam magna quamque multa in his quatuor exercitiis dulcedo, in lectione, in meditatione, in oratione, in actione!

[But all of these seem far inferior and minor compared to this singular delight [*suavitas*], in which you exult and rejoice — this joy, this sweetness, this merriment, this liveliness, this pleasantness, this serenity, this sincerity, this pleasure, everything to which we yearn ultimately (to cut this long speech short [*sic*]), the fullness of goodness and the beatitude and similarity to the celestial image. Oh, how much and how great a sweetness there is in these four exercises — reading, meditation, prayer, and action!][1]

This un-hedonistic celebration of pleasure comes from the stylus of Adam of Dryburgh (d. 1212), a Scottish monk who had exchanged in midlife the Premonstratensian communal life for the more eremitical and harsher Carthusian discipline. He is the author of a little-known treatise on the virtues and advantages of solitary monasticism. What is remarkable about his description of the 'exercises', or rather, practices, of the cell, a term he uses to

[1] Adamus Scottus, *De quadripartito exercitio cellae*, E1015: 828. All translations, unless otherwise specified, are my own.

Esther Cohen (esther.cohen1@mail.huji.ac.il) is professor emerita of Medieval History at the Hebrew University of Jerusalem, Israel. She is the author of monographs and articles on crime and justice, on animals, and on pain.

Pleasure in the Middle Ages, ed. by Naama Cohen-Hanegbi and Piroska Nagy, IMR 24 (Turnhout: Brepols, 2018), pp. 3–20 BREPOLS PUBLISHERS 10.1484/M.IMR-EB.5.113459

describe the entire Carthusian mode of life, is not the intensity of devotion or the harshness of asceticism. Such regimens of monasticism have of course been known before.[2] What is remarkable is the pleasure he derived from his mode of life. His description, laced with frequent allusions to the Song of Songs, exhausts an entire thesaurus of terms describing pleasure, joy, contentment, and harmony. And all this in a bleak, solitary Scottish Carthusian cell! Although I will return to the pleasures of solitude later in this paper, let me now point out that he was not unique in his time: the pseudo-Augustinian author of *De spiritu et anima* wrote, roughly during the same decades, of the enjoyment of the Trinity as pleasure (*delectatio*), joy (*gaudium* and *laetitia*), happiness (*felicitas*), and delight (*suavitas*): 'Munus Patris et Filii Spiritus sanctus est. Usus ergo in munere est, id est, delectatio, gaudium, laetitia, felicitas, suavitas' (The gift of the Father, the Son, and the Holy Ghost is sacred. The habit in the gift is pleasure, joy, happiness, and delight).[3] These quotations, quite common in monastic writings of the twelfth century, sit very awkwardly with modern ideas of pleasure. We tend to consider pleasure as originating largely within the sensory realm and proceeding thence to a sympathetic sensation. The motive force may or may not be sensory — after all, we can derive pleasure from a good novel as easily as from a painting or a concert — but even the pleasure of reading an enjoyable book will be translated in us into a sensation of well-being, a pleasurable sensation. We use here the term 'sensation' when discussing an experience that is not really recognized, according to present knowledge, through the senses, but directly in the brain. In other words, we mentally identify pleasurable sensations with sensory ones. We also are closet Epicureans, associating pleasure with hedonism. The perception that one might actually feel pleasure not through any sensation at all, but through intellectual activity alone, is alien to our post-Freudian world. Had we lived in the twelfth century, going beyond the pleasure principle would not be a search for 'Eros' (to quote Freud's own term), but for spiritual fulfilment.[4] So emphatic was the distinction between real spiritual pleasures and spurious physical ones in the twelfth century that some scholars created a contradiction between affect (to which I shall return) and understanding. Pleasure contradicted comprehension. Though this trend had no future, it was there in the twelfth century.

Pleasure — for the medievalist — is thus difficult to classify. It can be construed as a sensation or as an emotion or, more precisely, as a combination

[2] Evagrius of Pontus, *Traité Pratique, ou, Le Moine.*

[3] Anon. [Alcherus of Clairvaux, dub.], *De spiritu et anima liber unus*, ed. by Migne, col. 783.

[4] Freud, *Beyond the Pleasure Principle.*

of both with either serving as the source and the other the result. One can more easily disentangle emotional from physical pain than do the same with pleasure. How is one to distinguish the emotion of pleasure from sensual pleasure? It is as impossible a separation as that of the two meanings of the word 'feeling'. Though Adam of Dryburgh might have enjoyed asceticism, as he enthusiastically proclaimed in his treatise, was that pleasure purely intellectual? His words sound very much like those of nuns rejoicing in the ecstasy of sharing Christ's pain, an exquisitely sensory experience.[5] The pleasure of experience drips from the mind into the senses and cannot be disentangled. Pleasure, therefore, was and is essentially both emotion and sensation, both embodied and disembodied. If we wish to understand it, we must return to the language of the twelfth century: it is an *affectus*, a passion that touches all aspects of our being. The distinction of sensation and emotion is ours, not theirs. Though it comes from the outside and affects our inner self and formation of self, it becomes one with the recipient and changes him or her.

Much of the development of the idea of *affectus* as a positive force, as the writings of van 't Spijker show, is indebted to the work of the Victorine canons in twelfth-century Paris, especially Hugh of Saint-Victor (d. 1141). Hugh's analysis, I believe, marks the manner in which *affectus* came to be viewed and accepted at the time. In his explanation of *affectus* in the exegesis to Ecclesiastes, Hugh elucidates:

> Mens enim nostra in auditu malorum suorum quasi de quodam somno pristini temporis evigilans subito agnovit ubi esset [...] simul etiam considerare caepit de quanta sublimitate in hoc ipsum miseriae profundum cecidisset, et ad illam quia necdum effectu potuit miro quodam ardoris intimi desiderio suspiravit. Hoc ergo erat quod in illis verbis, quae nostram recitabant miseriam, nostrum traxit affectum.
>
> [by, as it were, waking us from a sleep, and drawing attention to where we have come from, [it] awakens in us the desire for that world that we cannot actually reach. Thus, in the words that recite our misery, the biblical author actually attracts our *affectus*.][6]

[5] The records of ecstasy during meditation on the crucifixion of Christ are far too numerous to cite. For a few examples of pleasure in mystical experiences of the crucifixion, see Julian of Norwich, *A Book of Showings*, ed. by Colledge and Walsh; Ebner, *Major Works*, trans. and ed. by Hindsley; Kempe, *The Book*, ed. by Windeatt.

[6] Hugo of Saint Victor, *In Salomonis Ecclesiasten Homilia XIX, homilia II*, ed. by Migne, col. 133. Cited from van't Spijker: '"Ad commovendos affectus"'. I thank Dr. van't Spijker for allowing me to see her work before publication.

In the work of twelfth-century intellectuals and exegetes, *affectus* became a merging of understanding, intellectual pleasure, suffering, and sensation. As in the times of Augustine (d. 430) there were four affects: fear and sadness, love and happiness.[7] Inevitably, it brought its unique meaning to bear upon pleasure as well.

In what follows, this article will attempt to delineate the pleasures of the monastic world of the High Middle Ages. Inevitably these pleasures differ from our expected or enjoyed pleasures. It is my argument, however, that the *affectus* of pleasurable experience is differently constructed from the post-Freudian one. Nevertheless, I have chosen to concentrate upon those feelings and experiences that we might recognize even nowadays as pleasure, though perhaps to a different degree. It is generally admitted that emotions and words of emotion change, as William Reddy has shown, even over a period of a few decades.[8] Pleasure recalled is for us a shadow, not a live, existent entity. It might well affect our present lives, but not to the extent that medieval authors found in their affects. They followed Augustine's view of memory as a storehouse one could enter at will to reclaim the original feeling, unsoiled by forgetfulness. Given this view, affects took a much greater place in the self-modelling of twelfth-century monastics. Thus, I will first address physical and spiritual pleasures; then I will talk about the supernatural pleasures of mystical visionaries, followed by the somewhat more mundane pleasure of monastic friendship and its relation to the pleasures of solitude, especially as experienced by mystical visionaries; and finally, I will talk about the pleasure of the quotidian routine of chanting the daily office, an experience that was a pleasure to many singers (and probably the audience, too). My argument, as these examples will hopefully make clear, is that *affectus* was a crucial component of the self, and much more powerful than what we consider pleasure. The redefinition of *affectus* reified new theories and experiences of pleasure, thus redefining the boundaries of the licit and the illicit while blurring the distinction of embodied and disembodied pleasures. In essence, one might hazard the view that the main distinction between pleasure in the Middle Ages and contemporary pleasure is that in the former pleasure overmastered us, while nowadays we are able to choose and dismiss our pleasures more freely. Such a distinction changes the entire character of pleasure, from an affect to an affection, and completely alters the relationship between the human and his or her emotions. The medieval reification of emotions depended upon various

[7] Augustine, *In Iohannis euangelium tractatus*, ed. by Willems, p. 479.

[8] Reddy, *The Navigation of Feeling*.

external factors and our inner self's reaction to them. We no longer make this dichotomous distinction today: the emotion is us.

But first one must make a short linguistic and philological excursus. Looking for pleasure in the Middle Ages is difficult. There is no exact equivalent to 'pleasure' in Medieval Latin or other Western vernaculars that I know of. If we go back to late antique Latin, what terms should we look for? It appears that pleasure has so many Latin synonyms as to put even Adam of Dryburgh to shame. The examples of Adam and the author of *De spiritu et anima* alone provide us with eight quasi-synonyms: reading, meditation, prayer, action, pleasure, joy, happiness, and delight. The written texts rarely make clear semantic distinctions between the various meanings. The only outstandingly different terms are those limited to carnal pleasure — *voluptas*, *concupiscentia*, and *luxuria* — while all other terms that are commonly used to describe non-sexual pleasures (among them those I will forthwith discuss) appear together. Thus, spiritual pleasures were perceived as a full experience, indistinct from each other, excluding the carnal pleasures, which are distinct.

Within the Latin tradition, Augustine spoke of *delectatio* in a neutral sense; but when referring to spiritual pleasure he mostly used the term *frui*, which can probably be translated as 'enjoyment' — a word destined to become popular again only with the advent of the Victorines in the twelfth century. *Frui*, it seems, was meant more in the sense of the general benefit of humanity than in the sense of individual pleasure. Nevertheless, it was also the common term for positive *affectus*.

The confusion in terminology becomes clearest towards the end of the Middle Ages, when Lorenzo Valla (d. 1457) decided to write a dialogue about pleasure. The dialogue is an interchange between a Stoic, who naturally disapproves of all pleasures as passions, an Epicurean, who embraces them, and a Christian, who finds moderate virtues in the senses, but not necessarily in pleasure. Valla named it first challengingly *De voluptate*, and the name sufficed to create a great uproar among those who had not read the book but automatically assumed Valla espoused the Epicurean position. Valla, who had done no such thing, wisely changed the name in subsequent versions to *De vero falsoque bono*: 'concerning the real and false good'. In fact, the author was very careful not to support the position that various subsequent interpreters had attributed to him. They either accused him of hedonism (following the Epicurean) or praised him for his devout Christian orthodoxy.[9] The roots

[9] Lorch, 'A Defense of the Senses in Lorenzo Valla's Theory of Pleasure'.

of misunderstanding lie in the choice of words, for *voluptas* was invariably associated with carnal pleasure.

Was there, then, a clear distinction between virtuous spiritual pleasure and lascivious and depraved sensory delight? In the medieval clerical tradition, were carnal or sensory pleasures to be shunned, especially by the regular clergy, and only spiritual pleasures to be sought? It takes very little effort and no originality at all to prove that spiritual pleasures were transmuted, chemically as it were, as Caroline Walker Bynum has pointed out, into sensory joys. 'Digesting', as she says, or mouthing the words of the Bible could be an experience of sublime taste, rendering all other gustatory pleasure — or rather, as one preacher put it, all gluttonous pleasure — insipid.[10]

Nor is this a unique case of the commingling of spiritual and sensory pleasure. Much has been written of the pleasurable sensory experiences of mystics, especially women. Hildegard of Bingen's visions are multisensory experiences, with olfactory, auditory, and tactile pleasures.[11] There are fragrances, textures, tastes of sweetness, music, and colours, so much so that the term 'vision' fails to do justice to the experience. Again, one cannot differentiate in these cases between carnal and spiritual or between embodied and disembodied. Hildegard had insisted that she received her visions while awake and conscious, so even the excuse of a dream cannot divest them of their heavily sensory content.[12]

The case of Agnes Blannbekin (d. 1315), a thirteenth-century Viennese beguine, is probably an extreme and somewhat bizarre example of what Bynum terms the 'radical physicality' of medieval religiosity:

> Ista persona solita erat quasi a juventute semper in die circumcisionis anxie deflere [...]. Sic quoque compatiens et flens coepit cogitare de praeputio domini, ubinam esset [...]. Et ecce, mox sensit super linguam suam parvam pelliculam ad modum pelliculae ovicum praemaxima dulcedine, quam deglutivit. Quam cum deglutisset, iterum pelliculam sensit in lingua cum dulcedine ut prius, quem iterum deglutivit. Et hoc accidit ei bene centum vicibus [...]. Tanta fuit dulcedo in degustatione

[10] Anthony of Padua (1195–1231), *Sermones dominicales et festivi*, sermo in dominica I in quadragesima, pars unica, ed. by Costa and others, I, 61: 'In omni dicit, quia omnis saporis suavitatem habet Dei verbum et sapientia, cuius sapor gulae delectationem insipidam facit'.

[11] On Hildegard's visions, see within a rich literature, Kerby-Fulton, 'Prophet and Reformer'; Murray, 'Prophecy in Hildegard'; Newman, 'Christian Cosmology in Hildegard of Bingen's Illuminations'; Dezzutto, '"Visio" y "affectus" en Hildegarda de Bingen'; Santos Paz, 'Visiones hildegardianas del cosmos'.

[12] Hildegard of Bingen, *Epistolarium*, ed. by van Acker, pp. 258–65.

hujus pelliculae, quod in omnibus membris et membrorum articulis sensit dulcem immutationem.

[On the feast day of the Circumcision [...] crying and with compassion, she began to think about the foreskin of Christ, where it may be located [...]. And behold, soon she felt with the greatest sweetness on her tongue a little piece of skin alike the skin in an egg, which she swallowed. After she had swallowed it, she again felt the little skin on her tongue with sweetness as before, and again she swallowed it. And this happened to her about a hundred times [...]. And so great was the sweetness of tasting that little skin that she felt in all [her] limbs and parts of the limbs a sweet transformation.][13]

In fact, Agnes was enacting a theological issue that had already troubled Guibert of Nogent (d. 1124) more than a century earlier: When Christ rose to heaven, what happened to those parts of his anatomy already detached from his body, such as the umbilical cord and the foreskin?[14] Guibert was granted no supernatural answer, but Agnes was, both in symbolic sensory terms and by inner knowledge, and her answer was the orthodox one —all these *membra disiecta* arose with the resurrected Christ.

What we have in this extreme case of spiritual and sensory pleasure is much more than 'popular devotion'. By, so to speak, desexualizing Christ and elevating his corporeal relics to heaven, Agnes achieved a transcendent pleasure coupled with theological knowledge. In Guibert's earlier treatise, the fusion of embodied/disembodied broke down into two separate experiences.

Visions were not exclusively monastic pleasures; they crossed the religious/lay divide, though I will concentrate on divine visions and ecstasies of monastic visionaries. Here we are much better informed about the thirteenth and fourteenth centuries than about the twelfth, with many male and female visionaries who, like Agnes Blannbekin, had had their mystical experiences recorded. Like friendship, mystical experiences could be two-edged: some were painful, but many were pleasurable and, frequently, a mixture of both. The twelfth-century visions of Hildegard of Bingen (d. 1179) were prophetic and intellectual rather than affective, and their writing was more a painful obligation

[13] Blannbekin, *Leben und Offenbarungen*, ed. by Dinzelbacher and Vogeler, pp. 116–18; Blannbekin, *Viennese Beguine*, trans. by Wiethaus, p. 35.

[14] Guibert of Nogent, *Quo ordine sermo fieri debeat; De bucella iudae data et de veritate dominici corporis; De sanctis et eorum pigneribus; cum appendicibus*, ed. by Huygens, pp. 110–37. See also Bynum, *Wonderful Blood*.

than a pleasure to her.[15] In the following centuries, Mechthild of Magdeburg (d. 1282/84) wrote of her ardent pleasure in experiencing Christ; Margaretha Ebner (1291–1351), after struggling for more than three decades with painful experiences, began her delightful relationship with the infant Christ through the medium of a doll, deriving much pleasure from her conversations with him and the ensuing intimacy. They shared her room, and at one point she begged him to stop playing so that she could get some sleep.[16] The pleasure of intimacy with a playful baby (she addressed him as *Kindlein*) had replaced the agony of the imitation of the Crucifixion.

I would like to turn now to another aspect of the overlap/continuity/confusion between the physical and spiritual, namely paradise. The literature on the somatic pleasures of spiritual experiences has been written and rewritten. It amply exhibits the embodiment of the spiritual and the spiritualization of the physical. But many medieval authors went farther: the pleasures of the dead in paradise were also explicitly physical. From the earliest visions of the afterlife, those that actually achieve a visit to paradise dwell with astonished delight upon the beauty of the landscape, the fragrances, the music of the angelic choirs, and the brilliant sumptuousness of the robes of the saints.[17] Taste and touch have received less attention from scholars than vision or hearing, though later Thomas Aquinas considered that the glorious bodies resurrected in paradise after the Apocalypse were to enjoy all senses.[18] Less orthodox, but far more imaginative, Catherine of Genoa (1447–1510) saw in her otherworldly journey not only the dancing, singing, and enjoyment of the righteous in paradise, but even the joy of the struggling souls in purgatory, who knew that each moment of agony brought them one step closer to perfect happiness in paradise.[19]

It is important to note that these were no metaphorical or metonymic descriptions of states of mind. The authors describing those feelings of sensory pleasure meant them most literally. Senses being an inalienable part of the human soul, they could transmute spiritual experiences into corporeally sensed

[15] Hildegard of Bingen, *Scivias*, ed. by Führkötter and Carlevaris, pp. 3–6.

[16] Mechthild of Magdeburg, *'Das fliessende Licht der Gottheit'*, ed. by Neumann and Vollmann-Profe; Ebner and von Nördlingen, *Ein Beitrag zur Geschichte der deutschen Mystik*.

[17] See, for example, the visions translated in Gardiner, *Visions of Heaven and Hell before Dante*.

[18] Thomas Aquinas, *Summa Theologiae*, Suppl., q. 80, art. 1.

[19] Catherine of Genoa, *Purgation and Purgatory; The Spiritual Dialogue*, trans. and ed. by Hughes, pp. 71–72, 81–85.

pleasures. This position would satisfy our modern perceptions, according to which pleasure is sensory, but as we saw at the beginning, all sorts of experiences could be perceived as pleasure or pleasurable, including those that some of us would consider sheer penance.

Visions were granted to the lucky few. The majority of monastics enjoyed more mundane pleasures, especially one specific type of pleasure. Perhaps the most obvious pleasure to leave its traces behind was friendship. Nuns and monks, especially the cloistered ones, left behind them a treasure-trove of correspondence that testifies to long-standing friendships between people whose only contact sometimes was through stylus and parchment. We are familiar with the most famous and erudite letters — the impassioned and high-minded correspondence of Abelard (d. 1142) and Heloïse (d. 1164), the irate fulminations of Bernard of Clairvaux (d. 1153), the preoccupied kindnesses of Anselm of Canterbury (d. 1109), contrasted with his passionate writing to intimate friends (among them God!) — but those are little more than the tip of the iceberg.[20] Twelfth-century monks and nuns wrote copious correspondence from one monastery to another. Friendship, as Brian Patrick McGuire has pointed out, became popular and permissible in monasteries as of the twelfth century, and it left behind it eloquent testimonies in writing.[21] Earlier authorities had stressed the community as a group and feared that one-to-one friendships would lead to homosexuality. By comparison, twelfth-century monastic communities, especially Cistercian ones, tolerated binary spiritual friendships. As several students of medieval monasticism have shown, affective relationships among monks, especially Cistercians, were common, though the evidence for homoerotic relationships is sparse and dubious to the point of non-existence, given that the constraints of letter-writing rules make such assumptions difficult to prove. Just to give one example, Baudri de Bourgueil — monk, abbot, and bishop (subsequently deposed) — wrote a treatise against homosexuality, homoerotic letters, and a highly stylized love poem to a nun, Constantia.[22]

[20] Abelard, *Historia calamitatum*, ed. by Monfrin; the text includes Heloïse's first two, personal letters; for Bernard of Clairvaux, see Bernard de Clairvaux, *Lettres*, ed. by Leclercq, Rochais, and Talbot, trans. by Rochais; Anselm of Canterbury, *Letters*, ed. and trans. by Frölich.

[21] McGuire, *Friendship and Community*; McGuire, 'The Cistercians and the Transformation of Monastic Friendships'.

[22] On Baudri, see McGuire, *Friendship and Community*, pp. 245–52. See also Baudri de Bourgueil, *Carmina* ed. by Hilbert, p. 200.

The obvious place to start is with Aelred of Rievaulx's writings on friendship: *De speculo caritatis* and mostly *De spiritali amicitia*.[23] As the author avows, he was influenced by Aristotle and Cicero.[24] Real spiritual friendship, for Aelred, consisted in open and honest dialogue, an opening of hearts to one another. The entire cosmos, for him, was infused with divine love, translated into friendship among humans (by which he meant men, actually). The treatise *De spiritali amicitia*, written as a dialogue between Aelred and his friend Ivo, discloses a community of two minds joined by common thoughts. Ivo first rejected Cicero because he who did not know Christ could not know real friendship. Aelred still accepted Cicero's definition of 'a benevolent and loving consensus of human and divine things'. Spiritual friendship, it appears, is a loving twinning of minds: 'friendship is therefore such a virtue as to make souls join together in a pact of love and sweetness, and from several, become one'.[25] Nothing, declares Aelred, is sweeter, pleasanter, nor more useful than to love and be loved. Paradoxically, the treatise was written because, as Aelred wrote in his prologue, he could not achieve true spiritual friendship, so instead he wrote about it. This writing is inadequate, he admits in one of his sermons, for affects are intransmissible: 'Fear has its own language, understandable only to him who knows fear. Pain also has its own language that only the sufferer understands. Thus love also has its own language, understood only by him who loves'.[26] All the same, inexpressible as the pleasure of friendship is, it does exist, it has norms and rules, and it is one of the pillars of monastic life for a Cistercian abbot like Aelred.[27]

Most of Aelred's letters, alas, have not survived, so we know more about how he valued friendship than how he practised it. Perhaps, like Anselm of

[23] Aelred of Rievaulx, *De speculo caritatis*, ed. by Hoste, and Aelred of Rievaulx, *De spiritali amicitia*, ed. by Talbot.

[24] Aelred of Rievaulx, *De spiritali amicitia*, bk III, ed. by Talbot, p. 318; McGuire, *Friendship and Community*, p. 296.

[25] Aelred of Rievaulx, *De spiritali amicitia*, bk I, art. 21, ed. by Talbot, p. 292: 'Amicitia igitur ipsa virtus est qua talis dilectionis ac dulcedinis foedere ipsi animi copulantur, et efficiuntur unum de pluribus'.

[26] 'Habet timor linguam suam, quam non intelligit nisi qui timet. Habet linguam suam et dolor, quam non intelligit nisi qui dolet. Habet ergo et linguam suam amor, quam non intelligit nisi qui amat': Aelred of Rievaulx, *Sermon 51*, ed. by Raciti, p. 40.

[27] For a summary and a trenchant dismissal of the argument concerning Aelred's putative homosexuality, see Boquet, *L'Ordre de l'affect au Moyen Âge*, pp. 308–23.

Canterbury, he was careful not to involve himself too deeply in friendships.[28] Enough contemporaries of his, though, have left their correspondence and thus a record of the pleasures of friendship behind them. Hildegard of Bingen made sure her correspondence was preserved, and through her letters runs a network of friendships and acquaintances inside and outside the monastic world. For example, in a letter to Guibert of Gembloux, the monk destined to become her second secretary but unknown to her at the time of writing, she ends by adjuring him to speak with Lord Siger of Wavre, encouraging him not to depart from his present intentions whatever his wife may say.[29] While we know little more about the deservedly mysterious Siger (barring a few charters), the fact that, while answering a spontaneous letter from an anonymous admirer, she could pull a mutual acquaintance into her letter at the drop of a hat is telling. Very little of her correspondence is emotional at all, or about friendship, but friendship is indeed its basis. Though the rules of the *ars dictaminis* often trapped straightforward informational letters in pseudo-amical language, the very possibility of corresponding, even to chide, nag, or offer unsolicited advice (and Hildegard was very good at all three), was a pleasure often exercised in twelfth-century monasteries and convents. If one adds the pleasure of unrestrained vituperation to the list, some of Bernard of Clairvaux's letters must have caused him considerable delight. The powers of great abbots and abbesses to inflict shame upon a truant nun or monk, or even a stubborn bishop who objected to the singing of nuns, was a significant tool in establishing a supra-hierarchical position in political manipulations, as well as aggrandizing themselves as lawgivers. These were not necessarily positive pleasures, but in the monastic world, even if garbed in modesty and restraint (often overtly so), the writing and publication of such letters must have been pleasurable to the authors.

Monastic friendship, it seems, was no vice to be shunned in favour of solitude. It was a virtue, but more than that: as Thomas Aquinas was destined to make amply clear in his thorough reliance on Aristotle, friendship was a pleasure. It was unnecessary for Thomas to state that the *Nicomachean Ethics* (bk VIII), where this statement appears, was a virtuous and reliable source.

Yet, as seen through correspondence, friendship was equally a source of grief. Silences, curt answers, angry reproaches, and evasiveness (Abelard was very good at the latter) — all provide little pleasure and much pain through letters. For

[28] McGuire, 'Love, Friendship and Sex in the Eleventh Century'.

[29] Hildegard of Bingen, *Epistolarium*, ed. by van Acker, II, 264.

example, when John of Salisbury (d. 1180) became Bishop of Chartres in 1176, his stream of intense correspondence with Peter of Celle (d. 1183) dwindled under the weight of administrative duties. Peter's complaints elicited no renewed fervour, though the memory of an intense and pleasurable friendship remained.[30] The very pain is grounded in the pleasure of a past friendship betrayed.

If one is to seek pleasures in monastic life, it appears, friendship and correspondence were thus ambivalent. By the same token, Adam of Dryburgh and his fellow Carthusians derived much pleasure from their solitude, as opposed to the Cistercian gregariousness of Aelred. Friendship might have been a common twelfth-century monastic pleasure, but it was an uncertain one.

One should not, however, put the pleasures of solitude and ecstasies in opposition to the pleasures of friendship. While most of what remained of monastic licit mystical pleasures was transmitted in records of confessions or vernacular autobiographical writings, like Mechthild's and Ebner's, the solitude of ecstasy did not prevent intense friendships. Ebner mentions in the early stages of her spiritual journey two sisters who took care of her and were dear friends; later she enjoyed a long and fascinating correspondence with a 'friend of God' as she called the priest Heinrich of Nördlingen, who visited her occasionally and wrote her regularly from 1332 onwards. We have Heinrich's letters (and one of Ebner's!), and it is clear that the correspondence was unique and personal and provided a great deal of pleasure to both writers. Heinrich was deeply impressed with Margaretha's visions and revelations, and encouraged her to write them down. Nothing in the *Revelations* shows that the act of writing itself provided Ebner with pleasure, but the correspondence did. She records hungrily every rare visit and every conversation, and his letters record the very enjoyment of the correspondence.

But mystics, despite the tremendous amount of research devoted to them in the last few decades, were few and far between. Those who recorded the pleasures of their experiences are even fewer. I would like, therefore, to turn to a pleasure common to most members of monastic communities.

Standard monastic life — if there was such a common denominator — included a whole list of minor homely comforts and pleasures, such as evening time in the *calefactorium*, feast days, special food for the sick; in short, the sort of quotidian pleasures most humans shared. But all monks had one special activity which, judging by the sources, they considered both holy and pleasurable: the daily liturgy, which bound the disparate monks into one emotional community.

[30] McGuire, *Friendship and Community*, pp. 280–83.

There is no doubt that the daily office was a duty rather than a permissible voluntary pleasure for many monks, but we have clear indications that, for those who loved to sing, psalmody was a pleasure of the highest order. Leaving aside the theory of music as one of the highest human achievements, the practice of vocal human singing was central to the monastic affective experience. Perhaps one of the clearest examples of its importance was the correspondential tantrum of Hildegard of Bingen when her nuns were temporarily forbidden to sing in their choir. In her letter to the Archbishop of Mainz she stresses not only her grief at the prohibition but also the tremendous importance of the singing for the holiness of her daughters.[31] Monastic literature from the twelfth and thirteenth centuries presents also a peculiar phenomenon affecting liturgy: from the times of Abbot Odilo of Cluny in the eleventh century to the exempla collection of Caesarius of Heisterbach in the thirteenth century, it seems that demons took a special pleasure in disrupting the daily office by making monks sing either off-key or on different scales.[32] As the work of Boynton and Dillon shows, such demonic disruptions caused grave distress to the choir monks, cancelling all their pleasure in the harmony of the song. The demons' investment in disrupting this activity is a clear indication of its centrality and its role as pleasure-*inducing* when not corrupted by demonic cacophony.[33] The monastic attitude to music, as to other carnal pleasures, was ambivalent. On the one hand, music was what angels sang in the spheres, a part of the *Quadrivium*, and possessed of a long and laudable history both as sound and as theory. At the same time, music was perilously close to mimicry and acting, and a borderline no-man's-land between the celestial and the humanly corrupt.

The choir's pleasure in its singing earned more than once the disapproval of abbots and novice masters, bent more on the sense of the words than on the beauty of the music. Caesarius of Heisterbach (d. 1240) tells of a choir singing in a parish church 'loudly, not piously, and lifting tumultuous voices on high'. They were rebuked by a listening monk, who saw a devil standing nearby, holding a big sack in his left hand, grabbing the sounds of loud music in his right hand and putting them into the sack. The chapter is entitled 'There you will find how much demons rejoice if voices are lifted in psalmody without humility'.[34]

[31] Hildegard of Bingen, *Epistolarium*, ed. by van Acker, I, 67.

[32] Moore, 'Demons and the Battle for Souls at Cluny'.

[33] Emma Dillon, pers. comm., summer 2011. Boynton, '"The Devil Made Me Do It"'; Boynton, 'Work and Play in Sacred Music and its Social Context'. Hammerstein, *Diabolus in Musica*.

[34] Cited by Boynton, '"The Devil Made Me Do It"', p. 95; Caesarius of Heisterbach, *Dia-*

The most thorough condemnation of pleasure in the choir comes from the pen of Aelred of Rievaulx, recounting in his friend's name:

> Stans interea vulgus sonitum follium, crepitum cymbalorum, harmoniam fistularum tremens attonitusque miratur; sed lascivas cantantium gesticulationes, meretricias vocum alternationes et infractiones non sine cachinno risuque intuetur, ut eos non ad oratorium, sed ad theatrum, nec ad orandum, sed ad spectandum aestimes convenisse [...] in usum assumitur illicitae voluptatis. Non enim sensui praeferendus est sonus, sed sonus cum sensu ad incitamentum maioris affectus plerumque admittendus [...] cum me [...] magis cantus quam verba delectant, poenaliter me peccasse confiteor, et mallem non audire cantantem.
>
> [standing among the people dazzled, shaking and astounded by the sound of bellows, the clashing of cymbals, the song of pipes; but the lascivious gesticulations of the singers, the meretricious voice changes and breaks cause unrestrained laughter, as though you saw them not at an oratory but in a theatre, not praying but posing for show. [...] I also felt that the sound was privileged [that is, to the sense] [...] in practice it has become illicit pleasure (*voluptas*) [...] they prefer the chanting to the word, and thus they sin, and it is better not to hear the singing.][35]

So, sinful or praiseworthy, performing the liturgy was obviously a pleasure to the singers and very probably to the listeners too. But music did not stand alone and neutral in the scale of monastic values. Its beauty took second harmonic place to the words of the liturgy. Like paintings and statues of saints displayed in churches, the music was an ornament to the truth at best. It was not the end of prayer in itself, and monastic authorities repeatedly stressed this point.

* * *

Brian Patrick McGuire has termed the twelfth century 'the age of friendship'. It could just as easily be termed the age of the transmutation of monastic pleasure. It was an age of emotional transmutations throughout the literate world, and

logus miraculorum, 5:9, ed. by Strange, I, 181. 'in ecclesia quadam saeculari fortiter, id est, clamose, non devote cantantibus, et voces tumultuosas in sublime tollentibus, vidit homo quidem religious, qui forte nunc affuit, quondam daemonem in loco eminentiori stantem, saccum magnum et longum in sinistra manu tenere, qui cantantium voces dextra latius extensa capiebat, atque in eundem saccum mittebat. [...] Capitulo quinto, ubi invenies, quantum ex hoc daemones laetantur, si sine humilitate in psalmodia voces exaltentur'.

35 Aelred of Rievaulx, *De speculo caritatis*, ch. 23, ed. by Host, II, 97–98; trans. Boynton, '"The Devil Made Me Do It"', p. 96. This is probably the earliest mention of polyphonic music. I am indebted to Dr. Yossi Maurey for this comment on 'illicit pleasures' of different voices singing in harmony, rather than in one voice.

monastic friendship was only one of them.[36] The semantic richness is proof of preoccupation with the subject, even if not of wholehearted approval. The varieties of correspondence, the harmonization of ecclesiastical music, and the constant discussions of friendship and its meaning bear witness to the fact that friendship was a pleasure much valued in the twelfth century, perhaps as much as honour was a century earlier.

One should not contrast pleasure with asceticism. On the contrary: many of the new monastic orders of the twelfth century were far more harshly ascetic than the old-fashioned Benedictine houses. But even the eremitical ascetics praised their rigorous discipline in terms of pleasure, joy, and delight. Conversely, community-oriented Cistercians who enjoyed communal liturgy could disparage the same if it became first and foremost a pleasure rather than a solemn, dutiful ritual. The very difference between eleventh-century Gregorian chant and twelfth-century budding harmonizations shows the difference between the solitary monk, chanting his psalm like all others, and the choir as a separate entity.

Perhaps the key to the transformation is not the legitimation of pleasure, but the change of *affectus*. Twelfth-century *affectus* were neutral, neither intrinsically good nor bad. They moved the soul in different directions. And pleasure — whatever word was used for it — was an *affectus*. It could therefore be good, when it moved monks and nuns to spiritual friendships, or bad, when it pushed one towards lust or gluttony. Thus 'good' liturgy could bother demons to the point at which they felt compelled to disrupt it, while proud, noisy psalmody might have given the singers pleasure, but it was, so to speak, bad pleasure — *voluptas*. In and of itself, pleasure was neither good nor bad.

The moral of the story, of course, is that one ought to avoid two pitfalls: one is the dissociation of the concept of pleasure from its textual context. It is impossible to unpack medieval pleasure without examining it within one specific context — in this case, the monastic one. Most importantly, we should beware the assumption that what we term pleasure had its exact mirror image in the past. We use the same word, but the semantic content has shifted. I would guess that even within the twelfth century there were different affective communities that saw pleasure differently from each other. As L. P. Hartley put it: 'The past is a foreign country: they do things differently there'.[37]

[36] I am indebted for this insight to Dr Piroska Nagy.

[37] Hartley, *The Go-Between*, p. 1.

Works Cited

Primary Sources

Abelard, Peter, *Historia calamitatum*, ed. by Jacques Monfrin (Paris: Vrin, 1959)

Adamus Scottus, *De quadripartito exercitio cellae*, in Michael Lapidge and Richard Sharpe, *Bibliography of Celtic-Latin Literature, 400–1200* (Dublin: Royal Irish Academy, 1985)

Aelred of Rievaulx, *De speculo caritatis*, ed. by Anselm Hoste, in *Aelredi Rievallensis Opera Omnia*, CCCM, 1 (Turnhout: Brepols, 1971), pp. 3–161

——, *De spiritali amicitia*, ed. by Charles Hugh Talbot, in *Aelredi Rievallensis Opera Omnia*, CCCM, 1 (Turnhout: Brepols, 1971), pp. 287–350

——, *Sermon 51*, in *Sermones XLVII–LXXXIV*, ed. by Gaetano Raciti, *Opera omnia*, III, CCCM, 2B (Turnhout: Brepols, 2001)

Anon. [Alcherus of Clairvaux, dub.], *De spiritu et anima liber unus*, in *PL*, XL, cols 779–832

Anselm of Canterbury, *Letters*, ed. and trans. by Walter Frölich, 3 vols (Kalamazoo: Cistercian Publications, 1990–94)

Anthony of Padua, *Sermones dominicales et festivi ad fidem codicum recogniti*, ed. by Beniamino Costa, Leornardo Frasson, Joanne Luisetto, and Paulo Marangon, 2 vols (Padua: Messaggero, 1979)

Augustine, *In Iohannis euangelium tractatus*, ed. by Radbod Willems, CCSL, 124 (Turnhout: Brepols, 1954)

Baudri de Bourgueil, *Baldricus Burgulianus carmina*, ed. by Karlheinz Hilbert (Heidelberg: C. Winter Universitätsverlag, 1979)

Bernard de Clairvaux, *Lettres*, ed. by Jean Leclercq, Henri Rochais, and Charles Hugh Talbot, trans. by Henri Rochais, Sources chrétiennes, 425, 458, 556 (Paris: Cerf, 1997–2012)

Blannbekin, Agnes, *Leben und Offenbarungen der wiener Begine Agnes Blannbekin*, ed. by Peter Dinzelbacher and Renate Vogeler, Göppinger Arbeiten zur Germanistik, 419 (Göppingen: Kümmerle Verlag, 1994); English trans. by Ulrike Wiethaus, Agnes Blannbekin, *Viennese Beguine: Life and Revelations* (Cambridge: Brewer, 2002)

Caesarius of Heisterbach, *Dialogus miraculorum*, ed. by J. Strange, 2 vols (Cologne, 1851)

Catherine of Genoa, *Purgation and Purgatory; The Spiritual Dialogue*, trans. and ed. by Serge Hughes (New York: Paulist Press, 1979)

Ebner, Margaret, *Major Works*, trans. and ed. by Leonard P. Hindsley, Classics of Western Spirituality (New York: Paulist Press, 1993)

Ebner, Margaretha, and Heinrich von Nördlingen, *Ein Beitrag zur Geschichte der deutschen Mystik*, ed. by Philipp Strauch (Freiburg, 1882; repr. Amsterdam: P. Schippers, 1966)

Evagrius of Pontus, *Traité Pratique, ou, Le Moine*, ed. by Antoine Guillaumont and Claire Guillaumont, Sources chrétiennes, 170–71, 2 vols (Paris: Editions du Cerf, 1971)

Guibert de Nogent, *Quo ordine sermo fieri debeat; De bucella iudae data et de veritate dominici corporis; De sanctis et eorum pigneribus; cum appendicibus*, ed. by Robert B. C. Huygens, CCCM, 127 (Turnhout: Brepols, 1993)

Hildegard of Bingen, *Epistolarium*, ed. by Luc van Acker, CCCM, 91A, 3 vols (Turnhout: Brepols, 1993)

——, *Scivias*, ed. by Adelgundis Führkötter and Angela Carlevaris, CCCM, 43–43A (Turnhout: Brepols, 1978), 2 vols

Hugo of Saint Victor, *In Salomonis Ecclesiasten Homilia XIX, homilia II*, in *PL*, CLXXV, cols 113–225

Julian of Norwich, *A Book of Showings to the Anchoress Julian of Norwich*, ed. by Edmund Colledge and James Walsh (Toronto: Pontifical Institute of Mediaeval Studies, 1978)

Kempe, Margery, *The Book of Margery Kempe*, ed. by Barry Windeatt (Harlow: Longman, 2000)

Mechthild of Magdeburg, *'Das fliessende Licht der Gottheit': Nach der Einsiedler Handschrift in kritischem Vergleich mit der gesamten Überlieferung*, ed. by Hans Neumann and Gisela Vollmann-Profe (München: Artemis Verlag, 1990)

Thomas Aquinas, *Summa Theologiae*, ed. by Pietro Caramello, 3 vols (Torino: Mariotti, 1948–63)

Secondary Works

Boquet, Damien, *L'Ordre de l'affect au Moyen Âge: Autour de l'anthropologie affective d'Aelred de Rievaulx* (Caen: CRAHM, 2005)

Boynton, Susan, '"The Devil Made Me Do It": Demonic Intervention in the Medieval Monastic Liturgy', in *European Religious Cultures: Essays Offered to Christopher Brooke on the Occasion of his Eightieth Birthday*, ed. by Miri Rubin (London: Institute of Historical Research, 2008), pp. 89–106

——, 'Work and Play in Sacred Music and its Social Context, 1050–1250', in *The Use and Abuse of Time in Christian History*, ed. by Robert N. Swanson, Studies in Church History, 37 (Woodbridge: Boydell, 2002), pp. 57–79

Bynum, Caroline Walker, *Wonderful Blood: Theology and Practice in Late Medieval Northern Germany and Beyond* (Philadelphia: University of Pennsylvania Press, 2007)

Dezzutto, Flavia, '"Visio" y "affectus" en Hildegarda de Bingen: Perspectivas éticas acerca de la relación entre intelección y afectividad', in *Conociendo a Hildegarda: La Abadesa de Bingen y su tiempo. La Primera Jornada Interdisciplinaria*, ed. by Azucena A. Fraboschi (Buenos Aires: Educa, 2003), pp. 173–84

Freud, Sigmund, *Beyond the Pleasure Principle*, trans. James Strachey and Gregory Zilboorg (New York: Norton, 1975)

Gardiner, Eileen, ed., *Visions of Heaven and Hell before Dante* (New York: Italica Press, 1989)

Hammerstein, Reinhold, *Diabolus in Musica: Studien zur Ikonographie der Musik im Mittelalter* (Bern: Franke, 1974)

Hartley, Leslie Poles, *The Go-Between* (London: Hamilton, 1953)

Kerby-Fulton, Katherine, 'Prophet and Reformer', in *Voice of the Living Light: Hildegard of Bingen and her World*, ed. by Barbara Newman (Berkeley: University of California Press, 1998), pp. 79–90

Lorch, Maristella, 'A Defense of the Senses in Lorenzo Valla's Theory of Pleasure', in *Homo Carnalis: The Carnal Aspect of Medieval Human Life*, ed. by Helen Rodnite Lemay (Binghamton: Center for Medieval and Early Renaissance Studies, State University of New York at Binghamton, 1990), pp. 121–28

McGuire, Brian P., 'The Cistercians and the Transformation of Monastic Friendships', *Analecta Cisterciensia*, 37 (1981), 1–63

——, *Friendship and Community: The Monastic Experience, 350–1250* (Ithaca, NY: Cornell University Press, 2010)

——, 'Love, Friendship and Sex in the Eleventh Century: The Experience of Anselm', *Studia Theologica*, 28 (1974), 111–52

Moore, Michael E. Hoenicke, 'Demons and the Battle for Souls at Cluny', *Studies in Religion/Sciences religieuses*, 32.4 (2003), 485–97

Murray, Robert, SJ, 'Prophecy in Hildegard', in *Hildegard of Bingen: The Context of her Thought and Art*, ed. by Charles Burnett and Peter Dronke (London: Warburg Institute, 1998), pp. 81–88

Newman, Marsha, 'Christian Cosmology in Hildegard of Bingen's Illuminations', *Logos*, 5.1 (2002), 41–61

Reddy, William M., *The Navigation of Feeling: A Framework for the History of Emotions* (Cambridge: Cambridge University Press, 2001)

Santos Paz, José C., 'Visiones hildegardianas del cosmos: del Scivias al *Liber divinorum operum*', *Studi medievali*, ser. 3, 52.1 (2011), 213–39

Spijker, Ineke van't, '"Ad commovendos affectus": Exegesis and the Affects in Hugh of Saint-Victor', in *Bibel und Exegese in der Abtei Saint-Victor zu Paris: Form und Funktion eines Grundtextes im europäischen Rahmen*, ed. by Rainer Berndt, SJ, Corpus Victorinum, Instrumenta, 3 (Münster: Aschendorff, 2009), pp. 215–34

'It Is Full Merry in Heaven': The Pleasurable Connotations of 'Merriment' in Late Medieval England

Philippa C. Maddern*

When we encounter our sources, we historians of emotion are perpetually reminded that writing about pre-modern emotions involves a constant, and difficult, practice of translation. According to the *Oxford English Dictionary*, even the term 'emotion' in the sense of mental agitation or inner feelings and their expression does not occur in English until 1602.[1] Certainly other terms in late medieval English seem to denote emotions

* This research was supported by the Australian Research Council's Centre of Excellence for the History of Emotions (project number CE110001011). The editors wish to thank Andrew Lynch and Susan Broomhall who, following Philippa's untimely death, took it upon themselves to assist in bringing the article to publication.

[1] *OED Online*, 'emotion'. Note, however, that 'émotions' in the sense of civil unrest, uprising or riot, appears to have been well established in French in the fifteenth century. Nicole Hochner, for instance, has found it as early as 1429 in *La Chronique du Bon Duc Loys de Bourbon* — the king 'avoit tant a faire en son royaume, tant pour les esmotions d'aucunes ses communes appellés Jacques et Maillets, comme pour le roi de Navarre, et d'autres grandes compaignies, qui lui estoient contraires'. *La Chronique du Bon Duc Loys de Bourbon*, ed. by Chazaud, p. 5; cf. p. 88, where 'l'esmotion du duc de Bretaigne' leads to a siege of Troye. I am indebted to Dr Hochner, pers. comm., for this invaluable reference.

Philippa Maddern (1952–2014) read History and Indonesian Studies at the University of Melbourne, and completed her DPhil at Oxford in 1985. It was later published as *Violence and Social Order: East Anglia 1422–42* (Oxford: Clarendon Press, 1992). She joined the History Department at the University of Western Australia in 1989 and remained there as an outstanding researcher, teacher, mentor, and administrator. Philippa published widely on later medieval English social history, with an emphasis on the lives of women, families, and communities. From 2011 to 2014 she was director of the Australian Research Council of Excellence for the History of Emotions, Europe 1100–1800.

Pleasure in the Middle Ages, ed. by Naama Cohen-Hanegbi and Piroska Nagy, IMR 24 (Turnhout: Brepols, 2018), pp. 21–38 BREPOLS PUBLISHERS 10.1484/M.IMR-EB.5.113460

— for instance the 'passional love, hate, desijr, drede, gladnes, sorynes, reuþ, schame' — identified by Reginald Pecock, *c.* 1445, as existing both in 'the sensual appetitis and in the herte';[2] or the 'effecciouns of herte', including the 'sodeyne drede othir ioye', whose physical signs (blushing, turning pale) Bartolomaeus Anglicus convincingly described in his popular encyclopedia *De Proprietatibus Rerum* in the thirteenth century.[3] The Latin-English wordlist *Promptorium Parvulorum* (*c.* 1440) offers Latin equivalents of a number of English terms that may easily seem to describe emotions: 'A-ffrayd' (*Territus, uel terror percussus*); 'Angyr, or Wrath' (*Ira, Iracundia*): 'Ashamyd, or made ashame' (*Verecundus, Pudorosus*); 'Envy' (*Invidia, Inuidencia*); 'Enioyn, or makyn ioy' (*Exulto, Gaudeo*), to name only a few.[4]

Unfortunately, however, the briefest consideration shows that these words map only uneasily onto modern meanings of emotion. 'Passion' was perhaps more commonly used to refer to the sufferings of Christ and his martyrs than as an indicator of strong feeling. Individual 'passions' such as wrath or envy were often classified by medieval scholars as vices or virtues, and hence were discussed in what, to us, are unexpected ways, and in unexpected genres such as devotional and didactic texts. It is improbable that a late medieval lay person, sternly admonished that only to feel unrepentant anger against anyone was automatically to be assigned 'To helle [...] the ferst gre', or that to succumb to envy was to be 'Bownde wyth the deuels band', understood or experienced these emotional phenomena exactly as modern individuals do.[5] Similarly, medieval medical understandings of emotions, inflected by humoral theory, related the causes and expressions of emotions in ways that may at first sight seem surprising to us. Melancholy, for instance — an excess of black bile — could produce not merely irrational fear or depression, but also violent anger;[6] the *Promptorium Parvulorum* lists 'Malincolicus' as one translation for 'Angri'.[7]

[2] *OED Online*, 'passion'; Pecock, *The Donet*, ed. by Hitchcock, p. 37. Pecock identifies all these passions as necessary in the development of 'freendfiul, welwilling loue' of God.

[3] Trevisa, *On the Properties of Things*, ed. by Seymour, I, 196. I use John Trevisa's early fifteenth-century translation of the thirteenth-century Latin text the better to reflect knowledge and word-use in late medieval England.

[4] *The Promptorium Parvulorum*, ed. by Mayhew, page columns 6, 12, 16, 146 and 150.

[5] Mannyng, *Handlyng Synne*, ed. by Sullens, pp. 94 and 100; see pp. 94–107 for the whole section on anger and envy. See also *Jacob's Well*, ed. by Brandeis, pp. 99–100, for further cautionary tales on unbridled anger.

[6] Trevisa, *On the Properties of Things*, ed. by Seymour, I, 161–62.

[7] *The Promptorium Parvulorum*, ed. by Mayhew, page column 12.

In short, medieval emotion terms display to modern readers a mix of comprehensibility and strangeness. Bartolomaeus's 'dread' is recognizable as an inward mental and affective response to an outward stimulus, manifested in physical signs (such as turning pale), and hence behaves very much like what we would classify as fear; yet his melancholic 'anger' exceeds the range of common modern understandings of the word. To read these texts is a process akin to translating from a foreign language into English, in which, as everyone who has tried it knows, seeking a simple word-to-word synonym will not do, though rendering the meaning and structure of the whole passage to the second-language reader is nevertheless possible in varying degrees.

The peculiar qualities of translation derive (to a non-linguist like myself) from two phenomena. Firstly, as any good language textbook will acknowledge, each word in each language has no single meaning, but a set of definitions, connotations, and metaphorical usages, and that set of meanings is unlikely to be exactly replicated by any one word in another language.[8] Hence the translator needs to understand the culturally determined meaning-sets in both languages in order to be able to represent the one as meaningfully as possible into the other. Secondly, if we take a Barthesian approach to language, we must presume that many words (or simple word combinations) act not only as signifiers, but as signs. As Barthes notes, in European languages red roses have become neither simply roses nor simply passion, but a sign combining the two — '"passionified" roses'.[9] But such signs are themselves culturally variable — red roses in China, for instance, may signify not passion, but good luck. The translator, therefore, is constantly faced with the question of whether to translate the signifier (the word-synonym), which may be superficially accurate but leaches meaning from the text or produces entirely different significances, or the sign, which involves finding a comparable signifier-sign construction in the language to which one is translating, a combination of word and understood reference that will 'mean' the same — or nearly so — to the second-language reader. If no such brief equivalent can be found, then it is surely the translator's duty to be able to explain to the reader what set of connotations and signs comprise the meaning of the relevant term in the original text; and it is these explanations which, I believe, lie at the heart of emotions history and comprise a fundamental task of a historian of emotions.

[8] See, for example, Sweet, Craig, and Seligson, *Latin*, pp. xiii–xxx.

[9] Barthes, *Mythologies*, pp. 117–74, esp. pp. 121–24. Quote from p. 121.

Such slippery terms are sometimes called 'false friends', from their tendency to deceive us into thinking that we know what they mean. Yet this assessment is, I believe, unduly pessimistic. Looked at in the light of translation, the very difficulty of explaining late medieval emotions terms becomes a point of opening, a case where the necessity to understand not only the word but its surrounding set of cultural connotations and signification is so compelling that it forces us to undertake broader and deeper analysis of the most basic terms of our research. This paper, then, is an attempt to demonstrate such a process through a case study; a translation exercise surrounding the term 'merry', and its connotations and meanings in regard to pleasure, as it was used in England roughly 1400–1550.

At first sight, 'merry' seems an unquestionably 'friendly' term — easily comprehensible to modern readers, consistently and solely denoting a happy, light-hearted, quick-witted, hilarious, and unproblematically pleasurable emotional style. Early dictionaries seem to confirm its continuity of meaning — the *Promptorium Parvulorum* (*c.* 1440) gives the unambiguously cheerful Latin terms '*letus/a*', '*iocundus/a*', '*hilaris/e*', and '*iocosus/a*' as the correct translation of 'Myry in chere', and associates the two words 'mery' and 'Blythe' (also to be translated '*letus*' or '*hilaris*').[10] More than a century later, John Veron's English additions to the 1542 work of Robert Estienne, published as the *Dictionariolum Puerorum Tribus Linguis Latina Anglica & Gallica* (1552) perhaps emphasized slightly more the joking corollaries of the word by translating it as '*iocosus/a/um*', 'Full of sporte and iestynge', and by defining a merry person as a 'tellar of merry iestes, or a *railleur*'. But the unambiguously light-hearted connotation still reassures us that we know what Veron meant.[11] Consulting the *Oxford English Dictionary*, one similarly finds 'merry' meaning 'causing pleasure or happiness; pleasing, delightful', or, of a person, 'characterized by happiness or joy' (supposed to be obsolete) from the ninth to the sixteenth centuries; 'amusing, diverting, funny' (from 1390 to the present day); 'full of laughter or cheerfulness; joyous' (1325 to the present); 'happy, pleased or content' (1380–1634); 'jocular, humorous, witty' (1616–1833); 'festive, joyful, jolly' (1425 to the present); and (as in 'Merry Christmas') 'characterized by celebration and rejoicing' (1534 to the present).[12]

[10] *The Promptorium Parvulorum*, ed. by Mayhew, page columns 42 and 290.

[11] Estienne, *Dictionariolum puerorum tribus linguis Latina Anglica & Gallica*, *s.v.*

[12] *OED Online*, 'merry (adj)', etymology. All these meanings are said to derive from Old High German, Gothic, and ultimately from the Sanskrit 'muhur', meaning sudden, or short.

But how was the word most commonly used in late medieval England? One sign that its meaning may be less unambiguously related to pleasure, jocularity, and cheerfulness than it appears arises in a passage from the well-known correspondence of the Pastons, an important gentry family in Norfolk. In 1466 Elizabeth Clere of Norfolk wrote to Margaret Paston at a time when one of Margaret's young sons, probably William Paston III (then aged about seven) was paying Elizabeth an extended visit. The writer takes care to send his mother news of the child: 'my litel cosyn your sone is a faire childe and a mery, blessed be God'.[13] Why should this signify anything other than a comment on young William's cheerfulness? William's father, John, had died in May 1466, probably only a matter of weeks before the letter was written. Making all allowance for the (possible) phenomenon of the absent medieval father, and the (certain) tendency of late medieval prescriptive writers to characterize children's normative emotional style as light-hearted cheerfulness, even in the face of sorrow or danger,[14] 'merry' seems an odd description of a recently bereaved son. Our assumptions should be even more disturbed by the will made by Joan Bukley, a Norwich widow, in August 1496, in which she described herself as 'hool of mynde & gode and mery being'.[15] It is hardly credible that Joan regarded her will-making as a 'jocular, humorous, witty' occasion, or that she herself was 'full of laughter and cheerfulness' at the time. On the contrary, the succeeding document proceeds soberly to set out her pious, charitable, and familial bequests, as any other serious will would do. The phrase 'hool of mynde & gode and mery being', far from describing her emotional state, appears to be the clerk's vernacular rendering of the standard formula in contemporary Latin wills describing the testator as '*compos mentis et sane* [or *bone*] *memorie existens*' (of sound mind and healthy [or good] memory).

It is almost impossible, therefore, to read this usage of 'merry' as meaning anything but 'sound', 'whole', or 'healthy'. Hence it seems likely that Elizabeth Clere's message to Margaret Paston was meant to convey reassurances as to her child's physical health, rather than to his mood. That this was a common practice in late medieval correspondence appears from references in surviving collections. The Celys very commonly reported on the 'mery' (healthful) con-

The derivation may imply something that shortens the time, whiling it away pleasantly.

[13] *Paston Letters and Papers*, ed. by Davis, II, Letter nos 724 and 351.

[14] See Maddern, 'How Children Were Supposed to Feel; How Children Felt', pp. 121–40, esp. pp. 127–30.

[15] NRO, NCC, Wills, Multon fol. 79^{r}.

dition of the family to their recipients, sometimes in the explicit context of recovery of health, or in contradistinction to more general disease risk. Thus in 1480, Richard Cely the younger told his brother George that 'at the making of thys [letter] howr father ys aull hooll and ryght merry thankyd be God'. In 1479, Richard Cely the elder, also writing to George Cely at Calais (who had evidently been ill) noted that:

> Your moder and I desyer for to here of youre reperyng and amenyng as I tryste in god ye schall right wyll be as mery as ye can and spare for no coste of syche tyngke as may be good for you in good mete dryke and your fessychens doe be there consell.

Later in the same year he commented to George on the younger Richard's fortunate state of health, 'Rychard Cely youre broder ys wyt my lorde of Send Johnys at Sotton al mery I thanke God the sekenese ys sore yn London'.[16] Though the Plumpton family used the term less often, their correspondence likewise associated the meaning 'healthy' with the term 'merry'. In 1543, John Doddington, writing to William Plumpton, asked him to 'informe Mr. Birnand his son is mery and in good health, thanks be to Jesus'.[17] The connotation of 'merry' to mean 'thriving' or 'in good health' may even have been transferred from Middle English to Latin. Around 1380, Edmund de Stonor senior received a letter from one 'Brother Edmund', giving an eyewitness account of his schoolboy son's recovery from illness. Brother Edmund wrote consolingly that the boy's infirmity was decreasing day by day ('cujus infirmitas descrescit de die in diem'), adding that though the lad sometimes had to rest for a couple of hours, afterwards he would get up, go to school, eat, and walk about 'sanus et jocundus, ita quod nullum periculum in eo videtur' ('healthy and merry, so that no danger to him is apparent').[18] Finally, the famous Stonor collection letter from Thomas Betson to his young fiancée, Katherine Ryche, written 1 June 1476, clearly associates the term 'merry' with the concepts of good health, thriving, well-being, and growth. Katherine was under the legally marriageable age of twelve at the time, and Betson's affectionate letter half-jokingly refers both to his pleasure in her 'loffynge delynge to me wardes', and to his sorrow

[16] *The Cely Papers*, ed. by Malden, p. 35, no. 34 and p. 16, no. 17. For further examples, see pp. 34, 40, 46, 49–50, and 77.

[17] *The Plumpton Letters and Papers*, ed. by Kirby, nos 238 and 216.

[18] *Kingsford's Stonor Letters and Papers*, ed. by Carpenter, I, no. 30. *Dictionary of Medieval Latin*, ed. by Latham, p. 1506, gives no equivalent usage for *jucundus*. *Middle English Dictionary*, ed. by Kurath, conjectures that *miri(e)* (adj.) may mean 'prosperous' and 'strong, lusty, sturdy' in some instances: (1a) (d) and 7 (b).

at any delay in her growth to nubile status. His advice on how to speed her development ran as follows:

> And yff ye wold be a good etter off your mete allwaye, that ye myght waxe and grow ffast to be a woman ye shuld make me the gladdest man off the world, be my trough [...]. And seeth well that ye be none eteter off youre mete, the which shuld helpe you greately in waxynge; for south than ye make me veray hevy agayn. And therffore I praye you, myn nown swete Cossen, evene as you loffe me *to be mery and to eate your mete lyke a woman.*[19]

No doubt Katherine's state of health and speedy growth was meant to conduce to the couple's mutual pleasure. But the implication is clear: to thrive, Katherine must be merry, and this quality in turn both constitutes and produces good health.

Nor were letters the only late medieval genre in which merriment was closely associated with health and pleasure as opposed to death and sorrow, healing and renovation as opposed to illness or injury. A fifteenth-century lyric, written in the voice of the Virgin Mary holding her crucified son on her knee, contrasts her (and his) state with that of mothers and their live children:

> Youre childer ye daunce upon youre knee,
> With laghing, kissing and mery chere:
> Behold my childe, beholde wele me,
> For now lyeth dedd my dere sone, dere.[20]

The late medieval editor of the miracles attributed to King Henry VI tends to ascribe merriment to those miraculously healed or revived by the alleged saint. Thus, according to the scribe, a boy of four, healed of an otherwise incurable facial tumour by the intercession and direct action of the king, displayed himself, newly healed, to his mother 'vultu hilaris et iocundo' (with a joyful and merry face). Taken on a thanksgiving visit to the shrine of the supposed saint at Windsor, the boy likewise showed himself 'letus' and 'iocundus'. His merriment clearly appears as a sign of healing as well as pleasure, and such a reaction is taken by the editor of the miracles to be so natural that even a fifteen-month-old child, revived from drowning through the offices of King Henry, could demonstrate it — he was led by his parents to the royal tomb, 'hilaris et iocundus' (joyful and merry).[21]

19 *Kingsford's Stonor Letters and Papers*, ed. by Carpenter, II, 6–8, Letter no. 166; quote from p. 7 (emphasis mine).

20 *Medieval English Lyrics*, ed. by Davies, Lyric nos 112 and 210.

21 *Henrici VI Angliae Regis Miracula Postuma*, ed. by Grosjean, pp. 284–86, quotes from pp. 286 and 209.

The editor of the miracles wrote in highly educated (indeed, high-flown) Latin; but the association between health and merriment/pleasure was not restricted to the educated. Late medieval London ecclesiastical court records contain the depositions of the plebeian associates of two servants, Beatrix Smyth and John Crote, as to their alleged marriage. John had been ill and had moved from his master's house to a rented room; Beatrix was still living in her mistress's household. One of their neighbours, Alice Vaughan, testified that Beatrix had visited and tended John in his sickness, presumably as a wife should, and that John had said to her 'in good feith Beatres Wif I shal nevir be mery til we haue ihade an end of that mater [their marriage] & that I be in myn own house'.[22] Said by a sick man, the words suggest that he meant he could achieve neither happiness nor health until the marriage and residence in a house of their own had been achieved and recognized.

Even more loosely, Richard Cely the elder could use 'merry' to connote 'thriving and prosperous *in business*'. Urging his son George to deal with merchants who, he had found, consistently paid in full 'befor the day', he remarked 'that ys mery for to dele wyt syche men'.[23] Clearly the term 'merry', to him, implied not just personal physical health, but any sort of well-being and prosperity.

Why should health, well-being, and lightheartedness be involved together in this way? An excessively pragmatic and somatic reading might suggest that it was so rare for a late medieval subject to feel entirely free from lingering illness or injury that the sense of well-being itself might produce profound joy. But this explanation is hardly sufficient. It does not account for the non-physical senses of 'well-being' implied in Richard Cely's use of the term 'merry', nor does it account for the fact that in late medieval England the link between health and happiness was clearly seen to be not just one way. On the contrary, 'merriment' was held to produce, not merely result from, physical health. This theory appears most clearly in the work of Andrew Borde, the early sixteenth-century scholar and physician, who had studied in Montpellier but returned to England to write his *A Compendyous Regyment or A Dyetary of Helth*, first published in 1542. In the dedication to his patron, the Duke of Norfolk, Borde directly acknowledges that

> dyuers tymes in my wrytynges I do wryte wordes of myrth; truly it is for no other intencon *but to make your grace mery — for myrth is one of the chefest thynges of*

[22] LMA, MS 9065, *Liber examinationum*, fols 35^r and 35^v.

[23] *The Cely Papers*, ed. by Malden, nos 10 and 11 (1478).

> *Physycke, the which doth aduertyse euery man to be mery, and to beware of pencyfulnes.*[24]

Borde recommends mirth at any time, but particularly on going to bed, to ensure healthy rest and slumber: 'To bedwarde be you mery, or haue mery company about you, so that, to bedwarde, no anger nor heuynes, sorowe nor pencyfulnes, do trouble or disquyet you'.[25] Why was mirth so health-provoking? The answer appears in Borde's lengthy excursus on the correct siting and building of a house; because 'the commodyous buyldyng of a place doth not onely satysfye the mynde of the inhabytur but also it doth comforte and reioyseth a mannes herte to se it, specyally the pulcruse prospect'. Whereas if

> the eye be not satysfyed, the mynde can not be contented. And the mynde can not be contented, the herte can not be pleased: yf the herte & mynde be not pleased, nature doth abhorre. And yf nature do abhorre, mortyfycacyon of the vytall, and anymall, and spyrytuall powers, do consequently folowe.[26]

Merriment, comfort, and pleasure were thus not merely health-giving, but literally life-preserving. Borde, however, was by no means the earliest writer to recommend mirth as a preservative and promoter of health. In Avicenna's influential medical thought, for instance,

> the emotions of the soul, such as joy, distress, fear, and anger, are also called the emotions of the spirit, since they are accompanied by cardiac and spiritual changes. [...] When people experience the same emotion often, they become prone to have it because of the changes in the system of the spirits and humours and the habituation of the faculties which are induced by it.[27]

In accordance with this prevalent view, joy was considered good for the body, and its practice was thought to make one a healthier person.

The ordinances drawn up for the care and education of the three-year-old Edward V in September 1473 specified that before his 8:00 p.m. bedtime, his attendants were to 'inforce themselves to make him joyouxe and merry towards his bedde'.[28] Lydgate's fifteenth-century 'A Dietary, and a Doctrine for the

[24] Borde, *The Fyrst Boke of the Introduction of Knowledge*, ed. by Furnivall, p. 228 (emphasis mine).

[25] Borde, *The Fyrst Boke of the Introduction of Knowledge*, ed. by Furnivall, p. 246.

[26] Borde, *The Fyrst Boke of the Introduction of Knowledge*, ed. by Furnivall, pp. 234–35.

[27] Knuuttila, *Emotions in Ancient and Medieval Philosophy*, p. 222.

[28] Orme, 'The Education of Edward V', p. 127, 'Ordinances concerning the guiding of our

Pestilence', though it admittedly uses the term 'glad' more often than 'merry', also opens with the advice:

> Who will been holle & kepe hym from sekenesse
> And resise the strok of pestilence,
> *Lat hym be glad, & voide al hevynesse.*[29]

The reader is particularly advised to be 'Glad toward bedde and at morwe, bothe too'; while in general, of the three things that 'consarue a mannys myth', 'a glad hert' is ranked first.[30]

One of the strongest therapeutic aspects of merriment was evidently its power to counter melancholy; for to allow the dominance of the melancholic humour over one's constitution was to risk the gravest consequences, both mental and physical. Melancholy, the coldest and driest humour, interfered with the proper digestion of one's food, producing, instead of nourishment, severely toxic by-products of ingestion. Hence the melancholic subject, wrote Borde, was 'the receptacle and the dragges of all the other humoures'. Not only physical, but dire mental consequences ensued, including paranoia, suicidal depression, and irrational rage. As Bartolomaeus Anglicus vividly described it:

> al that hath this passioun withouten cause beth often dredeful and sory [...]. And so if men asketh of suche what they drede and wherfore thei beth sory, they haueth none answere. Somme weneth that they schulen dye anon vnresonabliche. Somme dredith enemyte of som oon. Som loueth and desireth deth [...] somme falleth into wel euel suspicions withouten recouere, and therfore they hatith and blameth [...] hire frendes and somtyme smytith and sleeth hem.[31]

Hence, as Lydgate warned his readers, anyone seeking good health should 'take good heed' to be 'Nat malencolius for non adversite', but instead 'Nevir grucchyng, mery lik thi degree'.[32] Clearly, then, if merriment could, as Andrew Borde put it, preserve the 'vytall, and anymall, and spyrytuall powers', prevent the build-up of dangerous toxins in the body, and avoid the complete physical and mental breakdown associated with melancholy, it was a powerful agent of well-being.

[...] sonnes person', printed from TNA, Lord Steward's Department, Misc. Books, LS 13/280, fols 277–79.

29 Lydgate, *The Minor Poems*, ed. by MacCracken, p. 702 (emphasis mine).

30 Lydgate, *The Minor Poems*, ed. by MacCracken, pp. 703–04.

31 Trevisa, *On the Properties of Things*, ed. by Seymour, I, 161–62.

32 Lydgate, *The Minor Poems*, ed. by MacCracken, p. 705.

This reading of 'merriment' as the counter to melancholic disease may make sense of the title of the famous Tudor work the *C Merry Tales* (published 1525). Modern readers, I suspect, often find the work bewildering, granted that most of the stories in the collection seem anything but merry today. Admittedly, the large number of alleged instances of jest and quick-wittedness which may be reduced to variants of 'Shit on you' and 'Kiss my arse' may be explained in terms of the particular sense of humour of the early sixteenth century. But what are we to make of the many tales that seem simply to be cautionary or salutary stories? Tale number 56, for example, concerns a Warwickshire priest, who, 'though he were no great clerk nor graduate of the university', diligently preached the twelve articles of faith on Sunday, telling his parishioners:

> These articles ye be bound to believe, for they be true and of authority. And if you believe not me than for a more sure and sufficient authority, go your way to Coventry and there ye shall see them all played in Corpus Christ play.

The moral of the story is said to be that 'by reading of this tale, they that understand no Latin may learn to know the twelve articles of the faith'.[33] Where is the laugh-out-loud factor? Does it not make more sense to understand these tales as 'salutary', rather than 'humorous' in the modern sense? Presumably, in that case, a collection of 'merry' tales might well include some whose accounts of jests, tricks, and quick-witted repartee would, according to sixteenth-century understanding, help to repel depression and melancholy; and others whose moral or ethical meaning would still act to produce 'merriment' — in the sense of mental and spiritual health — in their audience. It is also presumably in that sense that Chaucer's Parson, disdaining poetic fictions, calls his long discourse on sin and repentance 'a myrie tale in prose'.[34]

For it is also clear from late medieval texts that the final set of meanings associated with the word 'merry' concerned spiritual wholeness and well-being, not just physical health. Andrew Borde's dictum that without pleasure of the heart, 'mortyfycacyon of the vytall, and anymall, and spyrytuall powers, do consequently folowe' is particularly telling here. These three categories clearly refer to the three parts of the human soul commonly identified by medieval scientists and theologians: the vegetative soul (which gives only life to the body), the sensible soul (common to animals and humans, which enables feeling and sense-impressions), and the *intellectus*, or reasonable soul, which humans

[33] *A Hundred Merry Tales*, ed. by Zall, Tale 56, pp. 115–16.

[34] Chaucer, *The Riverside Chaucer*, ed. by Benson, Fragment X (I), *Parson's Prologue*, p. 287, line 46.

alone possess, and which alone allows humans to discern vice from virtue and to apprehend, as far as possible in the fallen world, the incorporeal and the divine.[35] Borde's point therefore, is that to be merry keeps not only the body, but the soul, in good health; conversely he also taught that the practice of virtue, and spiritual exercise, was essential to true merriment. His *Dyetary*, like most other late medieval English examples of the genre, recommended both physical and spiritual care and exercise to produce good health;[36] 'whan you do ryse in the morenynge, ryse with myrth, and remembre God'. The duties of a household head, he believed, included enforcing religious observance and moral behaviour on the whole household, 'refraynynge them from vyce and synne, [and] compellynge them to obserue the commaundementes of God'. To achieve this end, 'he must contynewe in shewynge good example of lyuynge; *than may he reioyse in God, and be mery*, the whiche myrth and reioysyng doth lengthen a mans lyfe, and doth expell syckenes'.[37] To Borde, it appears, physical health, spiritual well-being, salvation, and merriment were inextricably linked. This association of merriment with both health and salvation may also make sense of Margery Kempe's famous vision (or rather, supernatural aural perception) of the 'sownde of melodye so swet & delectable, hir thowt, as sche had ben in Paradyse'. This phenomenon caused her to 'styrt owt of hir bedde' and exclaim 'Alas, that euyr I dede synne, it is ful mery in Hevyn'. Thereafter, she claimed, 'whan sche herd ony myrth or melodye' she experienced

> ful plentyuows & habundawnt teerys of hy deuocyon wyth greet sobbyngys & syhyngys aftyr the blysse of Heuen [...] & euyr aftyr this drawt sche had in hir mende the myrth & the melodye that was in Heuen [...]. For, wher sche was in ony cumpanye, sche wold sey oftyn-tyme, 'It is ful mery in Hevyn'.[38]

Here, the merriment taken to be the quintessence of heaven, though it produces in its human observer tears of longing and dissatisfaction with the joys of this world, nevertheless conduces to merriment in the sense of her true spiritual health and welfare. Indeed it is noteworthy that in the first chapters of her Book, Kempe consistently associates genuine health and prosperity with spiritual

[35] Trevisa, *On the Properties of Things*, ed. by Seymour, I, 95–96.

[36] Cf. Lydgate's 'Dietary', which recommends daily prayers, alms-giving, and avoidance of all vices, as part of a healthy regimen. Lydgate, *The Minor Poems*, ed. by MacCracken, pp. 705–06.

[37] Borde, *The Fyrst Boke of the Introduction of Knowledge*, ed. by Furnivall, pp. 234, 243–44, and 248 (emphasis mine).

[38] Kempe, *The Book*, ed. by Meech and Allen, p. 11.

enlightenment (and vice versa). Thus, her introductory paragraphs relate how she was brought from a state of half-hearted and vacillating repentance, accompanied by superficially apparent, but in fact unreliable, worldly health and prosperity, to true devotion through the mercy of Christ, who exposed the temporary and ultimately unreal nature of her worldly well-being, turning 'helth in-to sekeness, prosperyte in-to adversyte'. In Kempe's reading of her post-partum illness, it was the devil's urging her to avoid confession and true repentance of her sins, and tempting her to unbelief, that ultimately led her to display what Bartolomaeus Anglicus would have considered the classic symptons of melancholic breakdown — the will to suicide, self-harm, and slander of her husband and friends. Only after Christ's kindly visit to her bedside, and her resumption of perfect faith in him, did she regain spiritual, mental, and physical health.[39]

If merriment was thought to be thus related so closely to spiritual and physical well-being, it becomes obvious that heaven must be its typical locale. In heaven there is no sin, and the souls of the just are in perfect harmony, both with God and with their resurrected bodies. Furthermore, according to late medieval theologians, resurrected bodies would reclaim in heaven the perfect, invulnerable physical state of Adam and Eve before the Fall, subject to neither disease, death, nor decay.[40] No wonder the mode of heavenly music is mirth; such merriment is both product and sign of the true, and ultimate, spiritual and bodily wholeness and renovation enjoyed by the heavenly hosts — together with their concomitant joy in the full knowledge and sight of God.

It follows that joy and merriment are, in some late medieval texts, particularly associated with moments of triumph in the salvation history of humans. The editor of the miracles of King Henry VI, for example, notes that just as the pious should be horrified and sorrowful ('horrescimus et tristamur') at any victories of the devil, so they should equally 'iocundamur et gaudemus' ('rejoice and be merry') when the wiles of the devil are frustrated by virtue. In an exordium on the excellence of Henry VI as a miracle worker, he declared that his motive for writing was the 'animi iocunditas' ('joy/merriment of spirit') that overwhelmed him at the thought of the dead king's power to bring the dead to both life and faith.[41] The association of merriment with salvation may also

[39] Kempe, *The Book*, ed. by Meech and Allen, pp. 1 and 7–9.

[40] See, for example, Irlande, *The Meroure of Wyssdome*, vol. I, ed. by MacPherson, pp. 62–64; and Irlande, *The Meroure of Wyssdome*, vol. II, ed. by Quinn, p. 79.

[41] *Henrici VI Angliae Regis Miracula Postuma*, ed. by Grosjean, pp. 203 and 215.

account for the fact that though the term 'merry' occurs in various contexts in late medieval English lyrics, its most typical place is in carols celebating the Nativity. In this context, 'merriment' is often attributed first to angels (who naturally recognize immediately the vital salvific implications of Christ's intervention in human history); but humans are then called on to imitate angelic mirth, in recognition of the revelation and incarnation of their own salvation. A brief survey of the lyrics and carols in Richard Hill's early sixteenth-century commonplace book demonstrates the point. The first lyric, on the magi, urges its hearers 'Be mery all that be present | *Omnes de Saba venient*'. Number 20 evokes the Annunciation to the shepherds, who 'So merylye [...] began to blowe' when 'Off angels ther came a company | With mery songes and melody'. Number 11 recommends 'Make we mery in hall & bowr | Thys tyme was born owr Savyowr'.[42] Earlier lyrics repeat the theme. 'Make we mirth | For Christes birth' proclaimed an early fifteenth-century carol, setting out the various holy days and their devotional significance, from the Nativity to the Presentation in the Temple. A carol in honour of Christmas (*c.* 1450) notes that at the coming of 'Sire Christemasse', everyone 'Is glad and blithe'; 'Ye come to save all mankinde', the text continues, so that 'Alle manner of merthes we wole make | And solas to oure hertes take'.[43] Even the theological justification for displaying merriment particularly at the Annunciation and Nativity is carefully spelt out by John Mirk in his template sermon on the feast of the birth of the Virgin. He explains that the Church celebrates only three birthdays — those of Mary, St John the Baptist, and Christ — because these three signify that every 'man, womman and schylde' who is to be saved must be born three times, firstly of their mother, secondly in baptism (essential for any individual's salvation), and 'the thridde tyme oute of this worlde to ioy passing'. What guaranteed that the death of the righteous would constitute a glad transition to heaven? Only Christ's birth, the symbol and foreshadowing of our resurrection. Hence at the Nativity, says Mirk, 'was grete murth seyon and herde'.[44] Christmas thus became, archetypally, 'merry'.

The perfect joy of the saved in heaven may seem far removed from the mundane health concerns of the Celys' letters, or the scatological humour and trickster stories of the *C Merry Tales*. But we should be cautious in assuming

[42] *Songs, Carols and Other Miscellaneous Poems*, ed. by Dyboski, pp. 1, 11, 7; cf. also pp. 8, 9, 12, and 15.

[43] *Medieval English Lyrics*, ed. by Davies, nos 78, 116, 167–68, and 214.

[44] *John Mirk's Festial*, ed. by Powell, p. 222.

that medieval readers apprehended only some of the shades of meaning of the term 'mery' at any one time. There are, instead, some indications that a late medieval audience might readily make associations even between the most spiritual and apparently most down-to-earth readings of the word. The second shepherd's pageant of the Wakefield mystery play cycle (*Secunda Pastorum*) for instance, has often puzzled scholars. This sharply ludicrous tale of a sheep thief attempting to deceive his victims into thinking that a stolen lamb is his newborn baby seems to spend most of its time parodying the Visitation of the Shepherds (though they do, at the end of the play, attend the birthplace of the real Lamb of God).[45] So what place has it in an otherwise serious sequence of biblical pageants? To what genre does it really belong? At first sight surprisingly, it most resembles some of the trickster stories in the *C Merry Tales* (produced at much the same date); even Mak the sheep thief's eventual fate (being tossed in a blanket by the enraged shepherds) has the typically physical humour of these stories. I suggest, then, that the Wakefield Master, author of the pageants, has produced here a kind of genre pun, dependent on the multiple meanings of the word 'merry'. Just as Christmas is quintessentially a time of merriment, so it may properly be represented and celebrated by a presentation of what the lexicographer Robert Estienne called 'merry iestes' — however rough-and-ready they may seem to be. The third shepherd expresses the play's connection between Christmas merriment on earth at the angel's news and the heavenly 'mirth' that is promised in eternity:

> Be mery and not sad
> —Of myrth is oure sang
> Euer lasstyng glad
> To mede may we fang.[46]

Collectively, the shepherds express their sense of this double 'mirth' in a three-part song that matches in its homely way the angelic 'Gloria'.

If 'mirth' can mean so much, then it is the responsibility of historians to remember, always, that the term 'merry' in the period *c.* 1400–1550 cannot simply be read as signifying 'pleasure' in the sense of jocular, quick-witted, light-hearted cheerfulness. Instead it irreducibly carried with it much more serious — yet still pleasurable — connotations of health, well-being, renovation,

[45] *The Towneley Plays*, ed. by Stevens and Crawley, I.

[46] *The Towneley Plays*, ed. by Stevens and Crawley, I, 154, lines 963–66. Lines 965–66 may be translated as 'We can [now] receive eternal joy as a reward'.

revival, and salvation of body, mind, and soul. Our translation exercise should lead us, therefore, to locate late medieval notions of pleasure or happiness into much broader contexts than we, nowadays, are accustomed to consider, if we are to represent rightly the emotional and sensory experiences and expressions of the late Middle Ages.

Works Cited

Manuscripts and Archival Sources

Kew, The National Archives [TNA], Lord Steward's Department, Misc. Books, LS 13/280

London, London Metropolitan Archive [LMA] (formerly held by the Guildhall Library), MS 9065, *Liber examinationum*

Norwich, Norwich Record Office [NRO], Norwich Consistory Court [NCC], Wills

Primary Sources

Borde, Andrew, *The Fyrst Boke of the Introduction of Knowledge made by Andrew Borde, of physycke doctor. A compendyous regyment; or A Dyetary of Helth made in Mountpullier*, ed. by F. J. Furnivall, Early English Text Society, Extra Series, 10 (London: N. Trübner, 1870)

The Cely Papers: Selections from the Correspondence and Memoranda of the Cely Family, Merchants of the Staple, A.D. 1475–1488, ed. by Henry Elliot Malden, Camden Third Series, 1 (London: Longmans, Green, 1900)

Chaucer, Geoffrey, *The Riverside Chaucer*, ed. by Larry D. Benson (Boston: Houghton Mifflin, 1987)

La Chronique du Bon Duc Loys de Bourbon, ed. by A.-M. Chazaud, Société de l'histoire de France, 175 (Paris: Librairie Renouard, H. Loones successeur, 1876)

Dictionary of Medieval Latin from British Sources, ed. by R. E. Latham (Oxford: Oxford University Press for the British Academy, 1975–2013)

Estienne, Robert, *Dictionariolum puerorum tribus linguis Latina Anglica & Gallica*, English experience, its Record in Early Printed Books Published in Facsimile, 351 (Amsterdam: Teatrvm Orbis Terrarvm; New York: Da Capo Press, 1971)

Henrici VI Angliae Regis Miracula Postuma, ed. by Paul Grosjean, Subsidia Hagiographica, 22 (Bruxelles: Société des Bollandistes, 1935)

A Hundred Merry Tales and Other English Jestbooks of the Fifteenth and Sixteenth Centuries, ed. by P. M. Zall (Lincoln: University of Nebraska Press, 1963)

Irlande, John, *The Meroure of Wyssdome composed for the use of James IV, King of Scots A.D. 1490*, vol. i, ed. by Charles MacPherson, Scottish Text Society, 2nd ser., 19 (Edinburgh: Blackwood and Sons, 1926)

——, *The Meroure of Wyssdome composed for the use of James IV, King of Scots A.D. 1490*, vol. II, *Books III–V*, ed. by F. Quinn, Scottish Text Society, 4th ser., 2 (Edinburgh: Blackwood and Sons, 1965)

Jacob's Well, an English treatise on the cleansing of Man's Conscience, ed. by Arthur Brandeis, Early English Text Society, Original Series, 115 (London: Kegan Paul, Trench, Trübner, 1900)

John Mirk's Festial, edited from British Library Ms Cotton Claudius A. II, vol. II, ed. by Susan Powell, Early English Text Society, Original Series, 335 (Oxford: Oxford University Press, 2011)

Kempe, Margery, *The Book of Margery Kempe*, ed. by Sanford Brown Meech and Hope Emily Allen, Early English Text Society, Original Series, 212 (London: Oxford University Press, 1940)

Kingsford's Stonor Letters and Papers, 1290–1483, ed. by Christine Carpenter, Royal Historical Society Camden Classic Reprints, 1, 2 vols (Cambridge: Cambridge University Press, 1996)

Lydgate, John, *The Minor Poems of John Lydgate: Part II, Secular Poems*, ed. by Henry Noble MacCracken, Early English Text Society, Original Series, 192 (London: Oxford University Press, 1934; repr. 1961)

Mannyng, Robert, *Handlyng Synne*, ed. by Idelle Sullens, Medieval and Renaissance Texts and Studies Series, 14 (Binghamton, NY: Center for Medieval and Renaissance Studies, 1983)

Medieval English Lyrics: A Critical Anthology, ed. by Reginald T. Davies (London: Faber and Faber, 1963)

Middle English Dictionary, ed. by Hans Kurath (Ann Arbor: University of Michigan Press, 1952–2001), online at <http://quod.lib.umich.edu/m/med>

Paston Letters and Papers of the Fifteenth Century, ed. by Norman Davis, 3 pts (Oxford: Clarendon Press, 1976), II

Pecock, Reginald, *The Donet*, ed. by Elsie Vaughan Hitchcock, Early English Text Society, Original Series, 156 (London: Oxford University Press, 1921; New York: Kraus Reprint, 1971)

The Plumpton Letters and Papers, ed. by Joan Kirby, Camden Fifth Series, 8 (Cambridge: Cambridge University Press for the Royal Historical Society, 1996)

The Promptorium Parvulorum: The First English-Latin Dictionary, ed. by A. L. Mayhew, Early English Text Society, Extra Series, 102 (London: Kegan Paul, Trench, Trübner, 1908)

Songs, Carols and Other Miscellaneous Poems, from the Balliol MS 354, Richard Hill's Commonplace-Book, ed. by Roman Dyboski, Early English Text Society, Extra Series, 101 (London: Kegan Paul, Trench, Trübner, 1907)

The Towneley Plays, ed. by Martin Stevens and A. C. Crawley, Early English Text Society, Supplementary Series, 13–14, 2 vols (Oxford: Oxford University Press, 1994)

Trevisa, John, *On the Properties of Things: John Trevisa's translation of Bartholomaeus Anglicus De Proprietatibus Rerum: A Critical Text*, ed. by M. C. Seymour, 3 vols (Oxford: Clarendon Press, 1975–1988), I (1975)

Secondary Works

Barthes, Roland, *Mythologies* (trans. selections printed London: Jonathan Cape, 1960; reprinted London: Paladin, 1962)

Knuuttila, Simo, *Emotions in Ancient and Medieval Philosophy* (Oxford: Clarendon Press, 2004)

Maddern, Philippa, 'How Children Were Supposed to Feel; How Children Felt: England 1350–1530', in *Childhood and Emotion across Cultures, 1450–1800*, ed. by Claudia Jarzebowski and Thomas Max Safley (London: Routledge, 2014), pp. 121–40

Orme, Nicholas, 'The Education of Edward V', *Bulletin of the Institute of Historical Research*, 57 (1984), 119–30

Oxford English Dictionary Online <http://www.oed.com> [accessed 18 January 2013]

Sweet, Waldo E., Ruth Swan Craig, and Gerda M. Seligson, *Latin: A Structural Approach* (Ann Arbor: University of Michigan Press, 1957; rev. edn, 1966)

The Pleasures and Joys of the Humoral Body in Medieval Medicine

Fernando Salmón*

In 2002 Barbara Rosenwein published her influential paper 'Worrying about Emotions in History' where she coined the notion of 'emotional communities'.[1] In the years that followed she carefully developed this concept and outlined a research programme to help understand how people 'articulated, understood, and represented how they felt'.[2] A medievalist herself, she was aware of and pointed out the scarcity of medieval sources for a history of emotions and the often dry nature of its narratives. Despite this fact, she has been able to suggest that theories about emotions appear to have arisen from psychological and physiological explanatory models which were themselves the reflection of wider social ordering principles. Rosenwein's call for careful

* I would like to thank Montserrat Cabré and the editors of the volume for their careful reading of the paper and stimulating comments. The research has been funded by the Spanish Secretary of Science (HAR2011-25135-HIST and HAR2015-63995-P MINECO/FEDER).

[1] Rosenwein, 'Worrying about Emotions in History', pp. 842–45.

[2] Rosenwein, 'Problems and Methods in the History of Emotions', p. 11 n. 37.

Fernando Salmón (salmonr@unican.es) is professor of the history of science in the medical school at the University of Cantabria, Santander (Spain). His research interests pertain to the history of the modern hospital and medicine in the Middle Ages. His latest publications include 'The Physician as Cure in Medical Scholasticism', in *Ritual Healing: Magic, Ritual and Medical Therapy from Antiquity until the Early Modern Period*, ed. by Ildikó Csepregi and Charles Burnett (Firenze: SISMEL/Edizioni del Galluzzo, 2012), pp. 193–216; and in collaboration with Michael R. McVaugh, vol. XIV of *Arnaldi de Villanova Opera Medica Omnia* (Barcelona: Universitat de Barcelona, 2014).

Pleasure in the Middle Ages, ed. by Naama Cohen-Hanegbi and Piroska Nagy, IMR 24 (Turnhout: Brepols, 2018), pp. 39–57 BREPOLS PUBLISHERS 10.1484/M.IMR-EB.5.113461

analysis that takes into account detailed chronological and regional specificities resulted in a richer and more changeable panorama of medieval emotions than expected. However, in this quest for analysing how medieval people understood emotions, it is striking how little attention was given, initially, to medical sources. More recently though, historiography has shown a growing interest in medical sources for a history of emotions and a more general interest in the relationship between emotions and health.[3] This connection should not be surprising if we recall that in the Middle Ages the material locus that sustained the lay and medical understandings of the workings of the emotions was a body conceptualized and experienced within a holistic framework — a framework provided by humoralism[4] — where there was no radical separation between the psychic and the somatic. In fact, in all medical texts, from those that circulated in the West in the early Middle Ages to those that were produced later at the universities, emotions such as wrath, sadness, or joy were described as bodily movements that could promote health or induce disease. Pleasure and pain were not considered emotions per se, but belonged to the experiential realm of the emotions. Furthermore, some emotions, like joy and sadness, would usually be accompanied by pleasure or pain — and vice versa.

In this article I would like to focus on some of the approaches to pleasure (*delicia*) and joy (*gaudium*) as developed in Latin in the medical schools of the thirteenth and fourteenth centuries. In so doing, I explore the possible uses of medical sources for a history of how emotions were understood in the past and also for reflecting on how some of these emotions were experienced.

After extensive archival research carried out over the last thirty years, historians of medicine have convincingly argued that Galenism, the learned medical tradition based on humoralism that was developed in the medieval universities, constructed an understanding of health and disease that had a widespread social dissemination from the late thirteenth century onward.[5] This particular knowledge of the body in health and disease was developed in Latin with materials deriving from a rich medical tradition that had been recorded in Greek

[3] See, for example, Casagrande and Vecchio, *Piacere e dolore*; Carrera, *Emotions and Health, 1200–1700*.

[4] In this paper I will use 'humoralism' (and the same applies to 'humoral') as a vaguely defined system of thought about the functioning of the body in health and disease that dominated the ancient and the medieval Mediterranean, characterized by the importance given to balance, processes of transformation, and the flow of certain qualities or constituents of the body. See Nutton, 'Humoralism'; Horden, 'Introduction'.

[5] McVaugh, *Medicine before the Plague*.

and Arabic in diverse chronological, cultural, and geographical areas within the Mediterranean basin.

Research into the complex processes of the circulation, appropriation, and transformation of ideas and practices concerning health and disease within the main Christian, Islamic, and Judaic medieval cultures has shaped a great deal of the historiography devoted to medieval medicine.[6] Emotions are human experiences heavily laden with cultural values, and it seems logical to assume that their medical conceptualization, and the practices of care developed around them in different places and times, might involve complex processes of cultural translation that could result in incommensurable fragmentation rather than continuity. Yet an analysis of medical texts that were read and produced in the medieval medical schools in the thirteenth and fourteenth centuries shows that this logic applies only partially to pleasure and joy in their relation to medicine and health.

Sexual pleasure has proved troublesome for the Christian Latin tradition. But this aspect of pleasure — which has been the focus of attention of most of the historiography devoted to the topic[7] — was only one aspect of a wider discussion around pleasure developed in the medical schools. Instead, the analysis of medical debates on the topic highlights the tension between the theoretical framework that medicine proposed for the understanding of pleasure as perceived by any of the five senses and the practices of care that were performed in the context of those experiences. This tension was not structured around the need for adjustment to the cultural sensitivity of a specific community, as in the case of sexual pleasure, since both understanding and practices were shared in a relatively unproblematic way by the various Mediterranean cultures. Thus, it seems that continuity over fragmentation can be stressed as the result of the analysis of pleasure at the medieval medical schools. The second part of the paper also seeks to show this continuity. It seeks to recover traces of the emotional lives of the past by reflecting on praise for the beneficial effects of joy in the practice of medical care. The promotion of joy and the recommendation to avoid sadness was a common theme in the humoral system that sustained the lay and medical understanding of the body within the Mediterranean basin and beyond. I will contend that in this wide area practitioners and their patients from diverse cultural, linguistic, and geographical locations were able to share a common

[6] Jacquart, *La Science médicale occidentale entre deux renaissances (XIIe s.–XVe s.)*; García Ballester, *Medicine in a Multicultural Society*.

[7] Park, 'Medicine and Natural Philosophy'.

experience of the lived body that helped to ensure an unproblematic transfer of knowledge and practices around the effects of emotions for a healthy life.[8]

Pleasure

Most historians that have researched the concept of pleasure in the medical sources of the Christian Latin tradition have focused on *delectatio*, which usually emerges as the kind of pleasure obtained or withheld when medieval women and men were engaged in sexual desires and practices. Usually framed within the wider scheme provided by natural philosophy, *delectatio* and its appropriate modes of expression emerged in medical discussions and texts as a powerful determinant of basic social divisions based on sexual difference, reproductive and non-reproductive sex, or healthy and unhealthy bodies and practices. No wonder that it was considered dangerous stuff that needed to be culturally tailored if it was intended to travel among communities with different religious and social values.[9]

However, Latin medical sources also provide us with another idea of pleasure, more usually referred to as *delicia*. *Delicia* can also be felt in the sexual encounter as perceived through the sense of touch in the genitalia. Yet this term is not limited to sex: in the Galenic economy of the senses, it encompasses a wider meaning, as the opposite of pain. In this context, *delicia* is defined as being in accord with the natural state of the sensory organ. And as such, *delicia* stands out more prominently than *delectatio* in the preoccupations of the medical masters of the thirteenth and fourteenth centuries. In *c.* 1285 Jean de Saint-Amand (*c.* 1230–1303), the Parisian medical master, collected some four thousand extracts from medical authorities discussed in the classroom. He set them out under more than five hundred headings, arranged alphabetically to serve as an aide-mémoire of the essentials of Galenic medicine.[10] There is no entry for *delectatio* but seven for *delicia*.[11]

[8] In this paper I will use 'the Mediterranean' as a geographical and cultural space of fuzzy boundaries characterized by fragmentation and connectivity, as discussed by Horden and Purcell. See Horden and Purcell, *The Corrupting Sea*; Horden, 'Mediterranean Excuses'.

[9] Jacquart and Thomasset, *Sexualité et savoir médical au Moyen Âge*, pp. 121–92; Cadden, *Meanings of Sex Difference in the Middle Ages*, pp. 134–65; Cadden, *Nothing Natural Is Shameful*.

[10] Jacquart, 'L'Oeuvre de Jean de Saint-Amand et les méthodes d'enseignement à la faculté de médicine de Paris à la fin du XIIIe siècle', pp. 257–75.

[11] Pagel, *Die Concordanciae des Johannes de Sancto Amando*, p. 76.

The difficulty presented to medical authors by *delicia* had nothing to do with the cultural metamorphosis needed for the safe travel of the concept through diverse Mediterranean communities, as was the case with the more often sexualized *delectatio*, but with the disentanglement of its intrinsic theoretical complexities.

By the second half of the thirteenth century Jean de Saint-Amand in Paris, like other contemporaries of his in the medical schools of Montpellier or Bologna, eagerly devoted his energies to mastering a bulk of new works by Galen that were not included in the traditional medical syllabus known as the *articella*. The so-called 'new Galen', in García Ballester's phrasing,[12] included the *De morbo et accidenti*, a compilation of Alexandrian origin of four of Galen's most important treatises on general pathology.[13] The *De morbo et accidenti* must have posed an interesting challenge for the university medical masters of the late thirteenth century, as shown by the fact that despite its theoretical complexity, it was the object of at least nine academic commentaries produced between *c.* 1290 and 1345. Two of the commentaries were produced at Montpellier by two masters of that *studium* (Arnau of Vilanova (*c.* 1240–1311) and Bernard of Gordon (*c.* 1258–*c.* 1320)), four in Bologna (by Bartholomew of Varignana (*c.* 1260–*c.* 1321), Dino del Garbo (d. 1327), Albert of Bologna (*c.* 1280 – after 1348), and Anthony of Parma (fl. 1315)), and one in Perugia (Gentile da Foligno (d. 1348)), and another two of the extant commentaries remain anonymous.[14] The contents of the *De morbo et accidenti* might also be considered of interest for the physician-to-be since the work was incorporated in the ordinances of the medical school of Montpellier in 1309.[15] It is in this work that the medieval scholar could find the longest medical discussion of *delicia* and its opposite, pain.

In the Arabic–Latin translation of the work most commonly commented upon in the classroom,[16] the student was able to learn that, after defining its

[12] García Ballester, 'Arnau de Vilanova (*c.* 1240–1311) y la reforma de los estudios médicos en Montpellier (1309)'.

[13] Durling, 'Corrigenda et Addenda to Diel's Galenica', pp. 467–68. For a modern English translation of the four treatises from Kühn's Greek text, see Galen, *On Diseases and Symptoms*, trans. by Johnston.

[14] A description of these commentaries, along with their attributions and their interconnections can be found in Salmón, 'Technologies of Authority in the Medical Classroom in the Thirteenth and Fourteenth Centuries'.

[15] *Cartulaire de l'Université de Montpellier*, p. 220.

[16] A working edition of the fourth book of Galen's *De morbo et accidenti* (based on Montpellier, Faculté de Médecine, MS H-18, fols 18rb–21vb, and Edinburgh, University Library,

contrary (*contrarium delicie*), Galen offered a definition of pleasure as 'an affection (*passio*) where what is out of the order of nature is suddenly brought back again to nature'.[17] This very same quote, slightly rearranged, was chosen by Jean de Saint-Amand to describe *delicia* as 'an affection where suddenly the members recover their natural state'.[18] It is interesting to note that in Galen's presentation and in the lectures and quotations made of the fourth book of the *De morbo et accidenti*, pain was often named, not as *dolor*, but as the opposite of pleasure (*contrarium delicie*). In fact, 'Delicia vero et contrarium eius …' is the opening sentence of the long exposition on the topic.[19] And most medical authors agreed with the idea that pleasure must precede pain because it was the natural or ordinary course of things.[20] However, a sequence that prioritized pleasure over pain would seem to contradict the standard definition of pleasure just outlined, where the emphasis is on the idea of pleasure as a recovery from a previous lapsed state.

This apparent contradiction led to questions about the ontological priority of these two affections. The problem openly raised in the medical classroom was solved by admitting the possibility of experiencing pleasure not only when recovering the natural state previously disrupted by pain but also when achieving what is best attuned to nature. Thus a healthy eye feels pleasure merely by seeing the colour green or sea-blue, intermediate colours between the two extremes of black and white.[21] A further argument in favour of the independ-

MS 166, fols 5ra–7va) and the commentary attributed to Arnau of Vilanova (based on the only extant copy: Kraków, Biblioteka Jagiellowska, MS 781, fols 131^{r}–157^{v}) is in Salmón, *Las teorías de la visión en la medicina universitaria bajo-medieval*. All the quotations from these works will refer to this edition.

[17] 'delicia autem est passio qua subito reducimur ad naturam; nam si paulatim existat, eam minime senciemus': Salmón, *Las teorías de la visión en la medicina universitaria bajo-medieval*, p. 83.

[18] 'Delicia est passio qua reducuntur membra ad naturam suam, quia si fiat paulatim nihil aut parum sentitur': Pagel, *Die Concordanciae des Johannes de Sancto Amando*, p. 76.

[19] Salmón, *Las teorías de la visión en la medicina universitaria bajo-medieval*, p. 83.

[20] See, for example, the argument developed by Peter of Spain in his long *questio De dolore et delicia* in his *Questiones super libro de crisi et super libro de diebus creticis*, Madrid, BN, MS 1877, fols 249^{ra-vb}.

[21] 'Sed advertendum quod non solum delicia [fit] ex reduccione disposicionis non naturalis ad naturalem, sed eciam ex reduccione naturalis ad naturalitatem, sicut oculus sanus existens, si occurrat viridis color, statim delectatur': Salmón, *Las teorías de la visión en la medicina universitaria bajo-medieval*, p. 95. Albert of Bolonia follows the same reasoning: 'non solum fit delicia ex reduccione disposicionis non naturalis ad naturalem sed eciam ex disposicione naturalis ad ampliorem naturalitatem'. Albertus Bononiensis, *Commentum supra tractatum*

ence of pleasure from pain was the idea that since a bodily organ free from damage feels better than one that is harmed, a pleasurable feeling (perhaps an even greater pleasure) could also be achieved within a permanent healthy state.[22] Daily experience was also cited to support the prior and independent status of pleasure in relation to pain, for example, in arguments that it was possible to feel a pleasurable sensation in the tongue when placing honey upon it, regardless of whether there had been previous harm.[23]

The definition of pleasure, however, involved another consideration, one that deals with the pace of the movement. Following Galen, most medieval authors understood that this needs to be sudden because if it is done slowly there is no pleasurable perception or it is very poor.[24] For some, it also needs to be intense.[25] And the medical student also learnt that the pleasurable sensation

Galieni de morbo et accidenti, BAV, MS Reg. lat. 2000, fol. 53rb. The adequacy of the sense and sensible is given by Antonius de Parma in his collection of questions on the *De morbo et accidenti* as supporting this possibility: 'Sed est intelligendum quod non solum causa delicie per se est reductio dispositionis innaturalis ad naturalem; sed eciam naturalis ad naturalem sicut proprie convenientia sensus cum sensibili'. Antonius de Parma, *Quaestiones supra tractatum Galieni de morbo et accidenti*, BAV, MS Vat. lat. 4450, fol. 86rb. In Galen's reading the eye able to enjoy the intermediate colour, in this case sea-blue, is healthy but tired: 'sed eo [oculo] sano existente, licet fatigato, nihil ei adeo ita erit iuvativum, utpote confortativum, velut venetus color et post eum lividus; hii namque colores non dividunt vel dispergunt visum, sicut facit albus et splendidus, nec coadunat eum et extingunt, velut facit niger'. Salmón, *Las teorías de la visión en la medicina universitaria bajo-medieval*, p. 87.

22 Gentile da Foligno asked: 'Dubitatur que sit maior delectatio an quando occurrit conveniens corpori sano, an quando fit motus a disposicione contra naturam ad secundum naturam' (Gentile da Foligno, *Notata super libro de accidenti et morbo*, München, BS, MS Clm. 62, fol. 85rb), and concluded that 'delectatio non est solum in quantitate distancie terminorum a quo ad terminum ad quem, sed in bonitate comprehensionis convenientis et ista magis fit in sano' (fol. 85va).

23 'Quod si ponatur mel supra linguam que prius non dolebat sed indiferentis erat, tunc adgeneratur in ea delectatio; ergo, prius dolebat falsum est'. The reflection is posed by Petrus Hispanus in a *questio* on the precedence of pleasure over pain ('Queritur utrum delectatio precedat dolorem'). Petrus Hispanus, *Questiones super libro de crisi et super libro de diebus creticis*, Madrid, BN, MS 1877, fol. 249va.

24 'Delicia est passio qua subito reducuntur membra ad naturam suam, quia si fiat paulatim nihil aut parum sentitur': Pagel, *Die Concordanciae des Johannes de Sancto Amando*, p. 76.

25 'Sed convenit cum eo in tribus: scilicet ex eo cui adveniunt quia in omni sensu; et ex parte eius a quo eveniunt, quia a re vehementer alterante; et ex parte modi sui proventus, quia tam delicia quam dolor subito eveniunt': Salmón, *Las teorías de la visión en la medicina universitaria bajo-medieval*, p. 103. A similar idea was expressed by Albert of Bologna: 'secundo ex parte obiecti causantis ea scilicet quia ambo proveniunt ex re vehementer alterante'. Albertus

needs a bodily organ in order to occur. In fact, the connection with a particular bodily part, for most medical authors, marked the distinction between *delicia* and *gaudium* since the first is linked to the body and the second to the soul.[26] The particular body part through which the *delicia* finds its expression was considered to be the organ of any of the five external senses.

Delicia could be felt by each of the five senses, but it is experienced more intensively by the sense of touch, the coarsest and basest of the group.[27] The intensity of the pleasurable sensation was conditioned by the materiality of the object proper to each sense: the lightest sensation occurs in the case of vision whose proper object, colour and light, were considered to be the subtlest. The strongest sensation occurs in the case of touch whose object was defined by four sets of opposing qualities of hot and cold, dry and wet, hard and soft, and rough and smooth.[28]

Complex theoretical discussions around the perception of pleasure by the senses abounded among medical circles, as witnessed by the rich diversity of problems posed by the commentators on the *De morbo et accidenti* and in other works when trying to grasp and reconcile the various medical and natural philosophical traditions and authorities that they invoked.[29] But their preoccupa-

Bononiensis, *Commentum supra tractatum Galieni de morbo et accidenti*, BAV, MS Vat. Reg. lat. 2000, fol. 53vb.

26 'Tamen advertendum quod si dolor et delicia corporis in hoc conveniant quod dictum est cum tristicia et gaudio, tamen in alio differunt: quoniam dolor corporis et delicia passiones sunt anime, ut ad aliquod organum corporale referuntur; sed gaudium et tristicia passiones sunt eius non relate ad aliquod organum corporale; ex quo patet quod dolor corporis et delicia non dicuntur esse corporis quia ab anima non fiant, quoniam ab ea fiunt, sed dicuntur corporis quoniam non sunt anime, nisi ut ad /146rb aliquod organum corporale referuntur; ulterius quia dolor et delicia sunt anime ut referuntur ad organum corporale, ideo maxime in sensu consistunt': Salmón, *Las teorías de la visión en la medicina universitaria bajo-medieval*, p. 122.

27 Salmón, 'A Medieval Territory for Touch', pp. 64–65.

28 'Item delicie odoratus magis sunt in manifesto, quia substancia eius grossior est, quia, sicut aer splendore grossior existit, similiter fumus aere grossior existit. Sensus autem visus non sentit nisi splendorem et lumen, auditus vero aerem, odoratus autem fumum, sicut gustus non sentit nisi substanciam humidam, tactus vero duram': Salmón, *Las teorías de la visión en la medicina universitaria bajo-medieval*, p. 88. The same idea is expressed by Galen in the other main treatise on general pathology, *De interioribus*: 'tactus vero crossior est ceteris; sicut visus omnibus est subtilior et post eum auditus. Similiter post tactum in crossitie gustus est, odoratus vero inter quattuor sensus est mediocris'. Galen, *Opera Galieni*, *De interioribus*, lib. IV, c. 2, fol. 127rb. The same reasoning occurs in Avicenna, *Liber Canonis tocius medicinae*, lib. I, f. 2, d. 2, s. 2, c. 23, fol. 32vb.

29 The fact that Gentile's commentary marks the terminus ad quem of this series of expositions and that he freely uses contemporary authors makes his own commentary especially

tions were not just aimed at theoretical issues. Establishing the degree of the pleasurable effect of the action of a particular sensible thing on the corresponding sense organ could furnish some pieces of therapeutic advice. This includes suggestions on how to provide care to patients who have been exposed to excessive bright light or excessive darkness, or to those who have had their fingers paralysed due to freezing and damp. A comfortable transition to a room in partial shadow in the first case would be advisable, and avoidance of exposure to violent heat, in the second.[30] These recommendations seemed to contradict the well-established medical theory of the effect of contraries, thus compelling further explanation in the classroom.[31]

Here the advice on how to obtain a pleasurable sensation was problematic for Latin Christian physicians, not because it needs to be attuned to the specific cultural and moral sensitivities of their particular community (as in the case of advice on how to obtain pleasure in performing sex), but because there was disagreement between the theoretical framework proposed and common practice.[32] Such disagreement was easily resolved by the efficacious technology developed by medical scholasticism, which was able to incorporate the practical findings of the experience of care without challenging its own theoretical discourse.

revealing of this complexity. Gentile da Foligno, *Notata super libro de accidenti et morbo*, München, BS, MS Clm. 62, fols 83ra–85vb.

[30] Salmón, *Las teorías de la visión en la medicina universitaria bajo-medieval*, pp. 94–95 and pp. 109–10.

[31] The contradiction is clearly expressed in the *questio* posed by Antonius de Parma: 'Utrum cum visus patitur a tenebris debeat subito duci ad lucem. Et videtur quod sic quia omnis cura fit per contrarium; eciam quia est subita revocatio dispositionis innaturalis ad naturalem, per nos videmus quod visus que patitur a luce debet subito duci ad tenebras et fit tunc deliciam; ideo <…> etcetera'. Antonius de Parma, *Quaestiones supra tractatum Galieni de morbo et accidenti*, BAV, MS Vat. lat. 4450, fol. 87ra.

[32] 'Sed hic est dubitacio utrum visus paciens ex tenebris subito debeat reduci ad lucem. Videtur quod sic, quia ex mente Galieni in littera visus paciens a luce subito duci debet ad nigrum colorem vel tenebram; Quare et econtrario eodem modo. Item: quia omnis cura fit per contrarium equale sibi; Lux autem tenebrositati est contraria; Quare <…> etcetera. In contrarium argumentaur per illud quod patet ad sensum quoniam tunc visus minime videbit': Salmón, *Las teorías de la visión en la medicina universitaria bajo-medieval*, p. 109. Gentile posed a similar question ('Dubitatur an qui stetit in obscuro debeat subito venire ad lumen') to his students while advising of the danger of bringing someone to a bright light after a long exposure to darkness. He used Galen's story of the cruelty of Dionysus the Tyrant to support his view: 'dicit Galienus quod ille Dyonisius tenebat homines in carceribus obscuris longo tempore deinde subito faciebat eos duci ad unum locum valde luminosum et ibi subito perdebant visum'. Gentile da Foligno, *Notata super libro de accidenti et morbo*, München, BS, MS Clm. 62, fol. 83va.

If extreme heat was the theoretical recommendation for obtaining a pleasurable sensation in the case of the freezing of any body part, common practice showed that it should be avoided, because it would only intensify the painful sensation. Medical scholasticism did not reject this experiential truism despite the fact that it contradicted its theoretical model for the causes of pain and pleasure. But the contradiction needed to be solved by a logical explanation, and thus, some medical authors would argue, the use of heat should be avoided in the alleviation of pain in a freezing member, because the heat pushes the cold deeper, or towards a different location in the affected member, and this would produce a new and more intense pain instead of the pleasure that might have been expected.[33] Then the heat, according to this reasoning, would only be accidentally responsible for producing pain instead of pleasure, because of its effect on the unbalanced humoral complexion caused by the freezing.[34] It seems that this was considered to be a sound solution among university-trained physicians, since various lectures given not only on the *De morbo* but also on Galen's *De malicia complexionis diverse* and Avicenna's *Canon* offered a similar line of argument.[35] Thus, the medical student could learn how to incorporate into his own practical armoury what experience teaches (the fact that the contrary quality — extreme heat — cannot produce pleasure by bringing back to the natural state a member affected by extreme cold) without challenging the theoretical framework built upon pleasure.

[33] 'Tamen est quod quandoque per accidens in tali reduccione fit tristicia, racione reducciones contrarie sibi anexe, sicut in exemplo de quo dictum est; tunc tamen fit dolor, quoniam frigus ad partes digitorum pervenit quibus prius non ocurrebat propter calorem fortem qui, condempsans partes illas digitorum in quibus prius erat frigus, fugat frigidum ad partes alias': Salmón, *Las teorías de la visión en la medicina universitaria bajo-medieval*, pp. 94–95; 'quando ignis subito approximatur ipsis extremitatibus cum tunc unum contrarium fugiet ut frigus existens in superficie fugiet in profundo et profundatur magis ideo partes interiores leduntur et causatur ibi magnus dolor': Gentile da Foligno, *Primus Avic. Canon cum argutissima Gentilis expositione*, fol. 109ra.

[34] 'ut si sit aliquis habens aliquod extremum frigidum et ipsum aproximet igni vel forti calido, statim fit in ipso tristicia et hoc non fit nisi per accidens quia mala complexio frigida equalis existens primo in illo membro per calidum advenientis fit diversa': Antonius de Parma, *Quaestiones supra tractatum Galieni de morbo et accidenti*, BAV, MS Vat. lat. 4450, fol. 86rb.

[35] See, for example, Gentile's commentary on the *Canon*, lib. I, fen 2, doc. 2. c. 23. Gentile da Foligno, *Primus Avic. Canon cum argutissima Gentilis expositio*, fol. 109ra; Arnau de Vilanova, *Commentum super tractatum Galieni De malicia complexionis diverse*, ed. by García Ballester and Sánchez Salor, pp. 277–79.

The medical discourse on pleasure just outlined was shared by the Greek Galen when working in Rome in the second century, by the Persian Avicenna when composing his *Canon* in the eleventh century, and by the Italian master Gentile da Foligno when teaching in fourteenth-century Perugia. Its practical advice could be shared too by their patients. Why should this be so?

Joy and the Avoidance of Sadness

The problems posed by sensuous pleasure outlined above were indicative of the continuity in the theoretical development of the topic within an all-encompassing humoral medical tradition, despite the various cultural, linguistic, and chronological differences between the authors that contributed to it.[36] The incorporation of practical advice derived from experience also pointed to continuity in the tradition of care. It also indicated the limits and possibilities that the humoral body offered, not just for the understanding but also for the experiencing of emotions in the Middle Ages. To bring the humoral body centre stage may help to clarify the cross-cultural appeal of the beneficial effects of joy in its relation to health.

I am not denying that medical systems are built with and reflect historically shaped cultural values and need to be attuned to religious and social mores. Feminist scholarship has provided us with stimulating research on this point.[37] I am aware also of the discontinuities, differences, and local specificities that characterized the transfer of knowledge and practices. In recent years, the historiography of science has been eagerly devoted to the exploration of these.[38] However, historiography must also answer to themes of continuity and stability. It is by no means obvious that the same narrative should function equally satisfactorily in explaining the positive effects of joy to a rich Kairouan patient from the ninth century and to King Jaume II of Aragon five centuries later.

We must bear in mind that the success of a medical model does not necessarily stand on the historical accountability of its therapeutic efficacy, but rather on current expectations and on a plausible explanation of the causes of the ailment and of the symptoms that are felt. A convincing rationale needs a shared common ground in order to allow communication between patient and physician.[39]

[36] Compare, for example, the analysis of pleasure as given in Galen (*De morbo et accidenti*), Avicena (*Canon*), and Gentile da Foligno (Commentaries on *Canon* and *De morbo et accidenti*).

[37] Park, *Secrets of Women*; Green, *Making Women's Medicine Masculine*.

[38] Secord, 'Knowledge in Transit'.

[39] Kleinman, *Patients and Healers in the Context of Culture*.

Galenic humoralism was built on this common ground by using a convincing imagery for the workings of the body that connected with a sense of the lived self that was shared by the peoples where it was developed as the dominant medical system. I suggest that this experiential dimension of Galenism helps to explain its cross-cultural acceptance and the long-term success of this medical narrative within the ancient and medieval Mediterranean. In turn, this success opens up the possibility for recovering traces of the emotional life of the past by analysing its extant sources. An analysis of the medical recommendation of the avoidance of sadness and the beneficial effects of joy, as expounded by one of the most influential university physicians of the time, Arnau of Vilanova (*c.* 1240–1311), will illustrate the phenomenological resonance of this medical system.

There is not much information available about Arnau's actual healing activities, although his success and his patrons' appreciation of his application of the art are well documented. In fact, some of Arnau's written production was an answer to the demands, intellectual and practical, of his clientele.[40] But what did Arnau offer to his illustrious patients? Not necessarily a cure through drugs or a resolute treatment such as surgeons offered. Rather, a convincing explanation of the ailment, its course and its causes, and recommendations for the preservation of health and the avoidance of disease through the monitoring of the so-called *res non naturales* (six non-natural things) — including joy, one of the accidents of the soul.[41]

How did Arnau de Vilanova understand the way emotions worked in the body? How did he explain the actions and possible beneficial effects of joy, and to which kind of bodily experiences was he appealing?

This is not the place to discuss the Galenic bodily economy, but I want to stress that the humoral body, the very locus where medieval medicine acted, was also the experiential body of the patients who used this model of medicine. It was not an abstract ideal, but a body that varied from individual to individual. It was a body mediated by sensuous experiences, which could be seen, but also smelt, touched, and listened to. A body where there was no separation between the somatic and the psychic and the different parts of which were in dynamic exchange with each other and with what surrounded them.[42]

[40] McVaugh, *Medicine before the Plague*; Paniagua, *Studia Arnaldiana*.

[41] García Ballester, 'On the Origin of the "Six Non-natural Things" in Galen'.

[42] For a recent reflection on various humoral systems, see Horden and Hsu, *The Body in Balance*.

In order to follow Arnau's thinking on the relationship between emotions and health, I will offer a brief sketch of the model he outlined in three of his works: an academic commentary, the *Repetitio super vita brevis* (1301);[43] a regimen of health, the *Regimen sanitatis ad regem Aragonum* (1306–07);[44] and a compendium on the theory of medicine, the *Speculum medicine* (1306–08).[45] These represent Arnau's thoughts on the topic and also the two different audiences that he had in mind when writing, lay and professional. In this case, his lay audience was a very special patient, the King of Aragon, and the professional, his students and colleagues of the medical school of Montpellier.

In the *Regimen sanitatis ad regem Aragonum*, which is aimed at literally putting the life of Jaume II into order, the King was able to learn that the accidents of the soul affected his body in important ways, and that, among those accidents, he should principally avoid anger and sadness,[46] sadness in particular, because it cools and dries the body, producing exhaustion and severe loss of weight. Because sadness contracts the heart, the spirit that emanates from it is darker and heavier, and thus sadness alters the sense perception, obscures good judgement, and weakens the functions of memory. Joy should be sought after to revive the diminished and damaged spirits.[47]

Speret qui metuit. Morituros vivere vidi, spe duce victuros, spe moriente mori. These little verses, promising life if led by hope, and death if hope failed, are quoted in an anonymous commentary on the Hippocratic *Aphorisms* of the thirteenth century.[48] However, its moral did not derive from medical tradition but rather from one of Aesop's fables, memorized in the grammar schools

[43] Arnau de Vilanova, *Repetitio super aphorismo Hippocratis 'Vita Brevis'*, ed. by McVaugh.

[44] Arnau de Vilanova, *Regimen sanitatis ad regem aragonum*, ed. by García Ballester and McVaugh.

[45] Arnau de Vilanova, *Speculum introductionum medicinalium*.

[46] On the accidents of the soul in this treatise and generally on the tradition of the regimes of health, see the detailed analysis offered by Pedro Gil in his introduction to Arnau de Vilanova, *Regimen sanitatis ad regem aragonum*, ed. by García Ballester and McVaugh, pp. 803–27.

[47] 'Tristicia vero corpus infrigidat et exsiccat; propterea maciem et extenuacionem inducit, et quia cor constringit et spiritus obtenebrat et ingrossat, ingenium hebetat, apprehensionem impedit, iudicium obscurat, et obtundit memoriam; et ideo vitanda sunt eius obiecta nisi quantum racio persuadet ad detestacionem viciorum et mentis pulcritudinem reformandam. Qui vero multis curis et sollicitudinibus distrahuntur et crebro punguntur, gaudio sepe vacare debent et honestis solaciis, ut animus refloreat et spiritus recreentur': Arnau de Vilanova, *Regimen sanitatis ad regem aragonum*, ed. by García Ballester and McVaugh, p. 436.

[48] *Commentarius in 'Aphorismos' Hippocratis*, UB Erfurt, MS Ea Q. 181, fol. 91v.

from the twelfth century onwards (contemporary Latin proverbs conveyed the same idea).[49] Biblical passages from Proverbs or Ecclesiastes made the same connection between sadness and the deterioration of health, or even death. Thus, Arnau did not need to incorporate further explanations to make sure that the King would accept the threatening consequences of negative feelings such as sadness and despair and would willingly avoid them, since this was commonly accepted knowledge and not just some theory confined to medical prescriptions.

Even if anger could occasionally be considered an emotion with positive physical effects, the emotion that was unanimously thought by medical authors to be positive was joy. A moderate joy that set the vital spirits and natural heat in motion expanded the heart, cooled it, and was beneficial for the whole body. Recommendations to slow down daily preoccupations and to enjoy the company of friends, music, or pleasant stories were frequent in medical advice for the maintenance of health.[50]

It would seem logical that if physicians were familiar with these recommendations and their underlying physiological rationale, the handling of those emotions that arose in the healing encounter — sadness, hope, fear, etc. — would be considered when teaching students how to plan the encounter with the patient and how to use therapeutically positive emotions in actual care. And, in fact, it was within this framework that the medical student learned, literally, how to move the patient's heart, as Arnau taught in his commentary on the Hippocratic first aphorism, '*Vita brevis...*'. A well-developed theory of the emotions provided the theoretical ground for discussions regarding the physical effect of positive feelings such as joy or hope in health, and the basis for the standardization of bedside manners in a certain direction.[51]

Arnau's ambitious *Speculum*, or any similar works by his predecessors and contemporaries, provided a theoretical framework that upheld the recommendation of avoiding sadness and promoting joy without entering into conflict with the bodily experience of the emotion.[52] According to the basics of

[49] It is the fable (XXVIII) 'De leporibus et ranis' that forms part of the collection known as *Anonymus Neveleti*.

[50] On the Galenic tradition of these recommendations for promoting joy and avoiding sadness, see Arcangeli, 'Gioia e tristeza nella tradizione galenica (*c.* 1275–1525)'.

[51] Salmón, 'The Physician as Cure in Medical Scholasticism'.

[52] Arnau de Vilanova, *Regimen sanitatis ad regem aragonum*, ed. by García Ballester and McVaugh, pp. 811–15.

Galenic medicine, the heart was the seat of the radical heat installed in the origin of each individual's life and of the vital spirit that derived from food intake through various transformations and refinements — most of them a process of concoction and filtering. The vital spirit, whether in its original state, or as converted into a more subtle animal spirit, runs through the entire organism by means of the arteries, veins, and nerves.

Within this humoral system of the understanding of the body, something that is thought to be positive warms the heart and produces a dilation that helps to spread the warming sensation through the body and at the same time helps to cool down the heated heart. It is not difficult to ascertain empirically that heat has a dilating or even melting effect on certain substances. But, what is more important, despite the various degrees of theoretical complexity that can be found in the various medical sources that deal with the topic, this basic explanation fits intuitively with the experience of the body that each individual has when he or she is happy, a feeling of expansion and irradiation of warmth. And the same applies if we focus on the experienced bodily effects caused by sadness.[53]

I want to stress three points here. First, that Arnau was able to enter into a dialogue with his patient because Jaume II understood the logic behind Arnau's recommendations and because it connected with somatic sensations that were not alien to him or to his contemporaries. Second, that what Arnau taught his students about the care of emotions at the bedside was not an abstract programme but something intended to work in their communications with future patients because the explanations, again, called upon a shared phenomenological understanding of the body. Third, that the theoretical framework built at the medical schools provided a logical explanation that easily mirrored what was felt.

I suggest that reading medical sources from this perspective of what they had to say about the emotions offers the possibility of unveiling traces of the emotional experiences of the body as it was lived in the past despite the normative or prescriptive nature of the sources.

It has been recently argued that the vagueness and adaptability of the Western humoral tradition accounts for its enduring persistence as a general framework with which to think about health and disease.[54] Indeed differences in what are thought to be the basic tenets of the system — humours, balance, qualities, temperaments, and flow — can easily be found in both theory and

[53] Arnau de Vilanova, *Speculum introductionum medicinalium*, fols 156–69.

[54] Horden, 'Introduction', p. 3.

practice in the ancient and medieval Mediterranean. However, it would also be fruitful to follow Barbara Duden's insistence on 'taking seriously the humours as experience'[55] and to explore further the appeal of this medical system, due to its capacity to echo the lived experience of the body-self.

I am aware of the dangers of presentism and essentialism when approaching the embodied experiences, such as pleasure and joy, of the men and women of the past. However, what I would like to suggest is that certain human experiences, despite being endowed with various individual and cultural meanings in different chronological and geographical locations, bring about certain interoceptive sensations that make it possible for them to be easily shared, at least by people from proximate cultural traditions. I have tried to show how pleasure and joy, as bodily experiences, could shape what the humoral medical system(s) (that dominated the ancient and medieval Mediterranean) could predicate about them. Reading medical sources in this light might help not just to understand how emotions were thought about in the past but also to reflect on how some of them were lived.

55 Duden, 'Fluxes and Stagnations', p. 54.

Works Cited

Manuscripts

Albertus Bononiensis, *Commentum supra tractatum Galieni de morbo et accidenti*, Vatican City, Biblioteca Apostolica Vaticana [BAV], MS Reg. lat. 2000, fols 28^{r}–73^{r}

Antonius de Parma, *Quaestiones supra tractatum Galieni de morbo et accidenti*, Vatican City, Biblioteca Apostolica Vaticana [BAV], MS Vat. lat. 4450, fols 73^{r}–93^{v}

Commentarius in 'Aphorismos' Hippocratis, Erfurt, Universitätsbibliothek [UB] Erfurt, MS Ea Q. 181, fols 91^{v}–122^{r}

Gentile da Foligno, *Notata super libro de accidenti et morbo*, München, Bayerische Staatsbibliothek [BS], MS Clm. 62, fols 70ra–104rb

Petrus Hispanus, *Questiones super libro de crisi et super libro de diebus creticis*, Madrid, Biblioteca Nacional [BN], MS 1877, fols 248^{r}–255^{r}

Primary Sources

Arnau de Vilanova, *Commentum super tractatum Galieni De malicia complexionis diverse*, ed. by Luis García Ballester and Eustaquio Sánchez Salor, vol. xv of *Arnaldi de Villanova Opera Medica Omnia* (Barcelona: Universitat de Barcelona, 1985)

——, *Regimen sanitatis ad regem aragonum*, ed. by Luis García Ballester and Michael R. McVaugh, introd. by Pedro Gil-Sotres, vol. x.1 of *Arnaldi de Villanova Opera Medica Omnia* (Barcelona: Universitat de Barcelona, 1996)

——, *Repetitio super aphorismo Hippocratis 'Vita Brevis'*, ed. by Michael R. McVaugh, introd. by Michael R. McVaugh and Fernando Salmón, in vol. xiv of *Arnaldi de Villanova Opera Medica Omnia* (Barcelona: Universitat de Barcelona, 2014)

——, *Speculum introductionum medicinalium*, in *Opera Omnia* (Basel, 1585), fols 1–238

Avicenna, *Liber Canonis tocius medicinae* (Venice, 1527; repr. Brussels: Medicinae Historia, 1971)

Cartulaire de l'Université de Montpellier, vol. i (Montpellier: Richard Frères, 1890)

Galen, *On Diseases and Symptoms*, trans., intro., and notes by Ian Johnston (Cambridge: Cambridge University Press, 2006)

——, *Opera Galieni, De interioribus* (Venice, 1490), ii, fols 114^{r}–138^{v}

Gentile da Foligno, *Primus Avic. Canon cum argutissima Gentilis expositione* (Papiae: Jacob de Burgofranco, 1510–12)

Pagel, Julius L., *Die Concordanciae des Johannes de Sancto Amando* (Berlin: Georg Reimer, 1896)

Salmón, Fernando, *Las teorías de la visión en la medicina universitaria bajo-medieval: estudio y edición crítica del Arnaldi de Villanova commentum supra tractatum Galieni de morbo et accidenti cum texto Galieni, lib. IV (c. 1288–1292/1295)* (Barcelona: Publicacions de la Universitat Autònoma de Barcelona, 1991) [Microfiche edition]

Secondary Works

Arcangeli, Alessandro, 'Gioia e tristeza nella tradizione galénica (*c.* 1275–1525)', in *Piacere e dolore: Materiali per una storia delle passion nel Medioevo*, ed. by Carla Casagrande and Silvana Vecchio, Micrologus' Library, 29 (Firenze: SISMEL/Edizioni del Galluzzo, 2009), pp. 171–85

Cadden, Joan, *Meanings of Sex Difference in the Middle Ages: Medicine, Science and Culture* (Cambridge: Cambridge University Press, 1993)

——, *Nothing Natural Is Shameful: Sodomy and Science in Late Medieval Europe* (Philadelphia: University of Pennsylvania Press, 2013)

Carrera, Elena, ed., *Emotions and Health, 1200–1700* (Leiden: Brill, 2013)

Casagrande, Carla, and Silvana Vecchio, eds, *Piacere e dolore: Materiali per una storia delle passioni nel Medioevo*, Micrologus' Library, 29 (Firenze: SISMEL – Galluzzo, 2009)

Duden, Barbara, 'Fluxes and Stagnations: A Physician's Perception and Treatment of Humours in Baroque Ladies', in *The Body in Balance: Humoral Medicines in Practice*, ed. by Peregrine Horden and Elisabeth Hsu (New York: Berghahn, 2013), pp. 53–68

Durling, Richard, 'Corrigenda et Addenda to Diel's Galenica', *Traditio*, 23 (1967), 461–76

García Ballester, Luis, 'Arnau de Vilanova (*c.* 1240–1311) y la reforma de los estudios medicos en Montpellier (1309): el Hipócrates latino y la introducción del nuevo Galeno', *Dynamis*, 2 (1982), 97–159

——, *Medicine in a Multicultural Society: Christian, Jewish and Muslim Practitioners in the Spanish Kingdoms, 1222–1610*, Variorum Collected Studies Series (Aldershot: Ashgate, 2001)

——, 'On the Origin of the "Six Non-natural Things" in Galen', in *Galen un das hellenistischen Erbe*, ed. by Jutta Kollesch and Diethard Nickel (Stuttgart: Franz Steiner, 1993), pp. 105–15

Green, Monica H., *Making Women's Medicine Masculine: The Rise of Male Authority in Pre-Modern Gynaecology* (Oxford: Oxford University Press, 2008)

Horden, Peregrine, 'Introduction', in *The Body in Balance: Humoral Medicines in Practice*, ed. by Peregrine Horden and Elisabeth Hsu (New York: Berghahn, 2013), pp. 1–21

——, 'Mediterranean Excuses: Historical Writing on the Mediterranean since Braudel', *History and Anthropology*, 16 (2005), 25–30

Horden, Peregrine, and Elisabeth Hsu, eds, *The Body in Balance: Humoral Medicines in Practice* (New York: Berghahn, 2013)

Horden, Peregrine, and Nicholas Purcell, *The Corrupting Sea: A Study of Mediterranean History* (Oxford: Blackwell, 2000)

Jacquart, Danielle, 'L'Oeuvre de Jean de Saint-Amand et les méthodes d'enseignement à la faculté de médicine de Paris à la fin du XIIIe siècle', in *Manuels, programmes de cours et techniques d'enseignement dans les universités médiévales*, ed. by Jaqueline Hamesse (Louvain-la-Neuve: Institut d'études médiévales de l'Université catholique de Louvain, 1994), pp. 257–75

——, *La Science médicale occidentale entre deux renaissances (XIIe s.–XVe s.)*, Variorum Collected Studies Series (Aldershot: Ashgate, 1997)

Jacquart, Danielle, and Claude Thomasset, *Sexualité et savoir médical au Moyen Âge* (Paris: Presses Universitaires de France, 1985)

Kleinman, Arthur, *Patients and Healers in the Context of Culture: An Exploration of the Borderland between Anthropology, Medicine, and Psychiatry* (Berkeley: University of California Press, 1980)

McVaugh, Michael R. *Medicine before the Plague: Practitioners and their Patients in the Crown of Aragon, 1285–1345* (Cambridge: Cambridge University Press, 1993)

Nutton, Vivian, 'Humoralism', in *Companion Encyclopedia of the History of Medicine*, ed. by William Bynum and Roy Porter (London: Routledge, 1993), I, 281–91

Paniagua, Juan A., *Studia Arnaldiana: Trabajos en torno a la obra médica de Arnau de Vilanova, c. 1240–1311* (Barcelona: Fundación Uriach 1838, 1994)

Park, Katherine, 'Medicine and Natural Philosophy: Naturalistic Traditions', in *The Oxford Handbook of Women and Gender in Medieval Europe*, ed. by Judith M. Bennet and Ruth Mazo Karras (Oxford: Oxford University Press, 2013), pp. 84–100

——, *Secrets of Women: Gender, Generation and the Origins of Human Dissection* (New York: Zone Books, 2006)

Rosenwein, Barbara H., 'Problems and Methods in the History of Emotions', *Passions in Context: Journal of the History and Philosophy of the Emotions*, 1 (2010), 1–32; online at http://www.passionsincontext.ed/

——, 'Worrying about Emotions in History', *American Historical Review*, 107 (2002), 821–45

Salmón, Fernando, 'A Medieval Territory for Touch', *Studies in Medieval and Renaissance History*, 3rd ser., 2 (2005), 59–81

——, 'The Physician as Cure in Medical Scholasticism', in *Ritual Healing: Magic, Ritual and Medical Therapy from Antiquity until the Early Modern Period*, ed. by Ildikó Csepregi and Charles Burnett (Firenze: SISMEL/Edizioni del Galluzzo, 2012), pp. 193–216

——, 'Technologies of Authority in the Medical Classroom in the Thirteenth and Fourteenth Centuries', *Dynamis*, 20 (2000), 135–57

Secord, Jim, 'Knowledge in Transit', *Isis*, 95 (2004), 654–72

Bodily Pleasures: Late Medieval Medical Counsel in Context

Naama Cohen-Hanegbi

This essay explores a trio that has a long, ongoing history: health, pleasure, and morality. For people living in the twenty-first century, bombarded as they are by daily health advice, it may be obvious that these three elements intertwine. Among the articles appearing in the health section of newspapers there is a category of 'joyous' studies which reveal that chocolate/coffee/regular sex is healthy as much as it is fun. Alongside their entertaining role, these news items provide legitimacy for activities otherwise considered 'naughty'. As a number of sociologists of health have shown, they connect to a deep-seated notion in contemporary society that one is ethically responsible to care for one's own health and that, moreover, well-being is generally valued in moral terms.[1]

Late medieval medicine grappled with this triad no less, but the conventions of culture determined that the negotiation took on different features. For learned medieval physicians, morality itself was a complex matter. Being educated by texts composed by Greek, Roman, and Arabic authors, their

[1] Conrad, 'Wellness as Virtue'; Williams, 'Health as Moral Performance'.

Naama Cohen-Hanegbi (naamaco@post.tau.ac.il) is a senior lecturer in the History Department of Tel Aviv University. She has published articles on the medical and religious treatment of emotions and on medicine within inter-religious encounter. She is the author of *Caring for the Living Soul: Emotions, Medicine and Penance in the Late Medieval Mediterranean* (Leiden: Brill, 2017).

Pleasure in the Middle Ages, ed. by Naama Cohen-Hanegbi and Piroska Nagy, IMR 24 (Turnhout: Brepols, 2018), pp. 59–75 BREPOLS PUBLISHERS 10.1484/M.IMR-EB.5.113462

understanding of health absorbed ethical concepts of a non-Christian world, and yet they were also reared in the Christian faith — and they were often rather devout.[2] Fernando Salmón presents the strong appeal of ancient theories on pleasure and their absorption among Latin medical scholars of the fourteenth century.[3] Alongside this avid conservation of the Galenic tradition there was also a continuous endeavour of medical teachers, throughout the twelfth to fifteenth centuries, to align these received teachings with the morality of the Christian world. This alignment was a necessary task in order to produce a medical approach applicable to their own and their patients' worldview.[4] How this pursuit was shaped with regard to the idea of pleasure is the question that guides this paper on a larger scale. In order to render the task suitable for the scope of a single paper, however, I focus on opinions about the pleasures of sexuality as they appeared in the practical literature and regimen advice to patients written in Italy in the fourteenth and fifteenth centuries. With these sources in mind, my interest here is not in the theories of sex and reproduction, but in how sexuality, as a bodily pleasure, relates to the medical discourses of health and well-being.

According to medieval medicine, taking pleasure in the body was an important part of the healthy life. Some medical treatises included chapters on cosmetics, offering make-up 'recipes' and other beauty tips that had no strict medical purpose but which cared for the body's well-being.[5] Other treatises recommend pleasing foods, clothing, music, etc., to ensure a patient's health. Often, it seems, physicians regard 'pleasure' or 'pleasing' as indicators of health. This association is most pointedly visible in the discussions about the six non-natural elements necessary for prevention of disease and the restoration of health. According to Galenic medical theory, the complexion of the body was affected by its basic activities: the intake of air, food and drink, sleep, movement, excretions, and the passions of the soul. Administering a suitable regimen in accordance with these activities was necessary to achieve and maintain the body's balance. Pleasure was inevitably involved in achieving a good and disease-preventing regimen, in the sense that it relied on compatibility

[2] The list of examples is long; see, for example, Ziegler, *Medicine and Religion*; Demaitre, *Bernard de Gordon*; Courtenay, 'Curers of the Body and Soul'.

[3] Salmón, this volume.

[4] Crisciani, 'Éthique des *consilia* et de la consultation'.

[5] Cabré, 'Beautiful Bodies'; Moulinier-Brogi, 'Esthétique et soins du corps dans les traités médicaux latins à la fin du Moyen Âge'; *The Trotula*, ed. and trans. by Green.

between the temperament of a person and the temperament of element consumed. The positive value, and therefore the pleasing qualities, of such 'agreement' between the patient and the six non-naturals was an established philosophical principal in late medieval thought. But alongside this 'accidental' pleasure of the individual humoral complexion, we also find that many items in the *regimina* lists are defined as having inherent, universal, healthy, and hence, pleasing properties. In other words, things of a moderate, temperate, proportional quality — which are always 'good for you' — also generate pleasure. All in all, feeling healthy, or the absence of pain and illness, was viewed as a pleasurable state in itself.

Nevertheless, and to reiterate some of the sentiments mentioned above, pleasure was only regarded as healthy when it was moderate, measured. In many medical texts, extreme and sudden joy was considered to be more fatally dangerous than other commonly conceived 'negative' emotions such as sorrow or anger.[6] The mid-fifteenth-century author of a popular medical regimen of health, Benedetto Reguardati da Norcia (1398–1469), highlights this danger of excess joy by recounting two incidents told by classical authors of parents whose over-excited joy in their children's success — one of the most morally suitable pleasures — ends in death.[7] Benedetto Reguardati, a celebrated physician in the humanist circle of Milan, placed these stories at the top of his rather long chapter on the *accidentia anime* (the medical term commonly used for the passions of the soul) to mark, from the outset, that bodily health is affected by the affairs of the soul and that even the good can affect one for the worse where it leads to imbalance. Benedetto Reguardati's words, with their humanist flare, were not groundbreaking, either to his medical colleagues or, most probably, to his readers. Not only was the medical worldview of emotions well transmitted by then to the elite he was serving, but the idea that pleasures and joys should be curbed for the sake of health, whether bodily, mentally, or spiritually, had circulated widely in late medieval culture either through medicine, literature, or didactic religious teachings.

Though medicine had more appreciation for earthly joys than some of the more severe preachers, the idea that health required the mitigating and curbing of pleasures deeply underlined the period's discourse. The countless sermons, commentaries, devotional treatises, and even laws that drew the connec-

[6] For the basic approach of medicine to emotions in the period, see Gil-Sotres, 'Introduction'; Gil-Sotres, 'Modelo, teórico y observación clinica'.

[7] Wroclav, BUW, MS III Q 19, fols 106^{v}–107^{r}.

tion between health of the body and health of the soul gave grounds to draw links between moral attitudes and basic guidelines to health. This association between health and righteousness, and more particularly between illness and sinfulness, has been explored by scholars of the medieval period in great detail. In devotional literature the health of the body is often regarded as dependent on and shaped by the health of the soul, but at times, the body's state of health stands as a metaphor for spiritual states. Philippa Maddern, for example, demonstrates through a lexicographical study of 'merriment' that late medieval English linked good health, joyous feelings, and divine grace. Her sources further show that the spiritual sense of the pleasures of health circulated beyond religious authors, shaping lay approach to health as well.[8] Following Maddern and others, we can conclude that there was an ongoing shift between the physical and spiritual registers which sustained a multilayered understanding of health in the later Middle Ages. Interestingly, this layering of meaning is not generally a characteristic of the medical sources themselves. Medical texts, in having a professional focus and typically aimed at fellow physicians, resort less to the poetics of allusion and tend to avoid the decorative language of metaphor. Invocations for the parallels and affinities between the health of the body and the health of the soul are most commonly left to dedications to patrons. As devotional allusions spread, however, it is likely that some readers were already prone to draw connections and imbue medical advice with moral meaning.

Moreover, medicine was not indifferent to the culture it catered to, even if this is expressed more subtly. The sources I study in this paper, intended as they are to offer medical assistance to patients and clients, required some negotiation between medicine and ethics. Among these practice-oriented texts one finds popular manuals instructing the correct regimen for the preservation of health and case studies, or *consilia*, which offer individual regimens of diet and medicine for a particular disease or complexional imbalance. It has been previously noted by scholars that these practical texts are engrained in theoretical thought and should be seen as a teaching tool written as an expansion of theoretical ideas. While this is certainly true, we should not ignore the two-directional cultural role of these texts, first for the community of physicians, and second for the community of patients. Most *consilia* — and certainly all *regimina* — were written for the service of patients who paid for the advice. Even if they could not read or follow every aspect of the prescribed advice, it was transmitted to them in some way or another (orally, through servants, cooks, other physicians, etc.), and there was certainly an expectation that this advice should be followed.

[8] Maddern, this volume.

In the western Mediterranean there was, from the thirteenth century onward, a notable respect for Galenic medicine and an eagerness to promote medical learning that subscribed to its premise.[9] Thus we can assume that in this region physicians' notions of health resonated within elite circles at least. As the medical texts surveyed here are all from a closely knit web of university teachers and court physicians active in northern Italy who provided counsel for an equally intricate network of nobility, courtiers, rich merchants, and high clergy, it is possible to use these findings as evidence for communal perceptions of emotional health.

Sex, Pleasure, and Love

Sexual pleasure was a topic of some interest for scholastic authors of the thirteenth century. Theologians, admittedly, considered the topic for centuries, for it was a source of great danger to the religiously inclined soul. Debates regarding the degree of celibacy required from clergy and demands to limit sexual activity of laity to certain days, positions, practices, and so on endured from the early days of Christianity. It was only in the thirteenth century, however, with the flourishing of natural philosophy and medical investigation that the nature and function of sexual pleasure came to be examined in more detail. In a sense, this new scientific avenue of discussion demonstrates the commitment of the period's scientific authors to their Christian worldview. As Joan Cadden notes, this issue was hardly mentioned by ancient scientific authorities.[10] The basic idea upon which scholars elaborated (first offered by Constantine the African) was that God designed sex to be pleasurable in order to encourage procreation. Yet for some thinkers such as Hildegard of Bingen, pleasure is part of the curse of the Fall that is designed to deter mankind from turning to God. For others, pleasure was associated with beneficial purgation of superfluous matter.[11] Further questions followed, looking most particularly at the differences in the experience of pleasure with regard to intensity, duration, and triggers among men, women, and beasts. As Cadden shows in detail, these analytical questions were methodical and aimed to establish a scientific account of human nature and of sexual difference.[12]

[9] McVaugh, *Medicine before the Plague*; Nicoud, *Le Prince et les médecins*.

[10] Cadden, *Meanings of Sex Difference in the Middle Ages*, p. 134.

[11] Cadden, *Meanings of Sex Difference in the Middle Ages*, p. 77.

[12] Cadden, *Meanings of Sex Difference in the Middle Ages*, pp. 140–43.

With respect to the more practical concern of the role of sexual intercourse in pursuing and preserving health, medical authors were faced with the challenge of reconciling the Christian ideal of celibacy with the medical view that saw danger in retention of semen (whether male or female), and recognized the pleasures of sex as good for both mind and body. The essential work by Joan Cadden, the equally important *Sexuality and Medicine in the Middle Ages* by Danielle Jacquart and Claude Thomasset, as well as the expansive scholarship that followed in the footsteps of these scholars expanded on the negotiation of these two rival theories and offered us a deep understanding of the approach Latin medicine took to sexual activity and behaviour.[13] Yet while much attention has been paid to the disparity between spiritual and physical concerns, I would like to suggest that by reviewing the emotional aspect of sexual pleasure, we see more clearly that health and morality were strongly attached and that measured pleasure, even if triggered by sexual activity, was encouraged and signified moral well-being.

Sexual Joy

As noted above, medieval medicine regarded sexual relations to be useful to health both as a means of purgation and in producing pleasure. This dual function made it possible for physicians to include advice on sexual relations in two categories of the six non-naturals: as purgatives or as *accidentia anime*. Although this may seem a mere structural consideration relevant only to problems of definition and genre within the discipline, the position of the category within the text sets the tone for the treatment of the topic as well. On the one hand, this association opened the way to regard sexual pleasure as a sensation of joy that corresponds to a range of states such as *gaudium*, *letitia*, and *delectatio* that undermines the argument that sexual pleasure is different from any other pleasure. The lack of terminological distinction undermines the uniqueness of sexual pleasure, both in terms of sensation and in terms of morality. On the other hand, appending sex to the accidents of the soul binds it to cognitive processes such as imagination and thought which in turn invited a more moralistic reaction by physicians. This was further accentuated by the crossover, to be discussed below, between sexual delight and love (*amor*).

[13] Jacquart and Thomasset, *Sexuality and Medicine in the Middle Ages*; Cadden, *Meanings of Sex Difference in the Middle Ages*; Cadden, *Nothing Natural Is Shameful*.

That sexual pleasure could be regarded equal to various other pleasures can be seen, for example, in Michele Savonarola's (1384–1466) elegant discussion in his vernacular regimen *Libreto de tutte le cosse che se magnano* (roughly translated as 'Booklet of All Foodstuffs'), written *c.* 1450:

> Il gaudio temperato molto conforta l'anima, ingrassa el corpo, fallo bello. Imperò dicono le done, quando se alamentano di suoi mariti, alegreza de core fa bella pelle de viso. Questo tale gaudio diversamente se recerca, chi cum canti, chi cum donne, chi cum dinari, chi cum signorie, chi cum oldire le cosse de Dio, e de tutto dè essere ben informato il medico et cetera.[14]

> [Temperate joy greatly comforts the soul; it fattens the body, making it beautiful. This is what women say when they feed their husbands — it gives happiness to the heart and makes the skin look beautiful. This joy could be sought in various ways: there are those [who are joyed by] songs, others by women, or money, others yet by dominions, or by hearing the words of God; and the physician should be well informed about all etc.]

Michele's words reiterate how the rudimentary classification of healthy and unhealthy sensations and emotions was demarcated along a binary division between pleasure and pain. The expressed tolerant approach of the *Libreto* specifically befits the addressee, the Duke of Ferrara. A court physician to Niccolo (1383–1441) and his son Borso d'Este of Ferrara (1413–1471), Michele supplemented the usual advice to listen to music or to enjoy other pleasurable activities suitable for the economic and political elite with a further source of pleasure: the enjoyment of money and power. Though in other circumstances such joys might be deemed sinful, Michele equates these to the joy of hearing sermons, and to sex. Such open-mindedness had its limits, however: for men, sexual pleasure may only be enjoyed with women. Masculinity is constructed here in relation to the means of obtaining joy: it can be somewhat varied, but it is always temperate.

In another regimen, written by the Milanese physician Maino de Maineri (d. 1368) in 1331, we find a fuller explanation of the emotional pleasure sex can offer. Maino informs us that it makes the soul cheerful, calms anger, removes worries, and heals melancholy.[15] For him, as well, the pleasures of sex are on the 'healthy' side of the binary divide. Pointedly, Maino notes that some

[14] Michele Savonarola, *Libreto de tutte le cosse che se magnano*, ed. by Nystedt, p. 175.

[15] Maino de Maineri, *Regimen sanitatis magnini mediolanesis*, fol. 142^{r}.

sexual activities are sinful and can generate diseases, but these caveats relate to practices, not the pleasure itself. Pleasure, in moderation, was healthy.

While such advice was good in times of health, illness required more caution. Examples from the *consilia* reflect this mode of thinking: the Sienese physician and teacher of medicine Ugo Benzi (1376–1439) instructed a man who suffered from hair loss and another, suffering from headaches, to refrain from too much intercourse.[16] A young Genoese man, Jerome de Grimaldis, whose cold and dry complexion harmed his digestion and kidneys was told by another celebrated physician and teacher from Pavia, Giovanni Matteo Ferrari da Grado (d. 1472), that sexual activity would be very dangerous in his state and that he should therefore proceed very cautiously in that area.[17] The language of the instruction implies that overexcited pleasure was the lesser concern of these physicians; the main risk to the patient's health was the seminal discharge. A study of *consilia* directed to female patients reveals that women were usually not advised to limit their sexual activity. Here, the practical cases adhere perhaps to the notion reiterated in a number of medical works that women's pleasure in sex is less hazardous because it is extensive, whereas men's pleasure is intensive. Unless inordinate sexual activity was in question (and one such case will be discussed below), the pleasures of sex were not considered to be harmful to women, only to men.

These restrictions were commonplace and were guided, it seems, by the preference for measured pleasure that was prevalent in medieval medicine. Yet some theoretical works bear witness to the influence or negotiation of the Christian endorsement of abstinence. The earliest example we have for an attempt to cope with this conflict appears in a work by a Salernitan master active at the end of the twelfth century, Bartholomaeus of Salerno. Commentating on Galen's *Tegni*, Bartholomaeus explicates Galen's words on sex in reference to the Christian view on abstinence. His argument is somewhat provocative, positing the inclination of one's desire as contingent upon complexion, remarking that even spiritual exercise and commitment cannot undo one's humoral nature. Moral moderation and a correct regimen can, however, alter a natural inclination if guided by a physician.[18] In a more elaborate manner, as Gijs Coucke has shown, the late thirteenth-century philosopher-physician Peter of Abano (1256–1316) commented on the pseudo-Aristotelian *Problemata* by inserting

[16] Benzi, *Consilia*, fols 5^{r-v}, 6^{v}.

[17] Giovanni Matteo Ferrari da Grado, *Consilia*, fol. 99^{v}.

[18] Wallis, '12th Century Commentaries in the *Tegni*'.

several reservations on sex for the sake of pleasure (rather than for the sake of procreation); in this he aligned the text with normative Christian thought.[19]

Returning to sources which reveal the norms of medical practice, only a handful of cases display a concern for Christian morality. Mostly these are brief remarks for patients of clerical status, stating that they should refrain from sexual activity because it is prohibited by Christian law. In his fifteenth-century *consilium* to an abbot named Raymonius, for instance, Christopher Barzizia of Bergamon notes that 'religion prohibits coitus'. His contemporary Giovanni Matteo Ferrari da Grado gives a similar view in a *consilium* concerning weight loss to Jacopo Borromeo, the Bishop of Pavia between 1446 and 1453, remarking that no advice concerning sex is necessary because this should be regulated according to Church law. Given the didactic nature of the *consilia*, it may well be that these notes serve to explain why fuller treatment of the topic is not offered. Yet these additions were also expected when treating men vowed for celibacy and can be read as an expression of sensitivity to the patient's habits that are primarily governed by their vocation.[20] Giovanni Matteo indeed continued this tone in the next sentence, opposing the medical position towards sorrow and anger (in Borromeo's view some is good) and the religious position (sinful).[21]

These terse comments aside, Michele's view — that sexual delights are healthy in the same way that songs and sermons are — seems in line with the majority of medical *consilia*. That is, except when something goes extraordinarily wrong.

Impotence, Satyriasis, and Excessive Nocturnal Emission

Before we venture into the extraordinary, let us consider the more common problems concerning the male reproductive organs brought to physicians: impotence, lasting erection, and nocturnal emissions. These problems are routinely addressed in the *consilia*, and it seems that they were considered among the basic situations physicians should be acquainted with. Luke Demaitre's similar findings with regard to the *practica* literature further supports this assumption.[22] In such cases it was often noted that the sensitive

[19] Couke, '*Non adeo est honesta ut delectabilis*. Sexual Pleasure in Medieval Medicine', p. 124.

[20] There are exceptions: the Bishop of Bologna did receive advice about coitus from Taddeo Alderotti. Perhaps the physician preferred a full regimen for the specific illness to one tailored to the lifestyle of the patient. Alderotti, *I 'Consilia'*, ed. by Nardi, p. 122.

[21] Giovanni Matteo Ferrari da Grado, *Consilia*, fol. 101^{r}.

[22] Demaitre, *Medieval Medicine*, pp. 302–13.

soul played an important part, primarily through the faculty of imagination but also due to the involvement of such emotions as timidity and shame. Again, in a similar vein of the *practica* discussion, the *consilia* cases are usually silent about Christian attitudes, but they advocate cures which conform to its spirit and reaffirm the cultural norms regarding masculinity.[23]

Nocturnal emissions and other kinds of involuntary emissions are treated as problems that could subside through exercise and a good regimen of sleep, but avoiding thinking or seeing anything related to sex is also suggested. One man, treated for nocturnal emissions accompanied by headaches (aggravated by forced celibacy due to his wife's recent childbirth), was instructed by the above-mentioned Ugo Benzi to be particularly cautious about his sleep, but with regard to the accidents of the soul the advice was quite simple: to avoid unpleasant feelings and pursue temperate ones.[24]

A piece of epistolary advice by Sozzinus Benzi (Ugo Benzi's son, 1397–1467) to a young man who suffered from impotence lists emotional hindrances as a possible cause. Sozzinus admitted that he was unable to offer a certain diagnosis because he has never seen the patient, and so alternative explanations are provided and the advice is less personal. Nevertheless, it captures medical understanding of impotence. Alongside a physical deficiency, Sozzinus suggested that the patient was inflicted by shame that may stem from timidity or from a physical condition of an overly cold heart. His suggested treatment includes speaking often to young women. A rare explanation for the advice is added: a wife has a special beauty when she is approached delicately.[25] Conversation would lead to affection which, in turn, assist to overcome impotence.

More detailed advice on how to divert the mind to healthy thoughts appears in a case of a young man from Cremona who was afflicted with satyriasis, a state of constant desire for sex. His physician, Giovanni Matteo, dedicates a long passage to the regimen of the 'animal passions', advising him to avoid any sound or thought of women or of the act of coitus. The patient himself is to restrict his sexual activity to as little as he can (once a fortnight, only with his own wife) and to guard his physical and cognitive movements during the act lest his desire arise too much. Finally, Giovanni added that such a case calls for moral guidance more than the administration of medicines. Thus the patient should strive to recall the

[23] Demaitre, *Medieval Medicine*, p. 309.

[24] Benzi, *Consilia*, fols 64^{v}–65^{r}.

[25] 'Consulo tamen quia uxorem habeat propriam pulchram cum qua delectabiliter uniat': Silvestre, '"Notice sur le manuscrit de medicine Bruxelles", Bibliothèque 3204–18', p. 557.

Last Judgement, his future death, the importance of refraining from vice and maintaining *bene moribus* (good behaviour), and that 'the soul should be ornate instead of in sin'.[26] The exact same admonition also appears in an account of nocturnal emissions.[27] Here, perhaps more vividly than in the other cases, we can see that the physician elects to incorporate Christian faith as medicine.

Common to all these cases is the notion that healthy masculine sexuality can be restored through the correct governing of desire and by the enjoyment of measured delights. The Paduan physician Bartolomeo Montanagna (1380–1452) articulated this point more bluntly. The case of a Florentine soldier (his name was concealed) who suffered from partial impotence (in addition to other ailments) allows Bartolomeo an extensive discussion of the topic in which he lists psychological and physical reasons that might prevent erection. Among the possible solutions he offers are the avoidance of dishonest thoughts and of various 'abominations'.[28] Furthermore, in several cases he warns patients that too much sex can turn a man effeminate, and in a *consilium* to Angelo Simonetta, the secretary of Francesco Sforza, he writes that powerful and illustrious men are prone to vehement desires and pleasures, but acting on such intensity is unhealthy.[29] All of our examples meld licit, measured sexual behaviour with masculine traits. While desire and seeking pleasure is demonstrative of 'great men', being able to control these passions and to follow them only in accordance with norms and tradition is a sign of healthy manhood.

The Unhealthy: Inordinate Sexual Behaviour

A few telling cases induced physicians to be more explicit than usual about normative expectations regarding sex. Broadly speaking they can be distinguished from those mentioned earlier in that they deal with visible, public, sexual activity, rather than private and perhaps secretive situations. These outrageous behaviours and loss of social boundaries were understood in the *consilia* as manic states in which the cognitive order failed.

A case of a young man suffering from melancholy with manic episodes was described by Bartolomeo Montagnana. The disease is described in complexional terms: a general warm complexion but a cold and humid liver, heart, and brain.

[26] Giovanni Matteo Ferrari da Grado, *Consilia*, fol. 63^{v}.

[27] Giovanni Matteo Ferrari da Grado, *Consilia*, fol. 63^{r}.

[28] Bartholomaeus de Montagnana, *Consilia*, fol, 39^{v}.

[29] Bartholomaeus de Montagnana, *Consilia*, fols 48, 238^{r}, 378^{v}.

According to Bartolomeo's analysis, this situation affected the patient's cognition, impairing his reason and leading him to imagine violent quarrels, trickery, and insult. The gravity of the situation seems to have caused Bartolomeo to doubt whether it was at all possible to heal the patient. Yet his advice was decidedly directed to comfort the patient and to fix, to the greatest extent possible, the melancholic imbalance.

Pleasure and comforting words that would ease the patient's mind were recommended to temper the vehemence of the movement of the patient's spirits. At the same time, stern reprehension was voiced against excessive sexual activity that might further debilitate the body. Bartolomeo stated that some activity might be useful to discharge the young man's marked timidity, but only as long as it was carried out in moderation and *moraliter regulatum*. Nevertheless, doing the 'shameful act' (Bartolomeo's words) with cheap and hateful morals ('vilius et destabilius'), fleeting lasciviousness and delectation ('per lasciviam et delectacionem') like a *muliercula* — that is, in a weak and womanlike manner — is thoroughly condemned. Sexual activity should be moderate and followed by sleep so that the corporal and imaginative faculties would be restored.[30] It is unclear why the specific case drove the physician to lodge such harsh criticism against immoral sexual behaviour. Perhaps there is a hint here that the patient engaged in homosexual acts: unfortunately, the text offers no further information. However, the choice of words shows the conflation of health and morality as it pertains to managing pleasures, particularly alongside gender norms.

In his strong rebuke, Bartolomeo offers a valuable case study for Joan Cadden's account of the way physicians regarded the moral implications of their patients' sexual habits. According to Cadden, medical works rarely advised abstinence, and when they did so, it was only with respect to general physical weakness. More broadly, her research suggests that medicine 'maintained an independent existence' in relation to sexual habits while not being 'insulated from its context'.[31] While her analysis of twelfth- to fourteenth-century medicine may reflect Michele Savonarola's approach as it appears in his regimen quoted above, both Bartolomeo and Giovanni Matteo present a less independent or idiosyncratic medical practice. Their remarks reiterate the gendered and religious notions about sexuality in the period, even if for the sake of accommodating their patients' beliefs and social positions. In adhering to these standards they formulated anew their professional role towards their patients' *bene moribus* as vehicles of these social and religious norms.

[30] Cambridge, Trinity, MS 1239 (O.4.8), fol. 93^{v}.

[31] Cadden, *Meanings of Sex Difference in the Middle Ages*, p. 276.

Finally, these elements are again merged in Giovanni Matteo's *consilium* to a German woman who was said to have an obsessive desire for sex. According to Giovanni, in former times the woman lived with her husband *pudicissime*, but then she started to become mad when she was not pregnant. Her entire body would tremble before becoming still, then voices emerged from her belly, and finally she became intensely desirous. This was to occur repeatedly when she was not pregnant; upon conception, the cycle would cease. Giovanni offers an explanation of her situation, namely, an abundance of generative semen and other material issues, and adds a cognitive analysis with regard to the loss of reason. Although discussed primarily in physical terms and through medical reasoning, the normative sexual boundaries underlie the narration of the case. The woman's ailment is said to result from too much sex with her husband in her youth, and the regimen instructs that she should avoid the company of *luxuriosae* women and anything that can incite her desire: stories, sights, and sounds. Above all, her thoughts should be turned — whenever she is of sane mind — to moral things ('circa morales considerationes').[32] Again, though nowhere expressed explicitly, it is clear that the state of *furia*, of excessive sexual desire and constant seeking of its pleasures, was considered deeply immoral. This singular case of a woman possessed by these passions demonstrates that women were not thought of as immune to the problem. It was, however, much more common among men.

Love

Another condition which permitted a consideration of emotions in gendered terms was *amor heroicus* (or *hereos*), known colloquially as lovesickness. The condition (whether or not it could be called a disease was an open question) is documented in medical literature from the first century BC on, but it entered Latin debate in the eleventh century through Constantine the African's *Viaticum* and its commentaries, later appearing also in some *practica* collections.[33] Lovesickness was characterized broadly as an unceasing obsession with a loved one which caused superfluous black bile and depleted energy and could

[32] I discuss this case also in Cohen-Hanegbi, 'The Emotional Body of Women'.

[33] See McVaugh, 'Introduction', pp. 13–15. McVaugh notes that there was interest in lovesickness among teachers in Montpellier in the fourteenth century. It is curious that the subject continued to appear routinely in the *practica* compendia, while it is absent completely from *consilia* literature.

induce the loss of the cognitive faculties. Active distraction and diversion of the mind from the object of thought was, therefore, the main remedy suggested. This included, above all, being in the company of women other than the object of love and even having intercourse with them. The association between love and intercourse was central to the discussion of *amor hereos* because such love was understood to develop out of the pleasures (or desired pleasures) of coitus.[34]

Mary Wack has pointed out that commentators of the *Viaticum* disagreed with regard to the possibility that women are susceptible to the malady as well. The thirteenth-century teacher of medicine Peter of Spain argued, for example, that it was one's predisposition to intense sexual pleasure, rather than one's gender, that was the determining factor. He thus directed attention to complexion rather than to sex.[35] Yet while some medical sources asserted that women could be afflicted, most of them linked the condition to men, pinpointing the generative organ as the source of disease, whose aetiology concerned superfluous humours that needed to be expelled.[36] To this, particular attributions of healthy and unhealthy masculinity were attached (though in certain cases these were inverted to represent more noble and delicate sensitivity), as well as characteristics indicative of moral demeanour.[37] Bernard of Gordon, for example, suggested to rebuke the patient for his false imaginations, to shame him for his thoughts, and to remind him of Judgement Day and the joys of paradise, implying that such obsession was a danger not only to health but also to salvation.[38] Bernard's advice thus reflects the merger of health with Christian morality and gendered thinking.

Amor hereos represented a distorted form of desirous love, but what about more moderate love? Interestingly, physicians have little to say about this passion in their texts. Most Italian authors ignore it altogether, but those who do mention it indicate that it has the potential to turn into a state of excess.[39] A mid-fourteenth-century admonition of a Valencian physician to his student-sons to refrain from *amor mulierum* implies that the period's medicine saw love as a euphemism for pleasure and the desire that guides it.[40]

[34] McVaugh, 'Introduction', p. 26.

[35] Wack, *Lovesickness in the Middle Ages*, pp. 113–16.

[36] McVaugh, 'Introduction', p. 34; Guglielmo da Brescia, *Ad unamquamque egritudinem a capite ad pedes practica*, p. 23r.

[37] Wack, *Lovesickness in the Middle Ages*, pp. 110–12.

[38] Bernard de Gordon, *Lilium medicine*, p. 216.

[39] Wroclav, BUW, MS III Q 19, fol. 107r; Benivieni, *De regimine sanitatis*, ed. by Belloni, p. 44.

[40] Thorndike, 'Advice from a Physician to his Sons'.

Conclusion

Admonishing male patients to refrain from becoming effeminate and to have sexual intercourse only with their wives reveals that in cases of illness physicians reported in medical language the values and customs of their period. In this they seem to identify health and healthy behaviour as synonymous with the Christian worldview. Such a position does not seem to have developed out of a philosophical or theological understanding of the 'inclination to the good' or ideas about divine creation, though most probably they were infused by such notions. Rather what guides them is a more mundane designation of the normal as healthy and abnormal as malicious. It is in this sense that learned physicians' views on the pleasures of the body (and emotions more widely) participated in constructing the competing *emotionologies* of late medieval culture.[41] In establishing norms and ethics of 'healthy feelings', they offer set guidelines for emotional behaviour. These guidelines are entrenched by gendered assumptions and recognition of social stature which are, in turn, reaffirmed. At the same time, as authors wrote to fellow physicians, and as they were influenced by and quoted previous works, the conversation of physicians among themselves also developed an emotional style that came to define the culture of writing about pleasure in medical texts. The examples assembled here call for further investigation of late medieval Italian learned physicians' 'emotional style', by which morality, health, and emotional decorum are adjoined.

[41] I rely here on Peter and Carol Stearns's definition of the term in Stearns and Stearns, 'Emotionology'.

Works Cited

Manuscripts

Cambridge, Trinity College, MS 1239 (O.4.8)
Wroclav, Biblioteka Univwesytecka we Wroclawiu, MS III Q 19

Primary Sources

Alderotti, Taddeo, *I 'Consilia'*, ed. by Giuseppe Michele Nardi (Torino: Minerva Medica, 1937)
Bartholomaeus de Montagnana, *Consilia CCCV in quibus agitur de universis fere aegritudinibus, humano corpori evenientibus, & mira facilitate, curandi eas adhibetur modus* (Venice, 1497)
Benivieni, Antonio, *De regimine sanitatis ad laurentium medicem*, ed. by Luigi Belloni (Torino: Società Italiana di Patologia, 1951)
Benzi, Ugo, *Consilia Ugonis Senensis saluberrima ad omnes egritudines…* (Venice, 1518)
Bernard de Gordon, *Lilium medicine* (Lyon, 1574)
Giovanni Matteo Ferrari da Grado, *Consilia* (Venice, 1535)
Guglielmo da Brescia, *Ad unamquamque egritudinem a capite ad pedes practica* (Venice, 1508)
Maino de Maineri, *Regimen sanitatis magnini mediolanesis* (Paris, 1483)
Michele Savonarola, *Libreto de tutte le cosse che se magnano: un'opera di dietetica del sec. xv*, ed. by J. Nystedt (Stockholm: Almqvist & Wiksell, 1988)
The Trotula: A Medieval Compendium of Women's Medicine, ed. and trans. by Monica H. Green (Philadelphia: University of Pennsylvania Press, 2001)

Secondary Works

Cabré, Montserrat, 'Beautiful Bodies', in *A Cultural History of the Human Body in the Middle Ages*, ed. by Monica H. Green (Oxford: Berg, 2010), pp. 127–47
Cadden, Joan, *Meanings of Sex Difference in the Middle Ages: Medicine, Science, and Culture* (Cambridge: Cambridge University Press, 1993)
——, *Nothing Natural Is Shameful: Sodomy and Science in Late Medieval Europe* (Philadelphia: University of Pennsylvania Press, 2013)
Cohen-Hanegbi, Naama, 'The Emotional Body of Women: Medical Practice between the 13th and the 15th century', in *Le Sujet des émotions au Moyen Âge*, ed. by Piroska Nagy and Damien Boquet (Paris: Beauchesne, 2008), pp. 465–84
Conrad, Peter, 'Wellness as Virtue: Morality and the Pursuit of Health', *Culture, Medicine and Psychiatry*, 18 (1994), 385–481
Couke, Gijs, '*Non adeo est honesta ut delectabilis*. Sexual Pleasure in Medieval Medicine: The Case of Pietro d'Abano', in *Piacere e dolore: Materiali per una storia delle passioni nel Medioevo*, ed. by Carla Casagrande and Silvana Vecchio, Micrologus' Library, 29 (Firenze: SISMEL/Edizioni del Galluzzo, 2009), pp. 117–48

Courtenay, William J., 'Curers of the Body and Soul: Medical Doctors as Theologians', in *Religion and Medicine in the Middle Ages*, ed. by Peter Biller and Joseph Ziegler (Woodbridge: York Medieval Press and Boydell, 2001), pp. 69–75

Crisciani, Chiara, 'Éthique des *consilia* et de la consultation: À propos de la cohesion morale de la profession médicale (XIIIe–XIVe siècles)', trans. by Marylin Nicoud, *Médiévales*, 46 (2004), 23–44

Demaitre, Luke, *Doctor Bernard de Gordon: Professor and Practitioner* (Toronto: Pontifical Institute of Mediaeval Studies, 1980)

——, *Medieval Medicine: The Art of Healing, from Head to Toe* (Santa Barbara: Praeger, 2013)

Gil-Sotres, Pedro, 'Introduction', in Arnau de Vilanova, *Regimen sanitatis ad regem aragonum*, ed. by Luís García-Ballester and Michael R. McVaugh, vol. X.1 of *Arnaldi de Villanova Opera Medica Omnia* (Barcelona: Universitat de Barcelona, 1996), pp. 803–27

——, 'Modelo, teórico y observación clinica: las passions del alma en la psicología médica medieval', in *Comprendre et mâtriser la nature au Moyen Âge: Mélanges d'histoire des sciences offerts à Guy Beaujouan* (Geneva: Droz, 1994), pp. 181–204

Jacquart, Danielle, and Claude Thomasset, *Sexuality and Medicine in the Middle Ages* (Princeton, NJ: Princeton University Press, 1989)

McVaugh, Michael, 'Introduction', in Arnaldus de Villanova, *Tractatus de amore heroico; Epistola de dosi tyriacalium medicinarum*, ed. Michael R. McVaugh, vol. III of *Arnaldi de Villanova Opera Medica Omnia* (Barcelona: Universitat de Barcelona, 1985), pp. 11–39

——, *Medicine before the Plague: Practitioners and their Patients in the Crown of Aragon, 1285–1345* (Cambridge: Cambridge University Press, 1993)

Moulinier-Brogi, Laurence, 'Esthétique et soins du corps dans les traités médicaux latins à la fin du Moyen Âge', *Médiévales*, 46 (2004), 55–72

Nicoud, Marilyn, *Le Prince et les médecins: Pensée et pratiques médicales à Milan (1402–1476)* (Roma: École française de Rome, 2014)

Silvestre, H., '"Notice sur le manuscrit de medicine Bruxelles", Bibliothèque 3204–18: Suivie de l'édition d'un *Consilium* inédit de Sozzinus Benzi de Sienne', *Latomus* 14.4 (1955): 548–60

Stearns, Peter N., and Carol Z. Stearns, 'Emotionology: Clarifying the History of Emotions and Emotional Standards', *American Historical Review*, 90 (1985), 813–36

Thorndike, Lynn, 'Advice from a Physician to his Sons', *Speculum*, 6 (1931), 110–14

Wack, Mary F., *Lovesickness in the Middle Ages: The 'Viaticum' and its Commentaries* (Philadelphia: University of Pennsylvania Press, 1990)

Wallis, Faith, '12th Century Commentaries in the *Tegni*: Bartholomaeus of Salerno and Others', in *L'Ars Medica (Tegni) de Galien: Lectures antiques et médiévales*, ed. Nicoletta Palmieri (Saint-Etienne: Publications de l'Universite de Saint-Etienne, 2008), pp. 127–68

Williams, Simon J., 'Health as Moral Performance: Ritual, Transgression and Taboo', *Health*, 2.4 (1998), 435–57

Ziegler, Joseph, *Medicine and Religion, c. 1300: The Case of Arnau de Vilanova* (Oxford: Oxford University Press, 1998

Visual Pleasure and the Illuminated Prayer Book

Maeve Doyle*

> Scimus namque, quod illi sapientibus et insipientibus debitores cum sint, carnalis populi devotionem, quia spiritualibus non possunt, corporalibus excitant ornamentis. Nos vero qui jam de populo exivimus; [...] qui omnia pulchre lucentia, canore mulcentia, suave olentia, dulce sapientia, tactu placentia, cuncta denique oblectamenta corporea arbitrati sumus ut stercora, ut Christum lucrifaciamus: quorum, quaeso, in his devotionem excitare intendimus?
>
> Bernard of Clairvaux, *Apologia ad Guillelmum Abbatem*, XII.28[1]

* This essay emerged from research supported by a Fulbright grant to France and by Bryn Mawr College. I extend my thanks to the staff of the Médiathèque municipale in Cambrai for their warm welcome and permission to publish images of the manuscript. I am grateful to the editors of this volume for their invitation to contribute and for their insightful comments. My thanks also go to Dale Kinney, Alex Brey, Johanna Gosse, and Shannon Steiner, who provided feedback at various stages of this project. I owe further thanks to Patrick M. Crowley for insights on the Latin translations; any errors that remain are my own.

[1] '[Bishops] stimulate the devotion of a carnal people with material ornaments because they cannot do so with spiritual ones. But we who have withdrawn from the people [...] we who regard as dung all things shining in beauty, soothing in sound, agreeable in fragrance, sweet in taste, pleasant in touch — in short, all material pleasures — in order that we may win Christ, whose devotion, I ask, do we strive to excite in all this?' Bernard of Clairvaux, *Apologia ad Guillelmum*, ed. by Migne, cols 914D–915A; translated in Rudolph, *The 'Things of Greater Importance'*, p. 10.

Maeve Doyle (doylemae@easternct.edu) is Assistant Professor of Art History at Eastern Connecticut State University. She received her PhD from Bryn Mawr College in 2015 with a dissertation entitled 'The Portrait Potential: Gender, Identity, and Devotion in Manuscript Owner Portraits'.

Pleasure in the Middle Ages, ed. by Naama Cohen-Hanegbi and Piroska Nagy, IMR 24 (Turnhout: Brepols, 2018), pp. 77–111 BREPOLS PUBLISHERS 10.1484/M.IMR-EB.5.113463

> She loved the fresh air and the various aspects of the country, and when her eyes and cheeks glowed with mingled pleasure she looked very little like a devotee. Riding was an indulgence which she allowed herself in spite of conscientious qualms; she felt that she enjoyed it in a pagan sensuous way, and always looked forward to renouncing it.
>
> George Eliot, *Middlemarch*

For a medievalist reader, the devout Dorothea Brooke's Protestant pleasure in renouncing the joys of riding contains echoes of Bernard of Clairvaux's critical aesthetic rhetoric in his *Apologia* of *c.* 1125. The sensual potency of such 'material pleasures' is infused within Bernard's screed against excessive ornamentation of monastic spaces. In the end, he acknowledges the utility of such luxuries to 'stimulate the devotion of a carnal people'. A series of historiated initials in a northern French prayer book of the late thirteenth century, today known as the 'Cambrai Hours', illustrates vividly the contradictions that such an appeal to carnal spirituality entails.[2] The six surviving initials of a seven-image cycle show a well-to-do laywoman rejecting a series of worldly temptations presented by monstrous figures (Figure 1; see also Figures 3 and 4, below). The series's theme of abstention from secular pleasures is clear, yet its setting within the illuminated pages of a deluxe manuscript, which also provide a type of pleasure, seems to undermine its ascetic moral. This essay probes the apparent disjuncture between the rejection of physical pleasures this image cycle enjoins and the pleasure that the manuscript, as a whole, must have provided its reader. In examining the various roles that pleasure plays in this unusual manuscript, I call upon the energetic discussions of pleasure and vision in feminist film criticism, particularly the work of Laura Mulvey, who cites pleasure as a potent mechanism for social control. Yet, while I argue that the Cambrai Hours offers pleasure in order to control the gaze of its female reader, a close reading of the physical state of the manuscript also testifies to the medieval reader's active participation in the pleasures of her book. Ultimately, my study of this illuminated manuscript shows that, in contrast to Mulvey's reading of narrative cinema, the acceptance of pleasure need not necessitate a surrender of agency. Attentiveness to the pleasure of the anonymous owner of this book allows for a reconstruction of her agency in asserting her own pleasures and desires on a worldly and on a spiritual scale.

[2] Cambrai, BM, MS 87, fols 29^{r}, 43^{v}, 47^{r}, 50^{v}, 53^{v}, and 60^{r}.

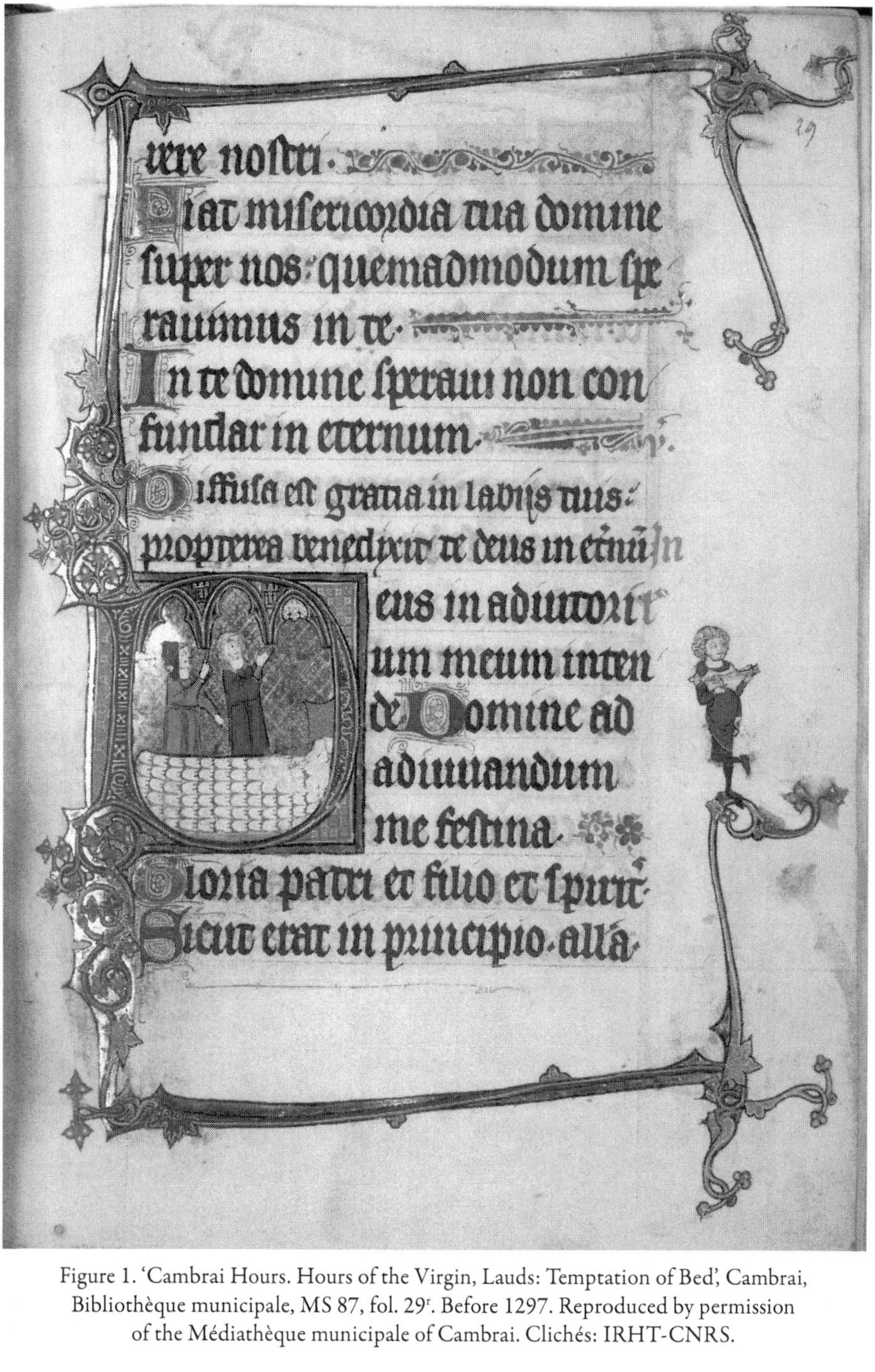

Figure 1. 'Cambrai Hours. Hours of the Virgin, Lauds: Temptation of Bed', Cambrai, Bibliothèque municipale, MS 87, fol. 29r. Before 1297. Reproduced by permission of the Médiathèque municipale of Cambrai. Clichés: IRHT-CNRS.

Seeking Pleasure in the Cambrai Hours

The 'Cambrai Hours' (so called for its current location in the municipal library of Cambrai) is an unusual, large-format book of hours for the liturgical use of Reims.[3] The style of the book's extensive illuminations date it to around the turn of the fourteenth century; the absence of Saint Louis in its calendar suggests that the book predates his canonization in 1297, though this dating is not conclusive. The 240 folios of the manuscript contain a variety of standard and non-standard books of hours texts in both Latin and French as well as numerous conventional and idiosyncratic illuminations. My analysis focuses on the illuminations and texts of three sections in the manuscript, all devoted to the Virgin Mary: the Hours of the Virgin, a Latin office illuminated with the temptation cycle mentioned above; the Five Joys of the Virgin in Latin; and the Nine Joys of the Virgin in French. Before I address these in greater detail, a brief description of the manuscript will serve to contextualize them within the work as a whole.[4]

The large size of the manuscript (the pages measure 250 × 180 mm), its generous margins, and its copious illumination mark the Cambrai Hours as a deluxe commission (see Figures 1 and 6). The manuscript opens with a Calendar, the localization of which is unclear.[5] Two full-page miniatures follow, one a composite of four fragmentary miniatures of Christ's Infancy, the second showing Christ and the Virgin enthroned within the heavenly city.[6] Next comes the Hours of the Virgin, the core text of a book of hours.[7] While the office begins with an initial showing the Annunciation, the subsequent initials break with its typical iconography to illustrate the temptation of a laywoman, which I reference above and describe in greater detail below. A second office, the Hours of the Cross in French, follows. The text returns to Latin (with French rubrics) with a prayer on the Passion and the Five Joys of the Virgin, which I also discuss

[3] For the manuscript's liturgical use, see Drigsdahl, 'Hore Beate Marie Virginis – Use of Reims (Rheims)'; Ottosen, *The Responsories and Versicles of the Latin Office of the Dead*, p. 145; Stones, *Gothic Manuscripts*, pt. 1, II, 417.

[4] For a detailed textual and iconographic description of the book, see Stones, *Gothic Manuscripts*, pt. 1, II, 417–20.

[5] Stones, *Gothic Manuscripts*, pt. 1, II, 417.

[6] Cambrai, BM, MS 87, fols 16^{v} and 17^{v}. For this latter miniature, see Stahl, 'Heaven in View'.

[7] For a succinct explanation of the Hours of the Virgin and books of hours generally, see Wieck, *Time Sanctified*. See also Leroquais, *Les Livres d'heures manuscrits de la Bibliothèque nationale*; Duffy, *Marking the Hours*; Reinburg, *French Books of Hours*.

below. Following these brief prayers are further standard book of hours texts: the Seven Penitential Psalms, Litany, and Suffrages. These are followed by a few more prayers in Latin, including the popular *O intemerata* and some specialized prayers, such as one to Veronica's Veil and another rubricated as 'pour les iex' (for the eyes).[8] While the Office for the Dead, next, is another book of hours mainstay, the eighty-five remaining folios that follow contain a selection of prayers in Latin and French of varying degrees of popularity and specialization. A number of these prayers address the Virgin, including the Nine Joys of the Virgin (a French variation on the Latin Five Joys appearing earlier in the book that I also discuss in detail), a French translation of *O intemerata*, two vernacular prayers attributed to Gautier de Coinci, and the Five Sorrows of the Virgin in French, a pendant to the prayers that highlight the Virgin's joys.

One of the many remarkable qualities of this book is the persistent presence of a thirteenth-century laywoman in prayer throughout its illuminations. This repeated figure corresponds to a type known in modern scholarship as an 'owner portrait', a representation of the person (or the type of person) expected to use the prayer book. While many devotional books contain one such owner image, this book represents its expected female owner over one hundred times in its margins and initials. Owner portraits establish a reflexive relationship between viewers and their images, one which simultaneously anticipates and dictates viewers' devotional performance. In calling attention to their viewers' acts of devotion, owner portraits further invite their viewers to reflect on their behaviour and to reshape themselves after the model of their exemplary images. Owner portraits in the two Joys of the Virgin texts, for example, pair the female owner figure with representations of the Virgin Mary. These illuminations at once demonstrate the process of modelling oneself against a divine exemplar and exhibit the reward of such piety.[9] The images of temptation in the Hours of the Virgin, on the other hand, comprise a unique use of the owner portrait type, as they show not the achievement of penance, but the consequences of its failure. Imagery of pleasure and pleasurable images run throughout these sections, playing various and surprising roles in their didactic programmes. Reading the texts and images of these sections together, I consider the interplay between the inherent visual pleasure the prayer book provides and the sensual and bodily pleasures its imagery depicts; further, I consider the reception of this pleasurable imagery by its likely thirteenth-century reader and its impact on her use of the book, whether for devotion, self-improvement, or self-fashioning.

[8] Cambrai, BM, MS 87, fol. 112^{r}.

[9] See Doyle, 'The Portrait Potential'.

Owner portraits and other distinctive elements throughout the manuscript suggest aspects of its expected owner's identity that are useful for considering the book's thirteenth-century reception. The owner figures depicted throughout the manuscript are predominantly female; furthermore, feminine word forms appear throughout the book's Latin and French texts in reference to their speaker, naming her a sinner (*peccatrix*, *pecheresse*) and a servant (*famulam*) and asking to be saved (*sauuee*).[10] These personalized elements suggest that its creators anticipated a female owner for this book of hours. Although, as I argue elsewhere, this does not preclude male readership or reception of the book,[11] my analysis here will assume the reception of a female reader positioned to recognize herself in its images.

Signs and suggestions of the owner's identity appear throughout the manuscript, although her name remains unknown.[12] The later quires especially contain numerous heraldic references; we may infer that the two blazons that appear quartered in the initials of a series of Marian prayers towards the end of the manuscript belong to the female owner and her husband (Figure 2). Alison Stones has identified the arms in the first and fourth quarters, *gules three pales vair, on a chief or a lion issuant sable*, as those of Gaucher de Châtillon d'Autresche, châtelain de Bar and avoué de Vic-sur-Aisne, who was active in the court of Philip the Fair between 1296 and 1311 and whose arms are recorded in seals of 1299 and 1302.[13] The primary position of the Autresche arms suggests that Gaucher was the husband of the book owner. Her arms, *sable a lion rampant argent, crowned or*, appear in the second and third quarters. This differenced version of the Brabant arms seems to reference a cadet branch, possibly that of Henri de Louvain, sire de Gaesbeck, whose arms appear in the Wijnbergen Armorial of *c.* 1280.[14] No documents relating to either family have

[10] Variations on *peccatrix* and *pecheresse* appear on Cambrai, BM, MS 87, fols 71^{r}, 108^{v}, 109^{v}, 112^{v}, 195^{v}, and 205^{v}; *famulum* appears on fol. 108^{r}; *sauuee* appears on fol. 195^{r}.

[11] Doyle, 'The Portrait Potential', ch. 3.

[12] Adelaide Bennett and Alison Stones are currently preparing a study of this manuscript, and I await their findings eagerly. Their latest work is published in Stones, *Gothic Manuscripts*, pt. 1, II, 417–34.

[13] *Les Manuscrits à peintures en France*, p. 37; Muzerelle, *Cambrai*, p. 16; Stones, 'Some Portraits of Women in their Books', pp. 12–13; Stones, *Gothic Manuscripts*, pt. 1, II, 432–33. For the Autresche arms, see Demay, *Inventaire des sceaux de la Flandre*, I, no. 741; Demay, *Inventaire des sceaux de la collection Clairambault*, I, no. 455.

[14] Muzerelle, *Cambrai*, p. 16; Stones, 'Some Portraits of Women in their Books', pp. 12–13; Stones, *Gothic Manuscripts*, pt. 1, II, 432–33. For the Gaesbeck arms, see Adam-Even and

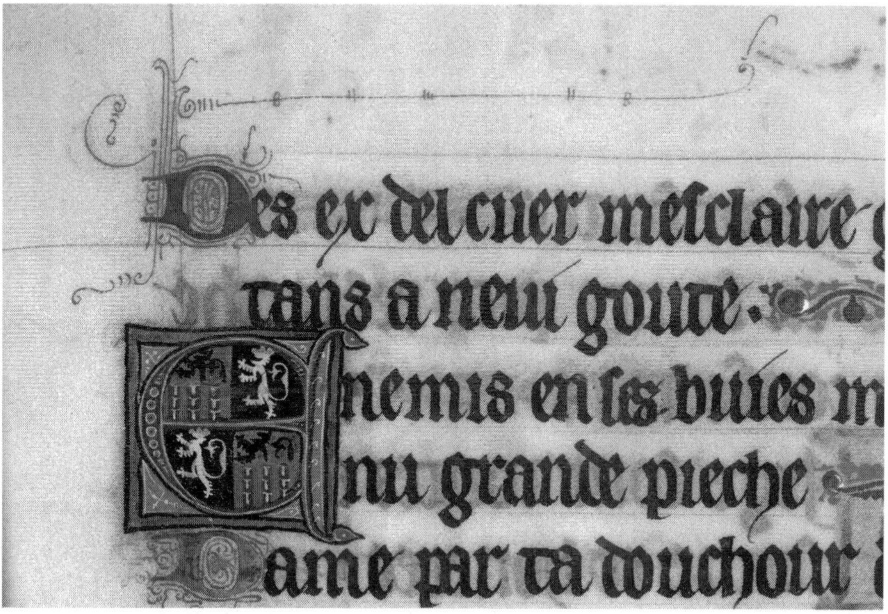

Figure 2. 'Cambrai Hours. Initial with quartered heraldry', Cambrai, Bibliothèque municipale, MS 87, fol. 211^{r} (detail). Before 1297. Reproduced with the permission of the Médiathèque municipale of Cambrai. Clichés: IRHT-CNRS.

been found to name a woman who can be associated with this manuscript.[15] Nevertheless, some details of her life experience can be gleaned from the manuscript itself. While she appears in certain portraits with her husband, there are no representations of children, either young or grown;[16] as is discussed

Jéquier, 'L'Armorial Wijnbergen', no. 1190. Misidentification of both arms has led other authors to attribute ownership of the book to one of two women, Mahaut de Brabant or Isabeau de Rumigny, who both married other members of the larger Châtillon family. For instance, Sydney Cockerell's account of the heraldry, published by Eric Millar, erroneously describes the secondary arms as having a red field rather than a black in support of an identification of the owner as Isabeau de Rumigny. Yet, as Stones points out, the secondary arms correspond with neither Mahaut's nor Isabeau's family devices, nor are their arms to be found anywhere else in the book. See Molinier, *Cambrai*, p. 22; Millar, *The Library of A. Chester Beatty*, II, 105; Plotzek, *Die Handschriften der Sammlung Ludwig*, p. 80; *L'Art au temps des rois maudits*, p. 310.

[15] Stones, 'Some Portraits of Women in their Books', p. 13.

[16] The contemporary Aspremont-Kievraing Psalter-Hours (Oxford, Bodleian Library, MS Douce 118, and Melbourne, Nationale Gallery of Victoria, inv. 1254–53) shows its owners with their grown children on select pages, while a book of hours from the diocese

further below, the owner's fertility is a theme of the illuminations, suggesting that, at the time the book was made, she and Gaucher did not yet have children, but expected to. The book of hours is bilingual, with prayers, offices, and rubrics in Latin, French, or both. The dispersal and balance of texts in the two languages suggests that its female user valued access to both. On the basis of the large script and the unusual suffrage for the eyes, Adelaide Bennett and Alison Stones have suggested that the book owner may have had poor eyesight.[17] As we know nothing about her outside of her prayer book, we cannot hope to fully contextualize her experience as a reader of its texts and images. We can, however, investigate the ways in which her manuscript worked to construct her gaze. Marks of use, furthermore, allow us to consider the pleasures that she, in turn, may have found within it.

Pleasure, as a subjective emotion or experience, resists either description or definition, especially in a historical context. Pleasures I consider here are the delight taken in an object of beauty or the fulfilment of a desire; the feeling of pleasure can be located in the body or in the mind. Pleasure is neither exclusively active nor passive: a subject may take pleasure, but pleasure might also be imparted to a subject. While I cite visual pleasure in my title, this is only one of the wealth of pleasures offered within this illuminated manuscript. In discussing the visual pleasure of this book, I am referring to the aesthetic pleasures its visual appeal affords its reader-viewers, with special consideration of the woman for whom it was made. The term 'visual pleasure' is a reference to Laura Mulvey's groundbreaking but controversial article, 'Visual Pleasure and Narrative Cinema', which has shaped feminist studies of visual culture since its appearance in 1975. Mulvey's essay isolated pleasure as an element for masking mechanisms of social control in Hollywood cinema. In Mulvey's account, the luminous beauty of images projected in the darkness of the movie theatre sets the stage for the repeated inscription of an eroticized scopic regime that privileges male subjectivity and desire. Through visual pleasure, cinema reinforces and normalizes a patriarchal social order that offers no room for female agency, subjectivity, or resistance.[18] Criticism of Mulvey's totalizing, psychoanalytic model has made 'visual pleasure'

of Thérouanne dated after 1318 (London, British Library, Add. MS 36684, and New York, Pierpont Morgan Library, MS M. 754) includes images of boys in prayer with the female owner. For representations of the book owners and their family in the former, see Morgan, 'Gendered Devotions and Social Rituals'.

[17] Cambrai, BM, MS 87, fol. 112^r; Stones, *Gothic Manuscripts*, pt. 1, II, 430.

[18] Mulvey, 'Visual Pleasure and Narrative Cinema', p. 8.

a charged concept.[19] Yet, despite the issues with Mulvey's approach (which I address further below), her attention to the political dimension of pleasure remains a valuable direction of inquiry. As a historical study of an object from a different culture, the goals of my work differ fundamentally: while Mulvey looked to the future possibility of feminist cinema and the chance 'to break with normal pleasurable expectations in order to conceive a new language of desire', my aim is, rather, to probe the subtle networks of agency legible in the creations and possessions of historical subjects.[20]

A digression into film theory might seem an unusual start for an essay on a medieval illuminated manuscript. My citation of Mulvey constitutes an exercise in what Madeline Caviness has termed 'triangulation'.[21] In Caviness's analytical model, the modern interpreter illuminates a historical object with metaphoric beams of light positioned at two different angles: on one side, details of the object's historical context illuminate it from a closer vantage, while the viewer's grasp of modern critical theory projects a more distant beam from a different angle. The aim of triangulation is not to collapse the two beams, but rather to establish a dialogue between the resulting analyses. Mulvey's concept of visual pleasure in modern cinema shines an intriguing light on the medieval reception of a deluxe book of hours. In this essay, I will probe further into the concept of visual pleasure and interrogate the role that visual and other sensory pleasures played in a thirteenth-century reader's experience of her luxuriously illuminated prayer book.

Like the cinematic projection, the illuminated manuscript presents a pleasurable and stimulating sight for its privileged viewer. But distinctions between the media of film and manuscripts provide the first point of departure for our triangulation. While film is a narrative spectacle for public display and entertainment, the devotional manuscript is a tool for semiprivate religious ritual, study, and self-improvement. Both manuscripts and movies are typically collaborative productions. Mulvey's suggestion, however, is that the eye of the camera exerts a strict control over the receptive gazes of the audience, modelling a specifically male gaze that oscillates between narcissism and scopophilia.

[19] See, for example, the multitude of short essays gathered in Bergstrom and Doane, *The Spectatrix*. For a critique of Mulvey's use of Freud, see Caviness, *Visualizing Women in the Middle Ages*, pp. 25–28.

[20] Mulvey, 'Visual Pleasure and Narrative Cinema', p. 8. L'Estrange, *Holy Motherhood*, p. 13, aptly characterizes the challenges of assessing women's agency in reading and devotion.

[21] Caviness, *Visualizing Women in the Middle Ages*, p. 31.

Under certain circumstances, an illuminated prayer book can produce a similarly totalizing effect: Madeline Caviness's reading of the Hours of Jeanne d'Evreux (*c.* 1324–28) demonstrated the potential for social control within a prayer book according to its authors' agenda.[22] Caviness argued that Jeanne's miniature prayer book exerted control through a denial or mitigation of pleasure, injecting frightening and intimidating hybrids, which she elsewhere terms 'freaks', into an object of otherwise utmost beauty.[23] Caviness's caveat that her interpretation was grounded in a specific biographical moment for Jeanne reveals a further key difference between film and manuscript.[24] A manuscript reader has a ritual relationship with the book, a relationship that entails both performative and repeated readings. This continued engagement with the book would have allowed the reader to shape her experience within and even beyond that provided by its authors through selective reading or the addition of content. A manuscript's visual pleasure plays a role in this return, enticing the reader back to the manuscript, just as a moviegoer is lured into the theatre. Unlike a film, however, a reader's return to a prayer book can also be selectively guided by her pleasure, as she can focus on favourite texts, sections, or images to the exclusion of others.[25] Within the performative use of an illuminated prayer book, pleasure can be a wellspring of resistance as well as a pathway for social control. This makes pleasure a generative thread along which to trace the competing signs of agency and submission within this prayer book.

While pleasure is the titular theme of Mulvey's essay, it lingers only in the margins of her argument and remains largely unexamined.[26] Mulvey's pleasure is monolithic and external. It is not an emotion to be felt as a subject, but rather one to be passively received from an outside source. Mulvey's understanding of pleasure thus shares in the same set of problems that plague her theory of the gaze, which one critic bluntly decried as 'too deterministic, ahistorical, rigid, abstract and not particularly sensitive to class, racial, age, ethnic, and other types of differences'.[27] Feminist film theorist Teresa de Lauretis provided

[22] Caviness, 'Patron or Matron?'; for the patrons, designers, scribes, and artists of a devotional book as its authors, see Sand, 'Picturing Devotion Anew', p. xiii.

[23] Caviness, *Reframing Medieval Art*, ch. 3.

[24] Caviness, 'Patron or Matron?', p. 41.

[25] See Huot, 'Polytextual Reading'.

[26] Mary Ann Doane critiqued Mulvey and subsequent authors' use of pleasure as 'an unthought term'. Doane, '[Untitled Response]', pp. 144–45.

[27] Marchetti, '[Untitled Response]', p. 227.

a useful revision of Mulvey's theory, inasmuch as her semiotic approach acknowledged that 'the relations between meanings and images exceed the work of the film and the institution of the cinema'.[28] Thus, while Mulvey agitated for the radical eradication of pleasure, de Lauretis argued that 'narrative and visual pleasure need and should not be thought of as the exclusive property of dominant codes, serving solely the purposes of "oppression"'.[29] Medievalists Anne Harris and Karen Overbey echoed this sentiment in a recent essay on the future of the 'material turn' in medieval art history, which meditated on pleasure's role in the power play between viewers, scholars, and objects. They noted that the aesthetic pleasures of 'connoisseurship and nineteenth-century formalism wrought *command* of objects, and teleologies of style and masters'.[30] Yet aesthetic pleasure itself cannot be controlled; it presupposes an ecstatic but 'unnerving' capitulation before the object's greater agency.[31] Harris and Overbey's object-oriented approach shifts the terms of submission and control. Pleasure becomes a democratizing force, negating (in their more Marxist formulation) any single person's ownership of an object through the ability of every beholder to take pleasure in it. Pleasure thus becomes a source of power, and 'moments of enjoyment can become moments of resistance to singular ownership and hierarchy'.[32] I posit that the same could be said for the first reader of the Cambrai Hours. The traces of the reader's pleasure within the manuscript's illuminated pages challenge the exclusive efficacy of pleasure as a medium for social control. This essay highlights the dialectic of pleasure within this book of hours, revealing not only its potential for social control, but also the opportunities for agency it provides.

Resisting Pleasure

This dialectic within pleasure is especially evident in the Cambrai Hours temptation cycle, which, as I mention at the beginning of this essay, situates its protagonist's rejection of material pleasures within the visually pleasurable medium of the illuminated book. The six surviving initials share a similar composition: at the left, a demonic personification of sin cloaked in the garb

[28] De Lauretis, *Alice Doesn't*, p. 69.

[29] De Lauretis, *Alice Doesn't*, p. 68.

[30] Harris and Overbey, 'Field Change / Discipline Change', p. 138.

[31] Harris and Overbey, 'Field Change / Discipline Change', p. 135.

[32] Harris and Overbey, 'Field Change / Discipline Change', p. 142.

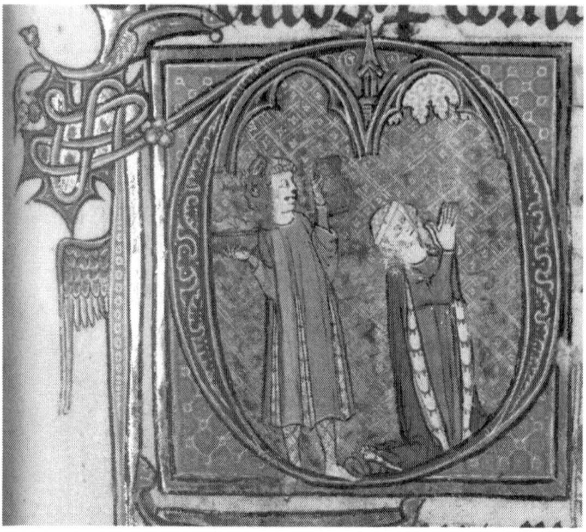

Figure 3.
'Cambrai Hours. Hours of the Virgin, Sext: Temptation of Food and Drink', Cambrai, Bibliothèque municipale, MS 87, fol. 47ʳ (detail). Before 1297. Reproduced by permission of the Médiathèque municipale of Cambrai. Clichés: IRHT-CNRS.

of earthly pleasures; at the centre, a female figure prays with her back to her tempter; and, in the upper right, pink and blue clouds denote her heavenly audience. The female devotee anticipates the reader's self-identification and models abstention from sin through constant prayer. This prescriptive series of images flags pleasure as a destructive force, disruptive to a woman's efforts to achieve salvation. Yet, in literally turning her back on worldly pleasures, she nevertheless reinforces their importance in a reader's path to salvation. Furthermore, the composition invites the viewer to consider the tempting pleasures that the devotee cannot or will not regard. In depicting for the viewer what her painted double cannot see, these initials establish the awareness of pleasure as an important element in the reader's salvation.

The six temptation initials illustrate the Hours of the Virgin, the central text of the book. They are preceded in the office's first hour, Matins, by a more traditional image of the Annunciation (see Figure 10, below). The temptation initials open the subsequent hours, and thus would have accompanied the reader's meditations over the course of her day of prayer. Opening the hour of Lauds, recited directly after Matins as the first waking act of the day, is an initial with two figures standing behind a well-appointed bed, complete with furred blanket and embroidered red pillow (Figure 1). A two-faced figure turns his human face towards the laywoman and gestures towards the bed, tempting her with its carnal pleasures. The woman, however, turns away from this tempter, sending a prayer, instead, to the upper right of the composition. A glimpse of heavenly clouds in the upper reach of the right-most arch indicates a favourable reception of the woman's actions.

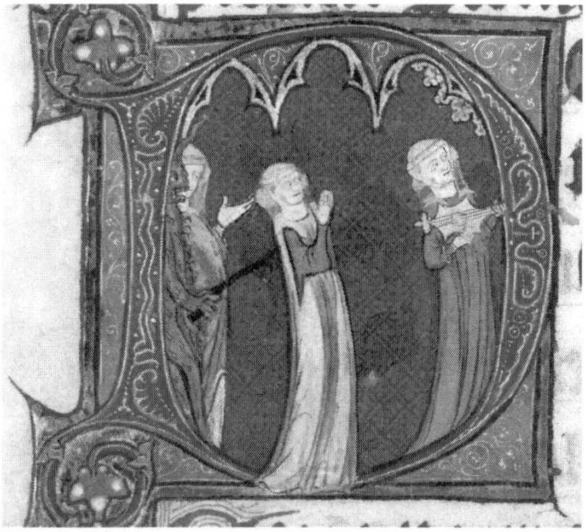

Figure 4.
'Cambrai Hours. Hours of the Virgin, Vespers: Temptation of Music', Cambrai, Bibliothèque municipale, MS 87, fol. 53ᵛ (detail). Before 1297. Reproduced by permission of the Médiathèque municipale of Cambrai. Clichés: IRHT-CNRS.

Similar scenes adorn the initials opening the subsequent hours. Although a missing page at the start of the next hour, Prime, renders the series incomplete, it is most likely that the office would originally have been illustrated with a total of seven scenes of temptation. Echoing the composition at Lauds, another two-faced figure — this time with the face of a cleric — offers the kneeling laywoman a coffer of precious items in the opening initial for Tierce; at the midday hour of Sext, a different two-faced figure tempts her with wine and meat (Figure 3). Eventually, temptations come mixed with threats: the initial at Nones shows a hairy demon aiming an arrow at the praying woman, imagery that evokes contemporary metaphors for both carnal love and disease. In the subsequent composition, at Vespers, a female musician to the right tries to distract the devotee while a second woman colludes with another hairy demon to hold a hooked weapon to the praying woman's back (Figure 4).[33] At Compline, the sixth and final initial in the series shows the woman stalwart against the pleasures of hawking.

The cycle shares some congruity with the seven deadly sins in its subject matter and original length. Although its iconography is distinct from any other contemporary representations, there does seem to be some overlap.[34] The initials to Tierce and Sext are unmistakable representations of avarice

[33] Stones, *Gothic Manuscripts*, pt. 1, II, 420.

[34] See Bennett, 'A Woman's Power of Prayer versus the Devil', p. 99, for a comparison with other, contemporary representations of the seven deadly sins. Bennett resists identifying this series with the seven deadly sins.

and gluttony, respectively; the identification of the others is less clear-cut and open to interpretation. The falcon and other implements of hawking carried by the demonic figure at Compline suggest noble pursuits, perhaps indicating pride. While Adelaide Bennett associates the Lauds initial with adultery, Alexa Sand suggests an interpretation of sloth — specifically, the hour-appropriate temptation to stay in bed and miss morning prayers.[35] The demon archer at the hour of Nones may signify lust or luxuria, as the arrow was a common metaphor for love or desire.[36] In the Vespers initial, the composition of women with a demon recalls a representation of female gossips encouraged by the demon Tutivillus on a misericord in Ely Cathedral;[37] perhaps the woman aligned with the demon to the left is tempting the devotee into envy of the oblivious musician. If the missing initial at Prime depicted the sin of anger, the set would be complete.

While a case can be made for identifying the initials with the seven deadly sins, many of the compositions also offer alternative readings. As already noted, the bedroom scene at Lauds could signify luxuria just as well as sloth. The falcon, which appears at Compline, could signify a wide range of sins: in the thirteenth-century *Bibles moralisées*, for instance, falconry seems to function as a catch-all indicator of sinful behaviour, appearing in compositions depicting avarice, gluttony, lust, and greed as well as pride.[38] Regardless of how closely the initials adhere to a conception of the seven deadly sins, each frames temptation in worldly, often bodily terms. Many present physical pleasures to be abjured, such as the luxury of reclining in a fur-covered bed or the exertions of hawking. If the Vespers initial with the group of women does connote envy, its source is implied to be the beauty of the musician's song. The ambiguity regarding the identification of the temptations as the seven deadly sins contributes to the cycle's didactic programme; the overlap between mortal sins and quotidian temptations encourages the reader to reconsider the severity of habitual indulgences. Whether the reader interprets the cycle as the seven codified mortal sins or a less formal selection of daily temptations, the emphatic theme of sensual pleasures frames the body and its senses as the site of sin. A sensually pleasurable temptation is lacking only in the composition with the demon

[35] Bennett, 'A Woman's Power of Prayer versus the Devil', p. 92; Sand, *Vision, Devotion, and Self-Representation in Late Medieval Art*, pp. 197–98.

[36] Sand, *Vision, Devotion, and Self-Representation in Late Medieval Art*, p. 198.

[37] See Armstead, 'Interpreting Images of Women with Books in Misericords', p. 65.

[38] Oggins, *The Kings and their Hawks*, pp. 130–31.

archer at Nones, which threatens, instead, the bodily integrity of the devotee. In their emphatic inclusion of the book owner type in their compositions, the illuminations implicate the body of the reader in the potential for sin and the obligation to resist it. While the placement of such a narrative within the opulent setting of a deluxe illuminated manuscript might seem to undermine its moralistic message, I assert that the visual pleasure the manuscript provides reinforces the cycle's didactic programme. This book, with its ostentatious size, opulent illuminations, and idiosyncratic iconography, was created on commission for an evidently pious woman. That it should employ such a degree of splendour in communicating a message of abstention suggests the need for a deeper exploration of the roles bodily and sensory pleasures might have played in its reader's penance.

Maternal Joys

Considering the apparent contradiction in the Hours of the Virgin illuminations between the rejection of sensory pleasures and their embrace, it is instructive to consider the role that bodily pleasures play in another section of the manuscript, the Joys of the Virgin. In contrast to the temptation cycle, this brief series of prayers addressed to the Virgin appears to explicitly mark out a space for pleasure. Yet, as we shall see, this section likewise engages in highly didactic visual and textual rhetoric. The licit pleasures of the Joys of the Virgin stand in contrast to the temptations of the Hours. Nevertheless, both underscore the critical role of the body in determining its subject's salvation.

The Joys of the Virgin, different versions of which can number between five and fifteen, highlight the happiest moments from the life of Mary and beg her intercession in remembrance of them.[39] Two versions of the Joys appear in this book of hours: the Five Joys, in Latin, and the Nine Joys, in French. In both its Latin and vernacular forms, the Joys of the Virgin is a short text meant to be recited in a single sitting. Although the specific Joys enumerated differ between the two versions, both texts emphasize Mary's joy in motherhood as the basis for her intercessory power. The illuminations of both sections, moreover, connect the maternal joys of the text with imagery referring to the owner's marriage: heraldic and figural references to Gaucher de Châtillon d'Autresche gloss both

[39] For the Joys of the Virgin, see Huot, 'Inventional Mnemonics, Reading and Prayer', pp. 106–07; Huot, 'A Book Made for a Queen', pp. 131–32; Winston-Allen, *Stories of the Rose*, pp. 38–41.

texts of the Joys of the Virgin. The illuminations of both texts mobilize Mary's maternal pleasures to model a similar role for her (perhaps newly) married devotee. Like the illuminations of the temptation cycle, the Joys emphasize the female body as a source of and a site for pleasure. In so doing, the illuminations distinguish between the licit pleasures of motherhood and devotion in the Joys and the illicit pleasures of the world in the temptation cycle. In establishing this didactic dichotomy and linking the reader's pleasure to her marital relationship, the manuscript articulates guidelines to regulate the pleasures and desires of its female reader.

The first of the two sections devoted to the Joys of the Virgin — the shorter, Latin version — covers only four manuscript pages.[40] The first two pages contain the joys themselves, while a collect, responsory, versicle, antiphon, and an additional collect follow. These brief texts emphasize Mary's bodily involvement in the miraculous events of her life and her son's. The five joys enumerated are Mary's conception of Christ through her ear at the Annunciation, her painless birth, the Resurrection of her son, his Ascension, and her own coronation in heaven. In this text, Mary's joys revolve almost entirely around her son, striking a balance between the events of Christ's infancy and those following his Resurrection. Each joy is a short statement of an event from her life: 'Gaude uirgo mat[er] xp[ist]i qui per aure[m] concepisti gabriele nuntio' (Rejoice, Virgin, mother of Christ, who conceived through the ear by means of Gabriel's annunciation). While this joy cites Mary's unusual means of conception through her ear, others also emphasize the Virgin's bodily experience of biblical history. The second joy remembers her delivery of Christ 'sine pena cum pudoris lilio' (without pain and with the lily of modesty). The fourth, remembering Christ's Ascension, specifies Mary's role as an empirical witness: 'Gaude xpo ascendente quod in celum te uidente motu fertur proprio' (Rejoice in the ascendant Christ, whom it was made manifest is in heaven through an extraordinary movement, as you saw). The prayers that follow the five joys emphasize Mary's bodily status as both Virgin and mother through the miracle of Christ's conception and God's preservation of Mary's virginity. The antiphon especially stresses the Virgin's body: 'Beatus uenter qui te portauit xpe et beata ubera que te lactauerunt dnm et saluatorem mundi' (Blessed is the belly that carried you, Christ, and blessed are the breasts that suckled you, lord and saviour of the world). The text of the Five Joys grounds Mary's intercessory abilities in her bodily experience. Her body likewise appears, by extension, as the seat of the 'ioies' (joys) that the French rubric primes the reader to see in the texts.

[40] Cambrai, BM, MS 87, fols 71^{r}–72^{v}.

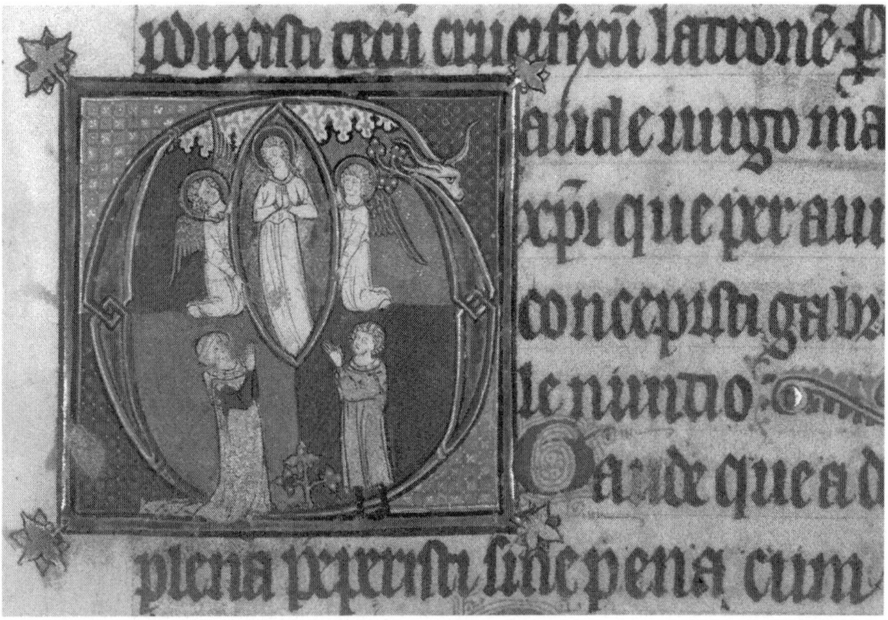

Figure 5. 'Cambrai Hours. Five Joys of the Virgin: Mary adored by book owner and husband', Cambrai, Bibliothèque municipale, MS 87, fol. 71r (detail). Before 1297. Reproduced with the permission of the Médiathèque municipale of Cambrai. Clichés: IRHT-CNRS.

The bodies of the Virgin and the reader also play a prominent role in the large illuminated initial initiating these brief prayers. The five-line initial shows a woman and a man, both clad in gold cloaks lined with vair, adoring the Virgin as she ascends to heaven, supported on either side by a kneeling angel (Figure 5). The quartered background of the initial divides terrestrial and heavenly spheres as well as feminine and masculine space. Only the Virgin transgresses these divisions. While her white garment matches those of the supporting angels, the gold background of her mandorla and her gesture of prayer resonate with the supplicants below. Mary looks down to her right, meeting the gaze of the woman. Although the book owner and her husband appear together in this initial, it is she who has the privilege to share the Virgin's gaze. While the painted book owner receives a vision of the Virgin Mary, her corporeal counterpart, the reader, perceives it through her embodied sight. The painted surface of the page mediates between the visible and the visionary, transforming the book into a bridge between the two. This is not to say, however, that the contents of the book are exclusively incorporeal.

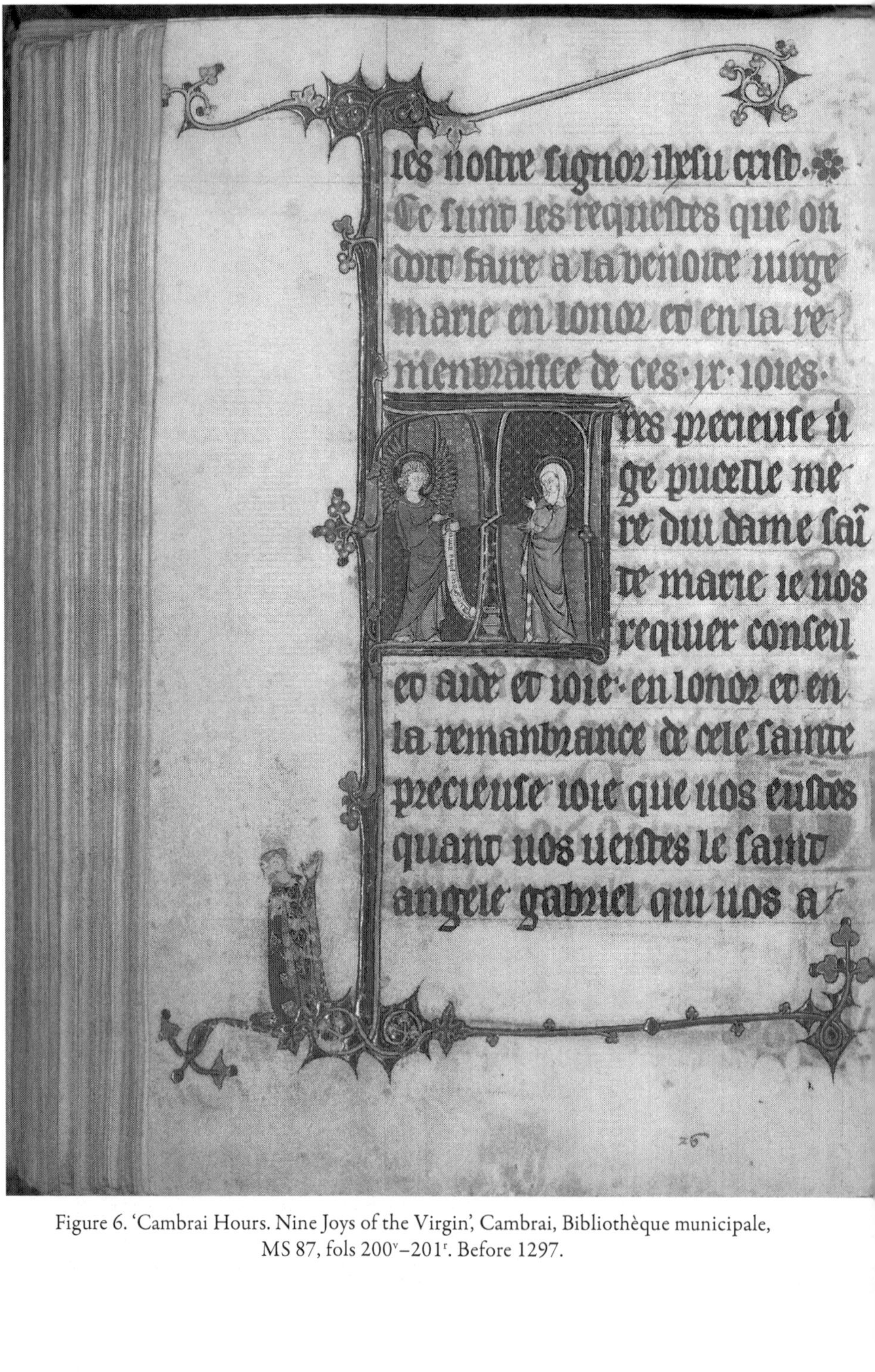

Figure 6. 'Cambrai Hours. Nine Joys of the Virgin', Cambrai, Bibliothèque municipale, MS 87, fols 200v–201r. Before 1297.

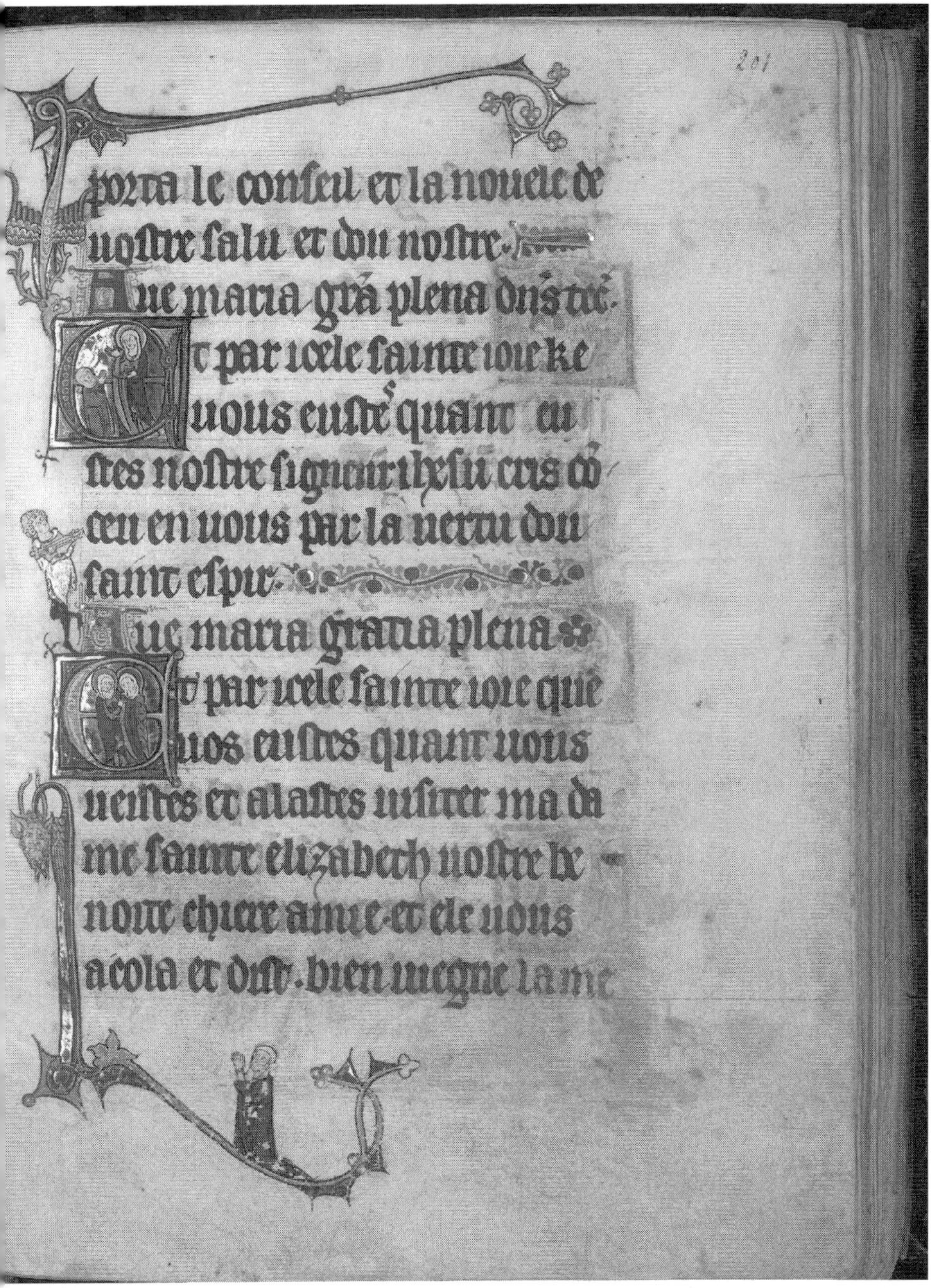
aporta le conseil et la nouele de
nostre salu et dou nostre.
Aue maria grā plena dn̄s tec̄.
Et par icele sainte ioie ke
uous eustes quant au
stres nostre signeur ihesu cris cō
ceu en uous par la uertu dou
saint espir.
Aue maria gratia plena
Et par icele sainte ioie que
uos eustes quant uous
ueistes et alastes uisiter ma da
me sainte elizabeth uostre be-
noite chiere amie et ele uous
acola et dist. bien uegne la me

Reproduced by permission of the Médiathèque municipale of Cambrai. Clichés: IRHT-CNRS.

While Mary's costume, her mandorla, and the supporting angels insulate the upper register of this initial from the corporeal realm, the text that follows dwells on the Virgin's humanity, as I describe above. The corporeal emphasis of the text and the shared gaze of the Virgin and the female devotee in the initial together undercut the incorporeality of the Virgin's painted figure and establish a parity between the two women depicted within the initial's frame. The presence, moreover, of the woman's husband in the initial resonates with the focus in the text that follows on the Virgin's motherhood and the parentage of her son. Text and illumination together establish motherhood as the shared experience of the Virgin and her female devotee, a pleasure situated explicitly in the materiality of the female body.

The vernacular variation on this text, the Nine Joys of the Virgin, reiterates the connection between motherhood, the body, and pleasure even more emphatically. The Nine Joys appears in the predominantly vernacular section of the manuscript that occupies its final quires (Figure 6).[41] The French text dwells somewhat longer on Christ's Infancy: the Annunciation, the Incarnation, the Visitation, the Nativity, the Adoration of the Magi, and the Presentation in the Temple comprise Mary's first six joys. The prayers then pass over the events of Christ's Passion and Resurrection to highlight his Ascension, Mary's reception of the Holy Spirit with the apostles at Pentecost, and her Assumption and Coronation. The format of the first joy, commemorating the Annunciation, exemplifies the eight that follow. Each prayer begins with a direct address to the Virgin, continues with a request for her aid in remembrance of a joyous event in her life, then ends with a prompt to the reader to recite an *Ave*:

> Tres precieuse v[ir]ge pucelle mere diu dame sai[n]te marie ie uos requier conseil et aide et ioie. En lonor et en la remambrance de cele sainte precieuse ioie que uos eustes quant uos veistes le saint angele gabriel qui uos aporta le conseil et la nouele de uostre salu et dou nostre. Aue maria gr[ati]a plena d[omi]n[u]s tec[um].[42]

> [Very precious virgin maiden mother of God Lady Saint Mary, I beg your counsel and aid and joy in honour and in remembrance of that holy, precious joy that you had when you saw the holy angel Gabriel, who brought you counsel and the news of your salvation and of ours. Hail Mary full of grace the Lord is with you.]

Two brief texts follow the recitation of the joys: the first reiterates the request for aid and intercession, pleading, 'iai grant besoig de uostre aide et de uos-

[41] Cambrai, BM, MS 87, fols 200v–203r.

[42] Cambrai, BM, MS 87, fol. 200v.

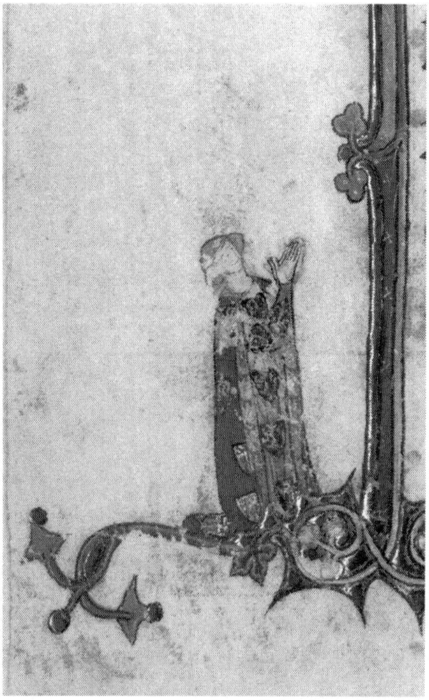

Figure 7. 'Cambrai Hours. Nine Joys of the Virgin: Book owner in heraldic garments', Cambrai, Bibliothèque municipale, MS 87, fol. 200v (detail). Before 1297. Reproduced by permission of the Médiathèque municipale of Cambrai. Clichés: IRHT-CNRS.

tre conseil en ame & en cors' (I have great need of your aid and your counsel in spirit and in body);[43] the second, rubricated text explains the efficacy of the prayers that precede it.

As in the Latin version of the text, illuminations work hand-in-hand with text to shape the reader's experience of her prayer and her relationship with its addressee, the Virgin. Each joy begins with a small historiated initial illustrating the appropriate scene from Mary's biography. While the Virgin appears in each of the prayer's initials, the female book owner is also present on every page, kneeling in prayer in the lower margin (Figure 6). Her placement at a remove from the Virgin replicates the processes of remembering and requesting that the text of the prayers describes; the narrative initials are also legible as illustrations of her thoughts and meditations in the course of completing her prayer. At the same time, their paired presence on the page's surface asserts their physical consonance.

The prominent depiction of the book owner on the opening page of the Nine Joys establishes the shared importance of the two women's figures in this section of the prayer book while framing both in terms of their procreative potential (Figures 6 and 7). The book owner kneels in the prominent lower left margin of the page in adoration of the Virgin, who appears in the Annunciation initial above. As Mary faces Gabriel in the initial, she is receiving, as the prayer reports, 'la nouele de uostre salu et dou nostre' (the news of your [Mary's] salvation and of ours). Mary's body is about to become a vessel for salvation; it will also become a conduit for a type of pleasure, the celestial joy of carrying the incarnate God.[44] The book owner's body, set in juxtaposition to the

[43] Cambrai, BM, MS 87, fol. 202v.

[44] For celestial and terrestrial joy, see Dybel, *Être heureux au Moyen Âge*, p. 18.

Virgin's at the bottom of the page, bears a different type of news: the dynastic union between the book owner and her husband. While the owner's mauve dress is covered with the differenced Brabant arms of her own family, shields bearing the arms of her husband, Gaucher de Châtillon d'Autresche, adorn the mantle that rests upon her shoulders. Here, as at the opening of the Latin Five Joys, the invocation of Gaucher relates the reader's marital aspirations and responsibilities with the Virgin's motherhood. As Mary takes on the salvation of humanity above, the devotee carries a different responsibility below: the continuation of her husband's lineage. The wear on this page, especially on the marginal figure of the book owner, suggests that it was consulted often. The parallel between the Virgin and her devotee seems to have resonated with the reader's hopes and desires for herself and her family.

The next initial in the Nine Joys series further reinforces the bodily relationship between the devotee and the Virgin. While the Incarnation was simultaneous with the Annunciation in the Five Joys, here it appears separately as the second joy in the series (Figure 8). The prayer opens with a two-line initial in which Mary holds a book, an attribute that at once denotes her piety while also recalling Christ's status as the Word made Flesh. The text describes Mary's conception of her son through the efforts of the Holy Spirit: 'Et par icele sainte ioie ke uous eustes quant eustes nostre signeur ihesu cris co[n]ceu en uous par la uertu dou saint espir' (And by that holy joy that you had when our lord Jesus Christ was conceived in you by the virtue of the Holy Spirit). In the context of the Incarnation, the book in the initial is a visual, external manifestation of the newly conceived saviour, hidden inside his mother's body. Yet, while the text of the joy cites the Holy Spirit in Christ's conception, no manifestation of the third member of the Trinity is visible in the initial. Instead, the kneeling book owner is present beside the Virgin. The devotee kneels to the left of the Virgin, and tilts her head back to address Mary; Mary, meanwhile, gesticulates as if speaking, but makes no other acknowledgement of the woman kneeling before her. The Incarnation initial is the only one of the series to incorporate the book owner into a narrative composition, breaking with the boilerplate iconography of the other initials, like the Visitation below. Unlike the Five Joys initial, where the composition and Mary's mandorla marks off the space of a sacred vision, nothing separates her from the devotee. They appear, instead, to be meeting face to face.

While the book owner's marginal position on the opening page of the Nine Joys framed her as a witness to the Virgin's joys, the incorporation of her form into the Incarnation initial elevates her from witness to participant. The devotee's bodily presence before the Virgin coincides with the moment

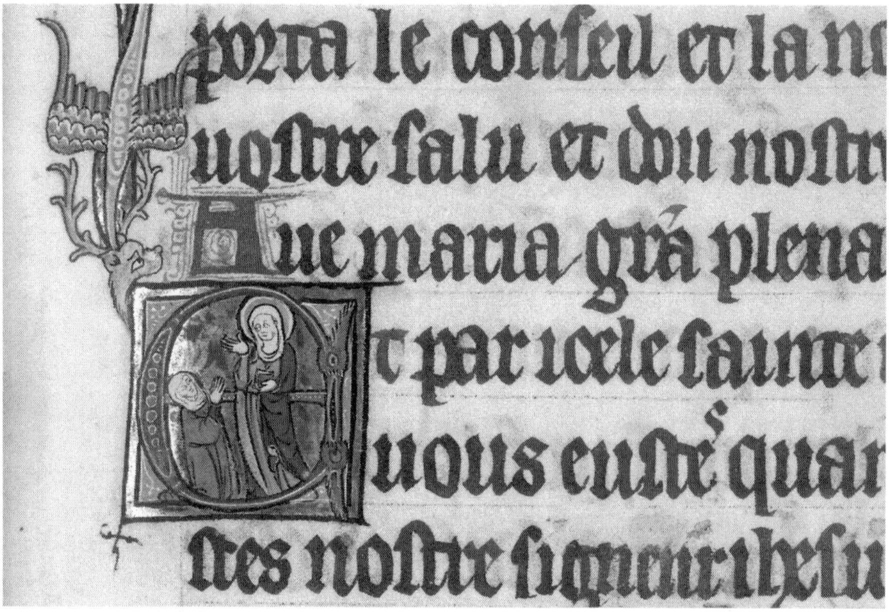

Figure 8. 'Cambrai Hours. Nine Joys of the Virgin: Incarnation', Cambrai, Bibliothèque municipale, MS 87, fol. 201r (detail). Before 1297. Reproduced by permission of the Médiathèque municipale of Cambrai. Clichés: IRHT-CNRS.

of Christ's bodily Incarnation, further elevating the significance of her privileged participation in the initial. Through the recursive properties of owner portraiture, this bodily participation spills over from the depicted book owner to her embodied counterpart, the viewer. The prominence of the book in the small initial casts a Christological significance on the book in which the initial appears, presumably open in the hands of the reader. This image collapses the reader's bodily experiences of holding and looking at her book with their mystical equivalents: gazing upon the Virgin Mary and holding the body of the infant Christ. The function of the book in the Incarnation initial as an externalized signifier of Mary's pregnancy reinforces the significance of the emblazoned shields depicted on the kneeling owner's garments in the margin of the opposite page. Just as the Virgin's body is a vessel for salvation, the owner's body is depicted here as the conduit for the continuation of both families' legacies. The reference to her husband overlays the book owner's witnessing of the conception and birth of Christ with her own responsibility to produce a male heir to bear the Châtillon arms. By referencing this responsibility within a recitation of the Virgin's joys, the manuscript frames procreation not as an obligation, but as an aspiration. The Virgin's joy at conceiving a son is a mirror in which the reader is encouraged to shape her own desire for offspring and anticipate her pleasure in a successful birth. The comparison with the Virgin elevates the stakes for the reader's procreation. As the text of the Nine Joys equates the Virgin's joyful conception of Christ with salvation, procreation is pictured as the route to both joy and salvation. This section presents the joys of motherhood and salvation together to produce and shape the contours of the reader's anticipatory pleasure in both.

This close reading of three sections of this book of hours — the Hours of the Virgin, the Latin Five Joys, and the French Nine Joys — demonstrates the illuminated manuscript's capacity to instil within its anticipated reader the social expectations of her rank and gender. The imagery of embodied pleasure in the two Joys of the Virgin and the luxurious materiality of the book in which they appear work together to present as desirable the expectations resting upon the body of a young, married woman at the end of the thirteenth century. This didactic capacity resonates with the potential that Laura Mulvey and others have isolated within narrative cinema to shape the desires and pleasures of its audience by controlling their gaze. I will now consider in greater depth what feminist film criticism can contribute to an understanding of this medieval object — and the limits of its applicability.

Central to my interpretation of this manuscript is a reconstruction of its gendered reception or, to borrow a set of terms from film theory, the female gaze. Mulvey's concern in 'Visual Pleasure and Narrative Cinema' was the definition of the male gaze. She described the male gaze as consisting of two modes: scopophilic (when turned on women) and narcissistic (when turned on other men). Troublingly, her model seemed to allow no role for a female spectator in the cinema audience. Mulvey's initial silence on the female gaze spurred critique among other scholars, who sought to remedy her oversight. Numerous later critics emphasized female objectification on screen as a challenge for the prospective female spectator. In Mary Ann Doane's view, identification with the objectified woman negated the possibility of a voyeuristic gaze, forcing women to choose between the extreme positions of either complicity in the objectification and degradation of women (that is, masochism), or narcissism, in which the viewer 'becom[es her] own object of desire'.[45]

Representations of the Cambrai Hours book owner in the three sections so far discussed appear to indulge both of Doane's spectatorial positions. The

[45] Doane, 'Film and the Masquerade', p. 87.

temptation cycle trades overtly in masochism: while the laywoman evades the threatened punishments, they still loom dangerously close, inviting the reader to imaginatively play out their execution. In their valorization of the penitent woman, with whom the reader performatively identifies, the temptation initials imply that a lesser woman would deserve the depicted tortures. However, it is not surprising that owner portraits more typically engage exclusively their subject-viewers' narcissism. Indeed, Doane's assessment of the cinematic viewer's transformation into the idealized 'object of desire' is apposite to the understanding of imagery within medieval devotional books, which functioned in part to guide the subject formation of their anticipated readers. The owner portraits of the Cambrai Hours model the performance of penance for their reader, an essential step in her progression from sin to salvation. Yet, as I argue above, the signs of the reader's familial circumstances, injected strategically in this book of hours into sections of vernacular Marian devotion, align this spiritual transition with the play of identities medieval laywomen regularly navigated: daughter, wife, mother, and teacher, as well as penitent. The owner portrait may be read as a mirror in which the reader-viewer is invited to compose herself on the twin models of the Virgin and her devotee.[46] This model complicates the image of the devotee, elevating it to an object of devotion even as it engages with the living reader's performance of prayer.

Thus the illuminations present the figures of the Virgin and the owner, together, not necessarily as objects of erotic desire, as Doane perceives in narrative cinema, but as objects of devotion. This devotion, however, bespeaks a different kind of desire: the desire for intimacy with the divine, which was often framed, in this period, in erotic terms.[47] In the illuminations accompanying the two texts of the Joys of the Virgin, the painted book owner, in addition to modelling devotion for her subject-viewer, also models a process of identification with and emulation of the divine. The book owner's relationship with the Virgin Mary in these two sections is grounded in their shared reproductive capabilities. The illuminations frame motherhood as a joy that transcends the earthly and the heavenly planes, a source of simultaneous physical and spiritual pleasure. In so doing, the illuminations strive to shape the desires of their anticipated female viewer with the promise of a pleasure

[46] See Smith, *The Taymouth Hours*, pp. 257–61; Sand, *Vision, Devotion, and Self-Representation in Late Medieval Art*, p. 4.

[47] Bynum, *The Resurrection of the Body in Western Christianity*, pp. 334–41; Easton, '"Was It Good For You, Too?"', pp. 2–5.

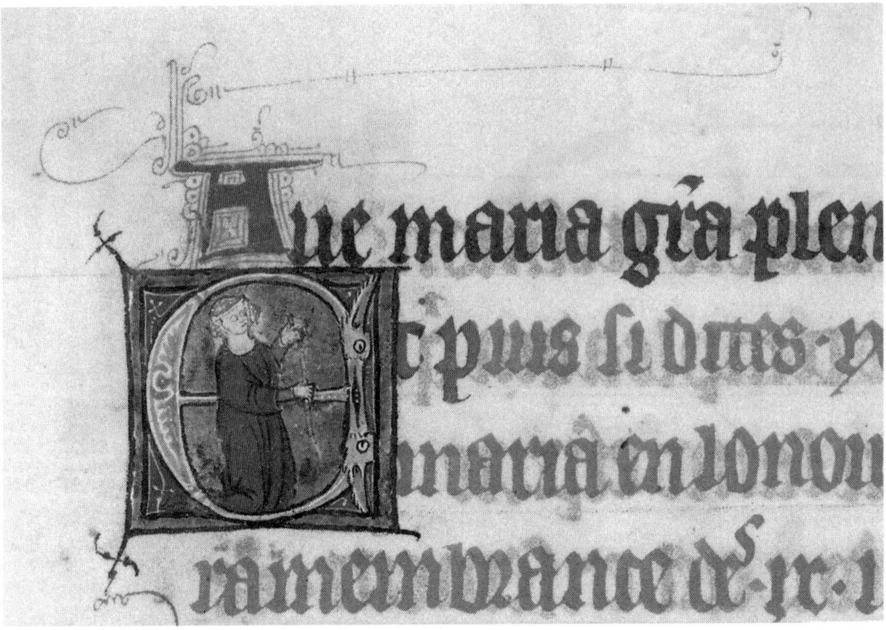

Figure 9. 'Cambrai Hours. Nine Joys of the Virgin: Book owner with a rosary', Cambrai, Bibliothèque municipale, MS 87, fol. 203r (detail). Before 1297. Reproduced by permission of the Médiathèque municipale of Cambrai. Clichés: IRHT-CNRS.

modelled and sanctioned by the Virgin. Thus, with her dual traits of sanctity and success in motherhood, Mary stands not only as an object of devotion, but as an object of desire.

While feminist film theory provides a useful framework through which to understand the didactic capacity of this prayer book's illuminations, it falls short in its approach to the viewer itself. This is due in part to the material differences between a film and a codex; while the former unfolds linearly for its audience, the latter is available for a variety of engagements: brief or prolonged; superficial or considered; singular or continued. Moreover, as the next section will show, this manuscript encourages multiple modes of engagement from its reader. Furthermore, it bears the traces of her engaged response, thus providing scant, but precious, evidence of her reaction to its offered pleasures.

Through their creative use of owner portraits in their illuminations, the Hours of the Virgin, the Five Joys, and the Nine Joys implicate the reader's body in either the embrace or the rejection of the pleasures each section offers. The final initial in the Nine Joys underscores the theme of embodied witnessing and participation established in the preceding pages while also introducing a critical new element to the reader's pious performance: sensory engagement (Figure 9). In this two-line initial, the book owner returns to the framed space of the composition, this time kneeling alone with a string of rosary beads. The initial precedes a rubric text that summarizes the effectiveness of the prayer: 'Et puis si dites.ix. fois Aue maria en lonor et en la ramembrance de[s].ix. ioies nostre dame et la benoite uirge marie uous aidera et conseillera & deffendra des temptations alanemi' (And if you say 'Hail Mary' nine times in honour and in remembrance of the nine joys of our lady, the blessed Virgin Mary will help you and counsel you and defend you against the temptations of the enemy).[48] The rosary in the devotee's hands identifies the focus of her prayer as the Virgin Mary and implies that she is performing the prayer that the reader has just completed. Yet this initial, together with the rubric text, reorients the reader's focus away from the Virgin and towards her own performance of remembrance and devotion. Moreover, the addition of a rosary to the book's standard owner portrait iconography calls the reader's attention to her physical performance. The owner portrait initiates a comparison between self and image that directs the reader's attention to the activities of her hands and the sensations beneath her fingers, whether or not she is actually using a rosary. The reader's attention to the sensations of her body is as much a part of the successful completion of the prayer as her attention to the affective material of the prayer itself.

Sensory Pleasures

Returning to the book's central text, the Hours of the Virgin, with this model of sensorially engaged reading in mind, we find much in the illuminations to tempt the reader's senses. Imagery of tantalizing food, as in the initial for Sext, engages the senses of smell and taste by activating the subject's prior experience of their pleasures (Figure 3).[49] Scenes of music and dancing — which appear prominently in marginal illuminations as well as in the initial for Vespers — evoke aural pleasures and the emotional stimulation they can provide (Figures 1, 4, and 6).[50] This imagery of sensory pleasures supplements the visual and tactile delights essential to the material manuscript. Within the illuminated book, these indulgences are no diversion; rather, they open its pages for the reader's complete sensory immersion. By couching the rejection of sensory pleasures

[48] Cambrai, BM, MS 87, fol. 203^{r}.

[49] See Carruthers, *The Experience of Beauty in the Middle Ages*, pp. 50–52.

[50] See Williamson, 'Sensory Experience in Medieval Devotion' for visual depictions of music.

within the stimulating medium of an illuminated book, the manuscript's authors exploit their reader's natural weakness to sensory stimulation, transforming the reader's weakness for temptation into a compelling avenue for her salvation.

The overwhelming beauty of this book of hours enlists its reader's inborn weakness to and desire for sensory pleasures to deepen her engagement with the content of the book. The temptation initials, while explicitly proscribing the range of worldly pleasures open to their affluent lay female reader, implicitly offer the book in which they appear as a source of sanctioned pleasure. These visual allusions to sensory stimuli reinforce the multisensory experience of using a medieval prayer book. Vision and touch work in tandem, each revealing and enabling engagement with the successive layered surfaces of the object. The reader must manipulate the book's cover and pages in order to see their contents and perform the devotions within; those contents, in turn, may inspire or require her touch. While sight and touch are the primary modes of contact, the use of a prayer book engages the other senses, as well. The open book scents the surrounding space with its particular animal odour, overlaid with the traces of its production and use.[51] The smell of the book recalls its material history as an animal product while also carrying the associations of its new, devotional function and marking the space as one for prayer.[52] A prayer spoken is metaphorically tasted in the mouth even as it is actually heard in the ears.[53] In presenting a variety of sensory stimuli within its illuminations, then, the book of hours provides visual amplification of its reader's total sensory experience of her performance of prayer. The multisensory experience of reading that this manuscript encourages resonates with earlier, twelfth-century conceptions of reading as an essentially sensory activity.[54] The emphasis on the senses may have a further significance for the role of the anticipated owner's gender in the manuscript since, as Helen Solterer has shown, women were considered exceptionally sensory beings in the later Middle Ages. Solterer suggests that this understanding coloured reading as an activity for which women had a

[51] Dugan, 'The Smell of Vellum', emphasizes parchment's vulnerability to environmental effects, including odours. My thanks to Professor Dugan for sharing this work with me before its publication.

[52] Kay, 'Legible Skins'.

[53] See also Camille, 'The Book as Flesh and Fetish in Richard de Bury's *Philobiblon*', pp. 40–41; Carruthers, *The Experience of Beauty in the Middle Ages*, pp. 7–8.

[54] Solterer, 'Seeing, Hearing, Tasting Woman', p. 130.

natural affinity.[55] An emphasis on sensory engagement is thus appropriate to a book made for a woman, as to read like a woman would be to read with all the body's senses engaged.

The vibrant illuminations in this book of hours explicitly play on their reader's appetite for sensory pleasures to lure her into the sustained engagement necessary for her salvation. In playing to its reader's pleasure, the illuminated manuscript unites salvation and desire within its pages. This lavish book, specifically, creates a space for female desire. Moreover, it configures female desire as an active force: while stock images of medieval romance frame women as passive recipients of devotion, the devotee within the prayer book takes on the active role of petition.[56] As noted above, the recipient of her petition, the Virgin Mary, stands not only as a model for emulation, but as an object of desire. While the eroticization of Christ in the texts and images of late medieval devotion, especially those associated with female mystics, has been a subject of scholarly inquiry, attempts to 'queer' devotion to his mother are, surprisingly, absent.[57] Yet the very qualities attributed to the feminized Christ of mystical devotion are the maternal qualities essential to Mary's identity within the faith. Christ's wounds, especially the side wound, were loci for devotion that focused on the saviour's generative, nourishing, permeable body.[58] A remarkable series of initials showing the female devotee adoring each of Christ's five wounds in turn demonstrates the currency of such affective, bodily devotion within the Cambrai Hours.[59] It is worth considering representations of the Virgin's body from a similar perspective.

The texts and images of the two Joys of the Virgin in the Cambrai Hours invite contemplation of the Virgin's reproductive body. While the text of the Five Joys lauds the womb and breasts that nurtured the infant Christ, the mandorla that frames the Virgin in the initial preceding it evokes at once the wound of Christ and the vaginal opening, connecting Mary's delivery of

[55] Solterer, 'Seeing, Hearing, Tasting Woman', pp. 129–31.

[56] See Smith, 'The Gothic Mirror and the Female Gaze' for the gendered dynamics of desire in representations of courtship in this period.

[57] Karma Lochrie briefly proposes a connection between Lollard criticisms of women's excessive devotion to religious images, specifically the Virgin Mary, and accusations of women's excessive sexuality. Lochrie, *Heterosyncracies*, p. 54.

[58] Bynum, 'The Female Body and Religious Practice in the Later Middle Ages', especially pp. 205–06; Lochrie, 'Mystical Acts, Queer Tendencies', p. 187. Lochrie critiques Bynum's reluctance to acknowledge homoerotic potential in descriptions of the feminized Christ.

[59] Cambrai, BM, MS 87, fols 177r–180v.

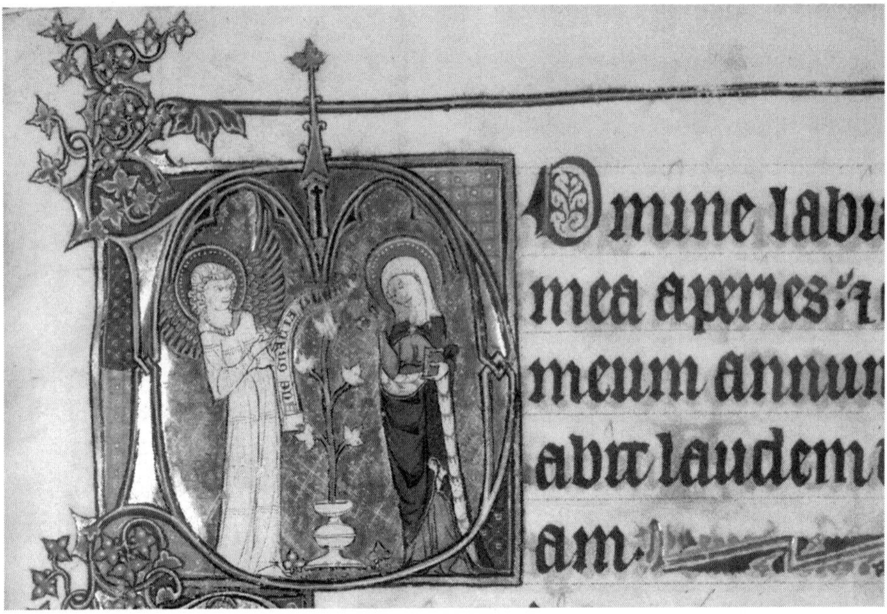

Figure 10. 'Cambrai Hours. Hours of the Virgin, Matins: Annunciation', Cambrai, Bibliothèque municipale, MS 87, fol. 19^{r} (detail). Before 1297. Reproduced by permission of the Médiathèque municipale of Cambrai. Clichés: IRHT-CNRS.

Christ with the promise of heavenly rebirth (Figure 5).[60] Already dressed in her celestial white robes, the Virgin appears fairly incorporeal in this illumination; other images, however, emphasize her corporeality. In the Annunciation initial opening the Hours of the Virgin, Mary draws her heavy, fur-lined cloak across her body, creating deep folds over and drawing attention to her abdomen (Figure 10). The artist has delineated the Virgin's breasts beneath the pink fabric of her dress, framing them with the blue cloak above and below. Mary's book, which she holds in front of her body, stands in for her pregnant womb, as it does in the Nine Joys Incarnation initial. The smudging on this illumination — on the Virgin's face and hand, the lily, and Gabriel's scroll — suggests repeated touching or kissing, revealing a reader's responsive touch.[61] Marks

[60] See Easton, 'The Wound of Christ and the Mouth of Hell', pp. 407–08. The almond shape of the mandorla similarly echoes the bloody wound through which Saint Margaret, the patron saint of childbirth, emerges from the beast in the illumination beside her suffrage in this manuscript (fol. 99^{r}).

[61] See Rudy, 'Kissing Images, Unfurling Rolls, Measuring Wounds, Sewing Badges and Carrying Talismans'; Rudy, 'Dirty Books'.

and wear such as this throughout this book suggest that this extraordinarily fine illuminated manuscript was not merely a show piece; it was a tool actively used in its owner's devotional practices. Whether made with lips or, more likely, fingertips, these smudges are a trace not only of the reader's repeated engagement with the book, but of her enactment of the desire for an intimate, bodily encounter with the Virgin.

The authors of this illuminated book of hours crafted its contents to capture the gaze and engage the senses of its anticipated female user. In controlling her gaze, its programme of illuminations worked to shape her desires, encouraging marital fidelity and procreation (in the Joys of the Virgin) while forestalling sins and other socially disruptive behaviours (in the Hours of the Virgin). Yet, through its status as a site (or sight) of pleasure, the book of hours ascribed agency and desire to its reader even as it controlled her gaze. Its illuminations inscribed her as the author of her own salvation, and its surfaces bear the traces of her desiring devotions. In her essay, Mulvey asserted that 'analysing pleasure [...] destroys it'.[62] When that analysis, however, can reveal the imprints of past pleasures, such as a loving and hopeful touch on the Virgin's painted face, it is much more difficult to reduce a complex, historical object to a mere instrument of patriarchy. Its study, instead, reveals some of the contours of gendered subjectivity at the end of the thirteenth century, the continued exploration of which is a certain source of pleasure for the modern scholar.

62 Mulvey, 'Visual Pleasure and Narrative Cinema', p. 8.

Works Cited

Manuscript

Cambrai, Bibliothèque municipale, MS 87; images available at Institut de recherche et d'histoire des textes, 'Bibliothèque virtuelle des manuscrits médiévaux', 2013, <http://bvmm.irht.cnrs.fr/> [accessed 22 May 2014]

Primary Sources

Bernard of Clairvaux, *Apologia ad Guillelmum, Sancti-Theodorici Abbatem*, in *S. Bernardi Abbatis primi Claræ-Vallensis: Opera Omnia*, *PL*, CLXXXII, cols 896–918

Secondary Works

Adam-Even, Paul, and Léon Jéquier, 'L'Armorial Wijnbergen', *Archives héraldiques suisses*, 68 (1954), 55–80

Armstead, Wendy, 'Interpreting Images of Women with Books in Misericords', in *Women and the Book: Assessing the Visual Evidence*, ed. by Lesley Smith and Jane H. M. Taylor (London: British Library, 1997), pp. 57–74

Bennett, Adelaide, 'A Woman's Power of Prayer versus the Devil in a Book of Hours of *c.* 1300', in *Image and Belief: Studies in Celebration of the Eightieth Anniversary of the Index of Christian Art*, ed. by Colum Hourihane (Princeton, NJ: Index of Christian Art, 1999), pp. 89–110

Bergstrom, Janet, and Mary Ann Doane, eds, *The Spectatrix*, special issue, *Camera Obscura*, 7.2–3, 20–21 (1989), <http://cameraobscura.dukejournals.org/content/7/2-3_20-21.toc> [accessed 30 May 2014]

Bynum, Caroline Walker, 'The Female Body and Religious Practice in the Later Middle Ages', in *Fragmentation and Redemption: Essays on Gender and the Human Body in Medieval Religion* (New York: Zone Books, 1991), pp. 181–238

——, *The Resurrection of the Body in Western Christianity, 200–1336* (New York: Columbia University Press, 1995)

Camille, Michael, 'The Book as Flesh and Fetish in Richard de Bury's *Philobiblon*', in *The Book and the Body*, ed. by Dolores Warwick Frese and Katherine O'Brien O'Keeffe, University of Notre Dame Ward-Phillips Lectures in English Language and Literature, 14 (Notre Dame: University of Notre Dame Press, 1997), pp. 34–77

Carruthers, Mary, *The Experience of Beauty in the Middle Ages*, Oxford-Warburg Studies (Oxford: Oxford University Press, 2013)

Caviness, Madeline H., 'Patron or Matron? A Capetian Bride and a Vade Mecum for her Marriage Bed', in *Studying Medieval Women: Sex, Gender, Feminism*, ed. by Nancy F. Partner (Cambridge, MA: Medieval Academy of America, 1993), pp. 31–60

——, *Reframing Medieval Art: Difference, Margins, Boundaries*, 2001; <http://dca.lib.tufts.edu/caviness/> [accessed 29 May 2014]

——, *Visualizing Women in the Middle Ages: Sight, Spectacle, and Scopic Economy* (Philadelphia: University of Pennsylvania Press, 2001)

De Lauretis, Teresa, *Alice Doesn't: Feminism, Semiotics, Cinema* (Bloomington: Indiana University Press, 1984)

Demay, G., *Inventaire des sceaux de la collection Clairambault à la Bibliothèque nationale* (Paris: Imprimerie nationale, 1885), I; <http://archive.org/details/inventairedessce01demauoft> [accessed 28 May 2014]

——, *Inventaire des sceaux de la Flandre recueillis dans les dépôts d'archives, musées et collections particulières du département du Nord*, 2 vols (Paris: Imprimerie nationale, 1873); <https://archive.org/details/inventairedessce01dema> [accessed 5 October 2017]

Doane, Mary Ann, 'Film and the Masquerade: Theorising the Female Spectator', *Screen*, 23 (1982), 74–88; <http://dx.doi.org/10.1093/screen/23.3-4.74>

——, '[Untitled Response]', in *The Spectatrix*, ed. by Janet Bergstrom and Mary Ann Doane, special issue, *Camera Obscura*, 7.2–3, 20–21 (1989), 142–47; <http://cameraobscura.dukejournals.org/content/7/2-3_20-21.toc> [accessed 30 May 2014]

Doyle, Maeve, 'The Portrait Potential: Gender, Identity, and Devotion in Manuscript Owner Portraits' (unpublished doctoral dissertation, Bryn Mawr College, 2015)

Drigsdahl, Erik, and Center for Håndskriftstudier i Danmark (CHD), 'Hore Beate Marie Virginis – Use of Reims (Rheims)', *Late Medieval and Renaissance Illuminated Manuscripts — Books of Hours 1300–1530*, 1997, <http://manuscripts.org.uk/chd.dk/use/hv_reims.html> [accessed 5 October 2017]

Duffy, Eamon, *Marking the Hours: English People and their Prayers, 1240–1570* (New Haven: Yale University Press, 2006)

Dugan, Holly, 'The Smell of Vellum', *Material Texts Network*, 1 May 2014, <http://www.materialtexts.bbk.ac.uk/?p=12> [accessed 30 May 2014]

Dybel, Katarzyna, *Être heureux au Moyen Âge: D'après le roman arthurien en prose du* XIIIe *siècle*, Synthema, 2 (Leuven: Peeters, 2004)

Easton, Martha, '"Was It Good for You, Too?" Medieval Erotic Art and its Audiences', *Different Visions*, 1 (2008), <http://differentvisions.org/issue1PDFs/Easton.pdf> [accessed 2 April 2013]

——, 'The Wound of Christ and the Mouth of Hell: Appropriations and Inversions of Female Anatomy in the Later Middle Ages', in *Tributes to Jonathan J. G. Alexander: The Making and Meaning of Illuminated Medieval & Renaissance Manuscripts, Art & Architecture*, ed. by Susan L'Engle and Gerald B. Guest (London: Harvey Miller, 2006), pp. 395–414

Harris, Anne F., and Karen Overbey, 'Field Change / Discipline Change', in *Burn After Reading*, vol. II, *The Future We Want: A Collaboration*, ed. by Jeffrey Jerome Cohen (Brooklyn: punctum; Washington, DC: Oliphaunt, 2014), pp. 127–43

Huot, Sylvia, 'A Book Made for a Queen: The Shaping of a Late Medieval Anthology Manuscript (B.N. Fr. 24429)', in *The Whole Book: Cultural Perspectives on the Medieval Miscellany*, ed. by Stephen G. Nichols and Siegfried Wenzel, Recentiores (Ann Arbor: University of Michigan Press, 1996), pp. 123–43

——, 'Inventional Mnemonics, Reading and Prayer: A Reply to Mary Carruthers', *Connotations*, 3 (1993), 103–09; <http://www.connotations.uni-tuebingen.de/huot 00302.htm> [accessed 8 January 2014]

——, 'Polytextual Reading: The Meditative Reading of Real and Metaphorical Books', in *Orality and Literacy in the Middle Ages: Essays on a Conjunction and its Consequence in Honour of D. H. Green*, ed. by Mark Chinca and Christopher Young (Turnhout: Brepols, 2005), pp. 203–22

Kay, Sarah, 'Legible Skins: Animals and the Ethics of Medieval Reading', *postmedieval: a journal of medieval cultural studies*, 2 (2011), 13–32; <http://dx.doi.org/10.1057/pmed.2010.48>

L'Estrange, Elizabeth, *Holy Motherhood: Gender, Dynasty and Visual Culture in the Later Middle Ages* (Manchester: Manchester University Press, 2008)

Leroquais, Victor, *Les Livres d'heures manuscrits de la Bibliothèque nationale*, 3 vols (Mâcon: Protat Frères, 1927)

Lochrie, Karma, *Heterosyncracies : Female Sexuality When Normal Wasn't* (Minneapolis: University of Minnesota Press, 2005)

——, 'Mystical Acts, Queer Tendencies', in *Constructing Medieval Sexuality*, ed. by Karma Lochrie, Peggy McCracken, and James A. Schultz, Medieval Cultures, 11 (Minneapolis: University of Minnesota Press, 1997), pp. 180–200

Les Manuscrits à peintures en France du XIIIe au XVIe siècle (Paris: Bibliothèque nationale, 1955)

Marchetti, Gina, '[Untitled Response]', in *The Spectatrix*, ed. by Janet Bergstrom and Mary Ann Doane, special issue, *Camera Obscura*, 7.2–3, 20–21 (1989), 226–30; <http://dx.doi.org/10.1215/02705346-7-2-3_20-21-226>

Millar, E. G., *The Library of A. Chester Beatty: A Descriptive Catalogue of the Western Manuscripts*, 2 vols ([Oxford]: Privately printed by J. Johnson at the Oxford University Press, 1930)

Molinier, Auguste, *Cambrai*, Catalogue général des manuscrits des bibliothèques publiques de France, 17 (Paris: Librairie Plon, 1885); <http://archive.org/details/cataloguegnr17fran> [accessed 22 May 2014]

Morgan, Nigel, 'Gendered Devotions and Social Rituals: The Aspremont "Hours" in the National Gallery of Victoria and the Image of the Patron in Late Thirteenth- and Early Fourteenth-Century France', *Melbourne Art Journal*, 6 (2003), 5–24

Mulvey, Laura, 'Visual Pleasure and Narrative Cinema', *Screen*, 16 (1975), 6–18; <http://dx.doi.org/10.1093/screen/16.3.6>

Muzerelle, Denis, *Cambrai*, vol. I of *Manuscrits datés des bibliothèques de France*, Catalogues des manuscrits datés des bibliothèques de France, ser. 2 (Paris: CNRS, 2000)

Oggins, Robin S., *The Kings and their Hawks: Falconry in Medieval England* (New Haven: Yale University Press, 2004)

Ottosen, Knud, *The Responsories and Versicles of the Latin Office of the Dead* (Aarhus: Aarhus University Press, 2007)

L'Art au temps des rois maudits: Philippe le Bel et ses fils, 1285–1328. Paris, Galeries nationales du Grand Palais, 17 mars–29 juin 1998 (Paris: Réunion des Musées Nationaux, 1998)

Plotzek, Joachim M., *Die Handschriften der Sammlung Ludwig*, vol. II, ed. by Anton von Euw and Joachim M. Plotzek (Köln: Schnütgen-Museum der Stadt Köln, 1982)

Reinburg, Virginia, *French Books of Hours: Making an Archive of Prayer, c. 1400–1600* (Cambridge: Cambridge University Press, 2012)

Rudolph, Conrad, *The 'Things of Greater Importance': Bernard of Clairvaux's 'Apologia' and the Medieval Attitude toward Art* (Philadelphia: University of Pennsylvania Press, 1990)

Rudy, Kathryn M., 'Dirty Books: Quantifying Patterns of Use in Medieval Manuscripts Using a Densitometer', *Journal of Historians of Netherlandish Art*, 2 (2010); <http://dx.doi.org/10.5092/jhna.2010.2.1.1>

——, 'Kissing Images, Unfurling Rolls, Measuring Wounds, Sewing Badges and Carrying Talismans: Considering Some Harley Manuscripts through the Physical Rituals They Reveal', *Electronic British Library Journal*, 2011, Article 5; <http://www.bl.uk/eblj/2011articles/pdf/ebljarticle52011.pdf> [accessed 2 April 2013]

Sand, Alexa, 'Picturing Devotion Anew in the Psalter-Hours of Yolande of Soissons (New York, Pierpont Morgan Library, M729)' (unpublished doctoral dissertation, University of California, Berkeley, 1999)

——, *Vision, Devotion, and Self-Representation in Late Medieval Art* (New York: Cambridge University Press, 2014)

Smith, Kathryn A., *The Taymouth Hours: Stories and the Construction of the Self in Late Medieval England* (London: British Library, 2012)

Smith, Susan L., 'The Gothic Mirror and the Female Gaze', in *Saints, Sinners, and Sisters: Gender and Northern Art in Medieval and Early Modern Europe*, ed. by Jane Louise Carroll and Alison G. Stewart (Burlington, VT: Ashgate, 2003), pp. 73–93

Solterer, Helen, 'Seeing, Hearing, Tasting Woman: Medieval Senses of Reading', *Comparative Literature*, 46 (1994), 129–45; <http://dx.doi.org/10.2307/1771574>

Stahl, Harvey, 'Heaven in View: The Place of the Elect in an Illuminated Book of Hours', in *Last Things: Death and the Apocalypse in the Middle Ages*, ed. by Caroline Walker Bynum and Paul Freedman (Philadelphia: University of Pennsylvania Press, 2000), pp. 205–32

Stones, Alison, *Gothic Manuscripts, 1260–1320*, Survey of Manuscripts Illuminated in France, part 1, 2 vols (London: Harvey Miller, 2013)

——, 'Some Portraits of Women in their Books, Late Thirteenth – Early Fourteenth Century', in *Livres et lectures de femmes en Europe entre moyen âge et renaissance*, ed. by Anne-Marie Legaré (Turnhout: Brepols, 2007), pp. 3–27

Wieck, Roger S., *Time Sanctified: The Book of Hours in Medieval Art and Life* (Baltimore: Walters Art Gallery, 1988)

Williamson, Beth, 'Sensory Experience in Medieval Devotion: Sound and Vision, Invisibility and Silence', *Speculum*, 88 (2013), 1–43

Winston-Allen, Anne, *Stories of the Rose: The Making of the Rosary in the Middle Ages* (University Park: Pennsylvania State University Press, 1997)

Abbasid Concubines and Slave Courtesans in *Adab* Discourse: Cultural Mediators for an Ethical Appreciation of Pleasure

Karen Moukheiber

Throughout history, female slaves have been turned into accessible sexual commodities. Islamic law conferred on the Islamic institution of female slavery its distinctive mark by legalizing concubinage. In Western societies, concubinage refers to an 'informal but semi-permanent sexual relationship between a man and a woman that is by definition outside the established laws of marriage and inheritance; [...] Islamic concubinage was a clearly defined legal institution [...]. While not all female slaves were concubines, all concubines were by definition slaves'.[1] The legalization of concubinage carried the potential for creating a context in which sexual relations and consequently sexual pleasure could take place outside the institution of marriage without any legal prohibition.

By the early Abbasid period, slavery — and more particularly female slavery — had become a main social force, notably in the capital cities of Baghdad and Samarra.[2] Two categories of slave women, namely the *jāriya* or concubine, and the *qayna* (generally referred to as a 'singing girl'), were increasingly perceived as embodiments of sensual and sexual pleasures. The concubine was mainly a sexual commodity which granted her owner legal access to sexual pleasure

[1] Marmon, 'Concubinage', p. 527.

[2] Bray, 'Men, Women, and Slaves in Abbasid Society', p. 125.

Karen Moukheiber (krm03@aub.edu.lb) currently holds a position of assistant professor in cultural studies at the University of Balamand. Her main interests are Abbasid female slavery, gender, sexuality and cultural studies.

Pleasure in the Middle Ages, ed. by Naama Cohen-Hanegbi and Piroska Nagy, IMR 24 (Turnhout: Brepols, 2018), pp. 113–130 BREPOLS PUBLISHERS 10.1484/M.IMR-EB.5.113464

outside the bonds of marriage. The *qayna* was a concubine trained in the arts of singing, music, poetry, and the seduction of men. She occupied very different positions in the wide spectrum of Abbasid female slavery ranging from the pleasure girls of the numerous taverns of medieval Baghdad to the highly educated and sophisticated courtesans of the caliphal court.

In the course of the third/ninth and fourth/tenth centuries, concubines and *qiyān* (pl. of *qayna*) were increasingly perceived as a potential source of moral and social depravation. In his *Epistle of Singing Girls* al-Jahiz (d. 255/868), a prominent protagonist of the *adab* genre, skilfully constructed the iconic portrait of the *qayna* as the deceitful seductress who masterfully appeals to sensual pleasures and traps hapless men into her snares. Al-Jahiz writes:

> Fa idha jā bāb al-qiyān ishtaraka fīhi thulsatun min al-ḥawās wa ṣāra al-qalbu laha rābi'an, fa l-il 'ayni al-naẓaru ila al-qayna al-ḥasna wa-l mushbaha [...] wa l-il sama'i minha ḥaẓẓu al-ladhi lā ma'ūnata 'alayhi wa lā taṭrabu ālatuhu illa ilyahi, wa li-l lamsi fīha al-shahwatu wa-l ḥanīnu ila al-bāhi, wa-l ḥawāsu kullaha rawādun li-l qalbi. [...] fa-yajtami 'u lahu fī waqtin wāḥidin thalāthu ladhdhātin lā tajtami 'u lahu fī shay'in qaṭṭu, wa lam tu'addu ilayhi mithlaha, fayakūnu fī mujālasatihi li-l-qaynati a'dhamu al-fitna.
>
> [When one comes to consider a singing girl, three senses are involved; and [the pleasure] of the heart makes the fourth. The eye has the sight of a beautiful attractive girl; [...] hearing finds its sole delight in listening to her voice, touching her leads to carnal desire and the longing for sexual intercourse. All these senses are there as if scouts for the heart. [...] In the presence of singing girls a man experiences concurrent pleasures such as he would not find conjoined in anything else and the like of which the individual senses could never give him. Thus in consorting with singing girls lays the greatest temptation.][3]

The *adab* genre refers to the literary discourse which embodied the culture of the humanist urban elite. *Adab* narratives from the third/ninth and fourth/tenth centuries demonstrate a strong awareness and concern for the potential lack of inhibition and indulgence in sexual pleasure associated with legal concubinage. Indeed, a recurrent rhetorical question in works of *adab* from the early Abbasid period concerns the nature of sexual relations linking free men to women, slave and free. Why, asks Ibn 'Abd Rabbih (d. 328/940), would a free man who has come to know slave women choose a free woman instead?[4] The question focuses primarily on the respective advantages and drawbacks of

[3] Al-Jahiz, *Risalat al-Qiyan*, ed. and trans. by Beeston, p. 31.

[4] Ibn 'Abd Rabbih, *al-'Iqd al-Farid*, VI, ed. by Amin, al-Abiyari, and Harun, pp. 83–142.

slave and free women as well as a potential double standard in men's attitudes towards slave and free women. It reflects, however, a certain male anxiety and concern for the role of sexual pleasure in masculine choices of female partners as well as for the values that these choices entailed. It reveals the emergence of a cultural ethos in need of an ethics for sexual pleasure.

In addition to providing an overview of the historical context witnessing the crystallization of the *adab* genre and its cultural significance, this paper investigates a selection of *adab* texts from the third/ninth and fourth/tenth centuries, namely *al-'Iqd al-Farid* or *The Unique Necklace* by the Andalusian writer and poet Ibn 'Abd Rabbih; *al-Faraj ba'da al-Shidda* or *Hardship and Deliverance* by the judge and litterateur al-Tanukhi (d. 384/994);[5] *al-Qiyan* or *The Slave Courtesans* and *al-Ima' al-Shawa'ir* or *The Slave Poetesses* by the Arab historian and poet Abu al-Faraj al-Isfahani (d. 356/967);[6] as well as *Risalat al-Qiyan* or *The Epistle of Singing Girls* by the famous Arab prose writer al-Jahiz. It argues that these texts used the juxtaposition of contrasting images of concubines and *qiyān* as sources of temptation as well as symbols of loyalty as a literary device and a rhetorical tool for the delineation of an ethical attitude towards sexual pleasure. This ethics of pleasure was further instrumentalized to construct a masculine code of conduct regulating men's sexual relations with women as well as relations of power with other men.

The Historical Context and the Cultural Significance of the Adab Genre

The instauration of the Abbasid dynasty favoured the crystallization of a number of structural changes underlying the formative period of Islamic history. The new capital Baghdad was rapidly transformed into a thriving metropolis centred on the caliphal court which concentrated much of the fabulous wealth of the sprawling empire. By the third/ninth and fourth/tenth centuries, the presence of slave women in the urban centres of the Abbasid Empire seems to have reached a critical mass. The emergence of the *qiyān* as a prominent and distinctive element of court culture was a reflection of these economic and social changes. Large sums of money, up to one hundred thousand dirhams, were spent on concubines and more particularly on *qiyān* by men belonging

[5] Al-Tanukhi, *al-Faraj*, ed. by al-Shalji.

[6] Al-Isfahani, *al-Qiyan*, ed. by al-'Attieh; al-Isfahani, *al-Ima' al-Shawa'ir*, ed. by al-Qaysi and others. These monographs are formed of fifty-seven and thirty-three chapters respectively with each chapter bearing the name of a *qayna* and providing a compilation of narratives about her.

mostly to the elite.[7] Numerous anecdotes convey the phenomenal numbers of concubines owned by the Abbasid caliphs who gradually abandoned the institution of marriage and replaced it by the legal institution of concubinage.[8] Al-Jahiz notes that only three Abbasid caliphs were the sons of free women.

Slave women acted in part as cultural intermediaries between elite and popular urban culture by introducing into the household an accessible feature of court culture.[9] Common household concubines could be bought for a price ranging from twelve dinars to one hundred and ten dinars rendering them accessible to families with more modest revenues than those of the notables.[10] If gender relations in the caliphal household did not answer to the same rules and needs of those of the wider urban population, the court did constitute the model as well as the centre of the intellectual and cultural life of Baghdad and of the empire at large.[11] The challenge to matrimonial gender roles and relations resulting from the increasing number of slave women at the caliphal court and more generally in the streets and households of the empire's capital turned slave women, mere concubines as well as the sophisticated slave courtesans, into 'the actual and symbolic centre of anxieties of tenth-century Baghdadi society'.[12]

The social significance of slave women was mirrored by their prominent presence in *adab* discourse. It was mainly in the course of the ninth century that the *adab* genre crystallized into a variety of textual discourse centred on man, his qualities, his passions, his pleasures as well as the material and spiritual culture created by him.[13] The *adab* genre embodied mainly the humanist ideals of the urban male elite, mainly Baghdadi court officials and civil servants, in an attempt to make them recognizable and reproducible. Julia Bray draws a parallel between the predicament of the men of the Abbasid elite in the third/ninth and fourth/tenth centuries and that of the elite in the early Roman Empire, as

[7] Cheikh-Moussa, 'Figures de l'esclave chanteuse à l'époque abbaside'.

[8] Kennedy, *The Court of the Caliphs*, p. 167. Kennedy gives the following numbers: al-Rashid is said to have had more than two thousand singing girls and servants in his harem; al-Mutawakkil is reputed for having had four thousand concubines and having had sex with all of them. After the death of Harun al-Rashid, caliphs, with rare exceptions, do not seem to have married.

[9] Bray, 'Men, Women, and Slaves in Abbasid Society', p. 1.

[10] Goiten, 'Slaves and Slavegirls in the Cairo Geniza Records'; Richards, 'Fragments of a Slave Dealer's Day-Book from Fustat', p. 92.

[11] Hodgson, *The Venture of Islam*, pp. 444–45.

[12] El Cheikh, 'Women's History', p. 135.

[13] Torawa, *Ibn Abi Tahir Tayfur and Arabic Writerly Culture*, p. 124.

it was described by Michel Foucault in *The Care of the Self*. Foucault suggests that 'If one wishes to understand the interest that was directed in these elites to personal ethics [...] it is not at all pertinent to speak of decadence, frustration or sullen retreat. Instead one should see in this interest the search for a new way of conceiving the relationship that one ought to have with one's status, one's functions, one's activities and one's obligations. [...] The new rules of the political game made it more difficult to define the relations between what one was, what one could do and what one was expected to accomplish'.[14] In a similar vein, in the face of structural social and political changes, the need to develop new codes of personal conduct was increasingly felt among the members of the Abbasid urban elite. They grew particularly wary of the court's seemingly excessive indulgence in sensual and sexual pleasures and engaged in reassessing the role of pleasure in delineating the boundaries of proper sexual relations between men and women as well as endurable relations of power among men.

The absence of free women from the 'public/masculine space' in addition to the norms of social propriety turned the concubine and the *qayna* into the privileged feminine interlocutors of *adab*'s discursive inquiry about pleasure and the masculine self. Janet Nelson points to the particular role of court women in 'the reproduction as well as the formation of courtliness, for the gendering of space and for a remodeling of aristocratic male psychology'.[15] Indeed, Gadi Algazi and Rina Drory describe the Abbasid court as a 'cultural laboratory' where the love for slave women was used to develop the self-discipline needed to produce a successful courtier.[16] Julia Bray also states that 'in the romantic literature, the luxury female slave plays a more complex role which is cultural, ethical even [...]. She is not a courtesan but a soul mate, who educates her lover in monogamous love. [...] These imaginative models were one of the means through which free men could reflect on their own moral identity and on what constituted tolerable relations of power'.[17] Consequently, the perception of slave women as the embodiment of sexual pleasure turned the respective representations of concubines and *qiyān* and the attitudes to adopt towards them into discursive means through which *adab* discourse articulated its own understanding of what constituted ethical behaviour in men's private sexual lives as well as in their public social roles.

[14] Foucault, *The Care of the Self*, p. 84; Bray, 'Men, Women, and Slaves in Abbasid Society', p. 125.

[15] Nelson, 'Gendering Courts in the Early Medieval West', p. 186.

[16] Algazi and Drory, 'L'Amour à la cour des Abbasides', p. 1271.

[17] Bray, 'Men, Women, and Slaves in Abbasid Society', p. 137.

Concubinage and the Regulation of Sexual Pleasure: Rejecting Double Standards and Supporting Loyalty

In their respective anthologies, namely *al-Faraj ba'da al-Shidda* and *al-'Iqd al-Farid*, both al-Tanukhi and in Ibn 'Abd Rabbih demonstrate that upholding a double standard towards sexual pleasure with slave and free women may threaten a man's happiness and the stability of the household. They thus seek to devise a legitimate attitude towards sexual pleasure which would allow men to avoid those pitfalls and insure their serenity in matters related to matrimony and concubinage.

An anecdote in al-Tanukhi's *Faraj ba'da al-Shidda* transforms turning points in the relation linking a man to his potential slave woman, namely the time preceding her acquisition through a sale transaction and the period of longing following their separation, into moments of thoughtful reflection assessing the role of pleasures in motivating his action.[18] The man asks himself about the motivations behind his desire to buy a slave woman and thus implicitly interrogates the ethical values, beliefs, needs, and emotions instigating his action.[19] This key moment of choice and decision making opens a literary space of discursive thought in which a hierarchy of values and codes of conduct are considered and discussed. That this internal questioning was triggered by a slave rather than a free woman is favoured by the woman's servile status which granted her owner a position of legal ownership and thus the possibility to exercise his power and authority with a margin of liberty which was not possible with the free. His relationship with the latter was bound by limits set by social propriety regarding female roles and positions. However, despite his margin of action and choice, the man is represented showing clear awareness that this legal capacity to act may have unwarranted personal consequences. Many anecdotes dwell on the detrimental consequences of concubinage. These include spending much money and becoming destitute, depriving a family of their needs, as well as losing one's profession and friends. Reflecting on whether he should buy the slave woman, the man comes to the conclusion that he will eventually get bored with the concubine and so refrains from buying her.[20] His projected potential boredom implies that he is acquainted with slave women and has come to realize that the pleasures that one enjoys with them eventually

[18] Van Gelder, 'Slave-Girl Lost and Regained'.

[19] Al-Tanukhi, *al-Faraj*, ed. by al-Shalji, p. 312.

[20] Al-Tanukhi, *al-Faraj*, ed. by al-Shalji, p. 310.

fade. The temporary and evanescent nature of these pleasures is thus suggested. The man then exerts self-restraint and abstains from buying the slave girl.

In the meantime the slave woman is sold, and the man comes to realize that his longing for her is not as temporary as he thought. Her absence gradually prevents him from working properly. His friends and employers are very disappointed with his behaviour, and he is about to lose his job when he again exerts self-control and forces himself to overcome his hardship and re-engages in his professional responsibilities. It is this double engagement in self-restraint and resilience which allows him to gain better knowledge of himself. His ability to abstain from what he perceived as temporary pleasures as well as to overcome his sadness eventually allows him to realize that the slave woman can become a source of long-lasting happiness if he approaches her not as a mere sexual commodity and thus as a punctual partner and source of pleasure but as a long-term companion.

Indeed, many anecdotes end with an implicit endorsement of lasting loyalty to one's partner. The relationship is often described as enduring until the death of the slave woman. In fact, in a large number of anecdotes, monogamy appears as the preferred practice whether through concubinage or marriage. Significantly, narratives of unrequited love are not limited to a free man and slave women but can also take place between a free man and a free woman or even between a free man and the wife that he loves who temporarily ignores him.[21] The implication of this choice is that the code of conduct that insures a man's needs and serenity in gender relations is to a large extent independent of the status of the woman involved. This is also illustrated by the fact that in some anecdotes men choose to leave their wives for a slave woman while in others the slave woman is abandoned in favour of the wife. These narratives express primarily a masculine concern with the factors motivating men's engagements with women and with the consequences of those engagements, regardless of the women's status. They put forth a man's ability to exert self-restraint when exposed to an accessible but temporary source of sexual pleasure as a means to a better understanding of his needs and of the means of ensuring long-lasting happiness as opposed to temporary and evanescent pleasure.

In a similar vein, Ibn 'Abd Rabbih develops a rhetorical strategy which prevents the establishment of a clear dichotomy between slave and free women

[21] Al-Tanukhi, *al-Faraj*, ed. by al-Shalji, pp. 306–08, relates the story of a man who is in love with his cousin. He also relates the story of a man who very insistently engages in asking his wife to forgive him, pp. 426–28.

and shifts the focus of discourse from one which associates sexual pleasure with legal status to one which links it to values and proper conduct. Ibn ʿAbd Rabbih establishes a comparison between the institutions of marriage and slavery by quoting a tradition from ʿAisha the wife of the Prophet in which she compares marriage to a form of slavery and advises men to carefully look into those to whom they enslave their daughters. Her words are echoed by those of the Prophet Muhammad who declares: 'I entrust you to care for your women for you hold them as your prisoners' ('wa ūṣīkum bi-l-nisāʾi fa-innahunna ʿindakum aʿwānun').[22] These narratives suggest that the differentiation between marriage and slavery is not associated with the institutions of marriage and concubinage but rather depends on the manners and code of conduct that men follow in the treatment of their female partners. These narratives also allude to two different masculine codes of conduct: one that befits free wives and another that would be demeaning to them by transforming marriage into a form of slavery. Masculine behaviour which is associated with slave women is not described as the proper way to treat slave women but rather as how not to treat free women. The implication is that the way men treat slave women is simply considered improper regardless of the status of women. The double standard regarding slave and free women is thus turned into a rhetorical tool used to distinguish between what is perceived as an ideal or desired masculine behaviour and an improper or detrimental one.

Despite their rejection of a double standard in sexual pleasure with slave and free women, Ibn ʿAbd Rabbih and al-Tanukhi express an awareness of the difficulty in upholding this stance, especially when marriage and concubinage are combined in the same household. Their narratives demonstrate a strong awareness of the threat that the unavoidable tensions resulting from the joined practice of concubinage and marriage implied to the peacefulness of the household. Ibn ʿAbd Rabbih relates an anecdote in which a man attempts to trigger his wife's jealousy by pretending to develop a liking for his slave woman; the wife responds by threatening to leave him. The man's response is to beg his wife to remain by his side and to offer her the slave woman as a gift, thus making the latter legally inaccessible to him.[23] Al-Tanukhi relates an anecdote which puts forth the inverse of this situation. A man feels a strong attraction for his wife's slave woman. The wife finds out and keeps the slave woman away

[22] Ibn ʿAbd Rabbih, *al-ʿIqd al-Farid*, ed. by Amin, al-Abiyari, and Harun, p. 82 (my translation).

[23] Ibn ʿAbd Rabbih, *al-ʿIqd al-Farid*, ed. by Amin, al-Abiyari, and Harun, pp. 105–06.

from her husband. Consequently, the man suffers great hardship. One night, he sees himself in a dream crying with the slave woman standing in front of him. A person then approaches them and recites to him a number of verses. He wakes up fearful and terrified and asks for a pen and a piece of paper to write down the poem. His wife who was lying next to him wakes up, inquires about his troubled state, and listens to him recounting his dream. She then says to him: 'All of this because of your love for my slave woman? I give her to you as a present' ('hādha kulluhu min ḥubbi fulanatin? qad wahabtuha laka').[24]

Put together, these anecdotes illustrate the anxiety associated with the perception of the concubine as an actual and symbolic embodiment of sexual pleasure. In real life, the concubine poses a threat to both the wife's and the husband's positions and thus to the stability of the household, as is shown in the first anecdote. This threat is represented as entailing, at times, a decisive choice between partners, revealing the intensity of the conflict that a concubine may trigger. The second anecdote reveals through a dream the situation that a man wishes for in real life, namely for his wife to wilfully grant him access to a slave woman that she owns in order to make her legally accessible to him. The wife is represented as the main obstacle in the realization of the fantasy as the man does not refer to her simply as his wife but as the slave woman's master. The solution to his dilemma lies in her hands. These anecdotes show that the authors of *adab* discourse were very much aware of the difficulties involved in combining pleasure through concubinage and marriage in the same household. Importantly, it also demonstrates a need or at least a desire for or an appreciation of an ideal household devoid of conflict.

Advocating a Circumspect Appreciation of Masculine Sexual Pleasure

The need to abate the perception of slave women as mere object of sexual pleasure is illustrated in Ibn 'Abd Rabbih's depiction of the role of the concubine as well as in his decision to discuss sexual relations and sexual pleasure with slave women in a separate section entitled *On Sexuality and What Has Been Said about It* located at the end of the chapter dedicated to women and not within the section dedicated to concubines.[25] His representation of women's sexuality conforms to what Fatima Mernissi describes as *fitna* which considers women's sexuality as a

[24] Al-Tanukhi, *al-Faraj*, ed. by al-Shalji, p. 393 (my translation).

[25] Ibn 'Abd Rabbih, *al-'Iqd al-Farid*, ed. by Amin, al-Abiyari, and Harun, pp. 139–42.

danger to the public order which needs to be contained.[26] It also illustrates what Ziba Mir-Hosseini refers to as the classical Islamic 'theory of difference in male and female sexuality'.[27] According to this view, women, whether slave or free, have greater sexual desire than men. Women's lust is described as insatiable, and men are advised to practice sexual intercourse with restraint.

Having shifted the focus from a discourse associating pleasure with status to one connecting pleasure to values, Ibn 'Abd Rabbih engages in contesting the popular representation of the concubine as a source of sexual pleasure. In what, initially, seems like a support for the role of the concubine as a provider of pleasure, Ibn 'Abd Rabbih grants the title *surriya* to the section devoted to concubines The term *surriya* refers to a slave woman within the domestic household with whom the master has sexual intercourse for pleasure and not for begetting children. However, this projected image of the concubine as an object of sexual pleasure is gradually undermined and replaced by her image as a procreator of famous men. Moreover, the high social and religious standing of the men who practiced concubinage throughout history is emphasized. Concubinage is thus granted both religious and historical legitimacy. Hajar, Abraham's concubine, is identified as having given birth to Ismail, and Mariah the Copt, the Prophet's concubine, is described as having given birth to his son Ibrahim. In other words the legitimacy of the practice of concubinage is illustrated by putting forth men who practiced concubinage and were held as models of behaviour to the Muslim community, namely the founder of monotheism, Abraham, and the founder of Islam, the Prophet Muhammad, and by pointing to the noble descendants begotten from such unions. This argumentation clearly locates concubinage as a practice taking place within the household with the purpose of begetting children and not as one where a man acquires a slave woman for sexual pleasure as the title of the section, *surriya*, seems to indicate. Ibn 'Abd Rabbih concludes this section by quoting verses which describe women, slave and free, as mere vessels for the bearing of offspring, implicitly negating their perception as objects of desire and pleasure.[28]

Ibn 'Abd Rabbih begins his section on sexuality and sexual pleasure with a statement attributed to Malik bin Anas who presents a very positive description of sexual pleasure comparing it to 'the light shining from your face'

[26] Mernissi, *The Veil and the Male Elite*, pp. 49–61, 180–88.

[27] Mir-Hosseini, 'The Construction of Gender in Islamic Legal Thought and Strategies for Reform', p. 10.

[28] El Cheikh, 'In Search of the Ideal Spouse', pp. 190–91.

('nūru wajhika') and leaving it up to the individual man to indulge in it or show restraint. This rather engaging approach to sexuality is mitigated by a saying attributed to Mu'awiya, who states that he can immediately spot a man with *nahim* (a voracious appetite) for sexuality from the look upon his face. The term *nahim* conveys a negative connotation which nuances Malik's supportive position. This negative attitude towards sexual behaviour is then emphasized by the sayings of Ibn Shammakh al-'Uqli and al-Mada'ini who both describe themselves as men who are able to greatly control their sexual drives, even when women are made available to them. Self-restraint when facing accessible pleasure is then implicitly encouraged.[29]

Ibn 'Abd Rabbih and al-Tanukhi engaged in defining not only men's attitudes towards sexuality but also women's sexual behaviour. A number of anecdotes show wives harbouring an excessive sexual appetite. A man who insists on being married to two women is advised to begin with marrying one. He quickly acquiesces having been married for just three days. Interestingly, the only identified woman engaging in vigorous sexual intercourse is a famous married free woman, 'Aisha bint Talḥa. The anecdote is presented as 'what has been said about 'Aisha bint Talḥa who was renowned for her beauty and the attraction she could exert on men'. The danger or *fitna* associated with beauty as a source of visual pleasure which may in turn trigger sexual attraction is again implicitly evoked. A woman from Kufa visits her and is told that 'Aisha is in the company of her husband. The visitor then listens to moans and sighs the likes of which were never heard before. Eventually 'Aisha comes out, her forehead dripping with sweat. The woman from Kufa tells her that she did not think that a free wife could act in this manner. 'Aisha answers: 'those horses of noble breed drink boisterously' ('inna al-khayla al-'itāqi tashrabu bi-l-ṣaffīri').[30] In other words 'Aisha describes her behaviour as a response to her husband's needs. She implicitly rejects the notion that ardour in sexual intercourse was triggered by the effect of her beauty on her husband or by her own initiative. Men, not women, are the initiators of sexual pleasure.

The feminine voices heard in this subsection are used to express what appears as the men's unwillingness to take heed of their need for sexual pleasure. The only time a slave woman is made to speak, it is to deprecate the sexual performance

[29] Ibn 'Abd Rabbih, *al-'Iqd al-Farid*, ed. by Amin, al-Abiyari, and Harun, p. 139 (my translation).

[30] Ibn 'Abd Rabbih, *al-'Iqd al-Farid*, ed. by Amin, al-Abiyari, and Harun, p. 140 (my translation).

of her partner. As for the free women, they mostly 'express' a need unfulfilled by their husbands. When, in an unusual reversal of roles, a man complains about his wife to the fourth caliph 'Ali bin Abi Talib because she keeps protesting that he extenuates her whenever he has sexual intercourse with her, the caliph advises him to do away with her.[31] The responses granted to feminine voices expressing their dissatisfaction regarding their sexual needs do not convey a concern for feminine pleasure. Women's excessive sexual desire or the lack of it are equally decried. Women voices are quoted but not heard. A woman, slave or free, is primarily meant to respond to her owner's/husband's needs.

Both Ibn 'Abd Rabbih and al-Tanukhi express straightforward support for the institution of marriage and a more cautious one for the institution of concubinage. However, they both implicitly argue that what differentiates marriage from concubinage does not reside in the institutions themselves but rather more fundamentally in how men treat their female partners. They propose that regardless of the nature of the institution of companionship that a man chooses to follow, his happiness and his serenity in gender relations ultimately rests in the code of conduct that he chooses to follow in sexual partnerships with women regardless of status. In other words, while both marriage and concubinage may be apprehended as commendable matrimonial relations, there is only one ethical way of treating women whether slave or free. This ideal code of conduct favours caution, moderation, and self-restraint towards sexual pleasures as well as resilience in the face of sexual longing. The values it endorses are loyalty to one's partner, as well as a tendency to endorse monogamy. This attitude does not necessarily emanate from a particularly high esteem that the authors of *adab* discourse held for women, but more fundamentally from a concern for masculine interests. It demonstrates a lack of concern for women's right to pleasure, with men acting both as the initiators and beneficiaries of sexual pleasure. It aims mainly at teaching men the proper behaviour that avoids the pitfalls of sexual relations and ensures social success.

Slave Courtesans as Pleasurable Instruments for the Mediation of Power among Men

The Abbasid institution of female slavery transformed the elite or highly educated *qiyān* or slave courtesans into a commodified form of pleasure with an exchange value that depended mainly on cultural investment. Legalized control of a slave woman's sexuality, exemption from veiling, and

[31] Ibn 'Abd Rabbih, *al-'Iqd al-Farid*, ed. by Amin, al-Abiyari, and Harun, p. 142.

access to leisure gatherings transformed her education in singing, music, and poetry into a lucrative endeavour. The most striking part of al-Jahiz's *Risalat* is unquestionably the one which contains eighteen clauses dedicated to the description of the *qayna*. It enshrines the popular image of the slave courtesan as an embodiment of sensual pleasures, a model of immoral behaviour, and a highly valuable commodity which could be legally bought and sold.

Nevertheless, *adab* discourse puts forth narratives which counter al-Jahiz's description. They demonstrate that elite slave courtesans were able to master the arts of poetry, music, and singing to a high degree of professionalism which granted them the appreciation of male poets and more importantly of the caliphs. This in turn conferred upon the slave courtesan and the pleasures with which she was associated legitimacy and an ethical dimension which they originally lacked. The *qayna* was thus able to accumulate a cultural capital bestowing upon her an authority which at times superseded her reputation for licentious activities. This official recognition transformed the *qayna* into a highly polished instrument of legitimate pleasure particularly conducive to mediating hierarchies of power. Pleasure and politics share parallel themes such as promiscuity and betrayal on the one hand, monogamy and loyalty on the other. Consequently, narratives on pleasures associated with the *qayna* were transformed into means through which men reflected upon not only private but also public masculine ethical codes of conduct.

Al-Qiyan of al-Isfahani includes the following anecdote.

> Jara bayna al-Amin wa bayna ʿammihi Ibrahim bin al-Mahdi kalāmun wa humā ʿala al-nabīdh. Fa-wajada al-Amin ʿala Ibrahim, wa bānat li-Ibrahim al-waḥshatu minhu. Fa-inṣarafa Ibrahim ila manzilihi qaliqan wa ḥajabahu al-Amin ʿanhu, wa balagha Ibrahim dhālika fa-baʿatha ila al-Amin bi-alṭāfin wa ruqʿatin yaʿtadhiru fiha. Fa-radda al-Amin al-hadiyya wa lam yujib Ibrahim ʿala al-ruqʿat.
>
> Fa-wajjaha Ibrahim ilayhi waṣīfatan malīḥatan mughaniyatan kāna rabbāha wa ʿallamaha al-ghinā' wa baʿatha maʿaha ʿūdan ma ʿmūlan min al-ʿūdi al-hindiyyi mukallalan bi-l-jawāhiri, wa al-basaha ḥillatan mansūjatan bi-l-dhahabi, wa qāla abyātan wa ghanna fiha, wa alqa ʿalayha abyātan ḥatta ḥafiẓatha wa akhadhat al-ṣawti wa aḥkmat al-ṣun ʿata fihi, thumma wajjaha biha ilayhi. [...] fa-surra biha al-Amin wa baʿatha ila Ibrahim fa-aḥḍarahu wa raḍiya ʿanhu wa amara lahu bi-khamsīna alfa dīnārin wa tammama yawmahu ma ʿahu.
>
> [An acrid exchange over a cup of wine irritates the caliph al-Amin who leaves his uncle Ibrahim ibn al-Mahdi anxious as to the intentions of the caliph. Attempts to conciliate al-Amin with graceful excuses are ignored. Ibrahim then sends the caliph Hadiyya, a *qayna* whom he trained and taught to sing, as a gift. He equips her with a jewel-encrusted lute made of Indian wood and with a dress embroidered with

> gold, and teaches her a set of eulogizing verses to sing before the caliph. […] This time the caliph is pleased with the gift; he calls for his uncle whom he rewards with fifty thousand dinars and spends the rest of the day in his company.][32]

The sensuality of the *qayna* and her cultural capital transform her into a highly appreciated and very pleasurable gift. The expression of regret through the mediation of the *qayna*'s voice impresses and flatters al-Amin and allows Ibrahim to regain the favour of the ruler. The slave courtesan flatters the masculine ego of the caliph and carries the potential to moderate the excesses of power. Pleasurable and cultural gifts were thus means through which ties of loyalty and positions of leadership were constructed.[33] They may be offered by caliphs to consolidate the loyalty of courtiers or by courtiers to secure the protection and favours of the caliph.

Pleasure, embodied in a courtesan offered as a gift, favoured mutual appreciation at court and mitigated the full exercise of power. The appreciation of self-restraint and moderation in the exercise of power appear again as key values in the exchange between the caliph al-Mutawakkil and two of his slave poetesses. Significantly, the story is related by the *qayna* Banan. She states that during a walk in the palace courtyard, in her company and that of another slave poetess the caliph addresses the latter by reciting the following verse: 'ta'allamtu asbāba al-riḍa khawfa sukhṭiha wa 'allamaha ḥubbī laha kayfa taghḍabu' (Fear of her wrath taught me to be content; and my love taught her how to tame her anger). The poetess responds by saying: 'yaṣuddu wa adnu bi-l-mawaddati jāhidan wa yab'udu 'annī bi-l-wiṣāli wa aqrubu' (When he rebukes me, I strive to respond smoothly; and when he moves away; I come closer with gentility).[34] If the seductive *qayna* is often portrayed as a source of tension and anxiety, the loyal *qayna* prompts feelings of security and tranquility as is illustrated in the stories of the *qiyān* Dananir al-Barmakiyya and Tajni.[35] The story of Dananir extols the value of loyalty to one's patron beyond death.[36] Having ordered the execution of Dananir's masters, the caliph Harun al-Rashid buys her and insists on having her sing and detach herself from her former patrons. She, however, chooses to wear a coarse garment and is unable to overcome her sadness until she dies. The name of the *qayna*, Dananir, is the plural of dinar. Her name and

[32] Al-Isfahani, *al-Qiyan*, ed. by al-'Attieh, p. 101 (my translation).

[33] Cutler, 'Gifts and Gift Exchange as Aspects of the Byzantine, Arab, and Related Economies'.

[34] Al-Isfahani, *al-Ima' al-Shawa'ir*, ed. by al-Qaysi and others, pp. 121–22 (my translation).

[35] Al-Isfahani, *al-Ima' al-Shawa'ir*, ed. by al-Qaysi and others, p. 131.

[36] Al-Isfahani, *al-Qiyan*, ed. by al-'Attieh, p. 83.

her attitude stand in contrast to each other, creating an opposition which only enhances the *qayna*'s rejection of the attraction of wealth for the sake of loyalty.

In the story of Tajni, al-Isfahani not only praises loyalty to one's patron but also points to the benefits associated with loyalty. In this narrative, the master of the *qayna* is al-Isfahani himself. He is surprised by an unwarranted sum of five thousand dinars sent to him by his patron al-Muhallabi. He cautiously asks his patron about the origin of the present. The latter explains that he had offered the money to al-Isfahani's *qayna*, Tajni, upon listening to her sing verses praising the Buyid leader Mu'izz al-Dawla. She had suggested, however, that the sum be sent as a gift to her master. Al-Isfahani expresses his gratitude to his patron not only for the sum of money but also for clarifying the cause of the unwarranted gift. Implicitly, the *qayna* teaches her master a lesson in the rewards reaped from circumspection, gratitude, and loyalty towards one's patron. Significantly, the name of the *qayna* matches her behaviour. Tajni means 'to harvest'. Located at the very end of the monograph, this narrative provides a double sense of closure. It may be read as a token of gratitude to the *qiyān* for making the highly competitive and unstable milieu of the court more pleasurable, and more importantly for granting pleasure, through the mastery of their craft, a legitimate and thus an ethical dimension transforming it into a powerful mediator of power relations among men.

Conclusion

In the early Abbasid period, concubines and *qiyān* formed an inherent part of urban and elite court culture. They were perceived as embodiments of sensual pleasures as well as agents of moral and social decadence. The *adab* genre, which embodied the cultural ideals of the Abbasid urban male elite, was part of a cultural trend centred in part on man, his passions, and his pleasures. The controversial status of slave women is expressed in *adab* textual discourse by a growing concern for the potential threat that concubines and slave courtesans posed to established social norms and values regulating sexual relations in the household as well as power relations at the caliphal court. The iconic portrait of the alluring and deceitful *qayna* put forth by al-Jahiz in *Risalat al-Qiyan* mirrors the contentious status of the slave women and their strong impact on the collective subconscious.[37] The necessity to construct a legitimate appreciation of sensual and sexual pleasures was strongly felt.

[37] Bouhdiba, *Sexuality in Islam*.

The works of *adab* investigated in this paper juxtapose narratives depicting concubines and slave courtesans as sources of temptation to narratives describing them as symbols of loyalty. These contrasting depictions of slave women opened a literary space for a discourse aimed at constructing a masculine code of conduct based on an ethical appreciation of pleasure. This discourse endorsed loyalty to one's partner as well as to one's patron. It contested the perception of women, slave and free, as objects of sexual desire by emphasizing their role as producers of offspring. Adopting a stoic perspective, it advocated self-restraint and moderation in men's consumption of sexual pleasures as well as resilience in the face of sexual longing. Feminine sexuality was perceived as a potential threat that needed to be contained. Legitimate access to sexual pleasure remained a masculine prerogative.

Works Cited

Primary Sources

al-Isfahani, Abu al-Faraj, *al-Qiyan*, ed. by Jalil al-'Attieh (London: Riad el-Rayess Books, 1989)

al-Isfahani, Abu al-Faraj, *al-Ima' al-Shawa'ir*, ed. by Nuri Hammudi al-Qaysi and others (Beirut: Maktabat al-Nahda al-'Arrabiya, 1984)

Al-Jahiz, *Risalat al-Qiyan*, ed. and trans. by A. F. L. Beeston (Warminster: Aris & Phillips, 1980)

al-Tanukhi, Abu 'Ali al-Muhsin bin 'Ali, *al-Faraj ba'da al-Shidda*, ed. by 'Abbud al-Shalji (Beirut: Dar Sader, 1978)

Ibn 'Abd Rabbih, *al-'Iqd al-Farid*, ed. by Ahmad Amin, Ibrahim al-Abiyari, and 'Abdel Salam Harun (Cairo: Maṭba'at Lajnat al-Ta'līf wa-l-Tarjama wa-l-Nashir, 1949)

Secondary Works

Algazi, Gadi, and Rina Drory, 'L'Amour à la cour des Abbasides: Un code de compétence sociale', *Annales: Histoire, Sciences Sociales*, 55 (2000), pp. 1255–82

Bouhdiba, 'Abdelwahab, *Sexuality in Islam*, trans. Alan Sheridan (London: Routledge, 1985)

Bray, Julia, 'Men, Women, and Slaves in Abbasid Society', in *Gender in the Early Medieval World*, ed. by Leslie Brubaker and Julia Smith (Cambridge: Cambridge University Press, 2004), pp. 121–46

Cheikh-Moussa, Abdallah, 'Figures de l'esclave chanteuse à l'époque abbaside', in *Figures de l'esclave au Moyen Âge et dans le monde moderne*, ed. by Henri Bresc (Paris: L'Harmattan, 1996), pp. 45–54

Cutler, Anthony, 'Gifts and Gift Exchange as Aspects of the Byzantine, Arab, and Related Economies', *Dumberton Oaks Papers*, 55 (2001), 247–78

El Cheikh, Nadia Maria, 'In Search of the Ideal Spouse', *Journal of the Economic and Social History of the Orient*, 45 (2002), 179–96

El Cheikh, Nadia Maria. 'Women's History: A Study of al-Tanukhi', in *Writing the Feminine: Women in Arab Sources*, ed. by Manuel Marin and Randi Deguilhem (London: I. B. Tauris, 2002), pp. 129–48

Foucault, Michel, *The Care of the Self*, vol. III of *The History of Sexuality*, trans. by Robert Hurley (New York: Vintage Press, 1986)

Goiten, S. D., 'Slaves and Slavegirls in the Cairo Geniza Records', *Arabica*, 9 (1962), 1–20

Hodgson, Marshall, *The Venture of Islam: Conscience and History in a World Civilization* (Chicago: University of Chicago Press, 1974), pp. 444–45

Kennedy, Hugh, *The Court of the Caliphs: The Rise and Fall of Islam's Greatest Dynasty* (London: Wiedenfeld and Nicolson, 2004)

Marmon, Shawn, 'Concubinage', in *Dictionary of the Middle Ages* (New York: Scribner, 1983), III, 527–29

Mernissi, Fatima, *The Veil and the Male Elite: A Feminist Interpretation of Women's Rights in Islam*, trans. by Mary Jo Lakeland (New York: Basic Books, 1987)
Mir-Hosseini, Ziba, 'The Construction of Gender in Islamic Legal Thought and Strategies for Reform', *Hawwa*, 1 (2003), 1–28
Nelson, Janet, 'Gendering Courts in the Early Medieval West', in *Gender in the Early Medieval World*, ed. by Leslie Brubaker and Julia Smith (Cambridge: Cambridge University Press, 2004), pp. 185–97
Richards, D. , 'Fragments of a Slave Dealer's Day-Book from Fustat', in *Documents de l'Islam médiéval: Nouvelles perspectives de recherches*, ed. by Yusuf Ragheb (Le Caire: Institut français d'archéologie orientale, 1991), pp. 89–98
Torawa, Shawkat, *Ibn Abi Tahir Tayfur and Arabic Writerly Culture: A Ninth-Century Bookman in Baghdad* (London: Routledge, 2005)
Van Gelder, G. J. H., 'Slave-Girl Lost and Regained: Transformation of a Story', *Marvels and Tales*, 18 (2004), 202–17

Courts and Pleasures: The Neuroscience of Pleasure and the Pursuit of Favour in Twelfth-Century Courts

William M. Reddy

Michel Zink recently remarked that William IX of Aquitaine (1071–1126), the legendary first troubadour, was possessed by an 'obsession with sex' and a 'wild sensuality' that he could only partly appease through the 'obscene representations' of his so-called 'ribald' songs.[1] Other scholars have agreed in seeing William IX's ribald songs as equating sexual dominance with political dominance,[2] or with an ironic celebration of 'sexual prowess'.[3] But such readings of his work are not at all culturally neutral; instead they rely on modern commonsense ideas about sexual craving and sexual identity that are direct descendants of twelfth-century clerical thinking. They obscure the intriguing possibility that William IX was reflecting on, via parody, a trend of his own time: a new clerical obsession with sexuality.[4]

[1] Zink, *Les Troubadours*, p. 76. These songs are referred to as 'ribald' by Bloch, *Medieval Misogyny and the Invention of Western Romantic Love*, p. 158.

[2] See the discussion of Song 1 by Bond, 'Introduction', p. xxv.

[3] See the discussion of Song 6 in Gaunt, *Troubadours and Irony*, pp. 23–24.

[4] Rita Lejeune's reading of the songs may be overworked, as Zink suggests (in *Les Troubadours*, pp. 54–55), but at least it has the merit of seeing William as, very probably, an observer and critic of clerical preoccupation with chastity. See Lejeune, *Littérature et société occitane au Moyen Âge*.

William M. Reddy (wmr@duke.edu) is William T. Laprade Professor of History and professor of Cultural Anthropology at Duke University; he is a fellow of the American Academy of Arts and Sciences, and author of *The Making of Romantic Love: Longing and Sexuality in Europe, South Asia, and Japan (900–1200)* (Chicago: University of Chicago Press, 2012).

Pleasure in the Middle Ages, ed. by Naama Cohen-Hanegbi and Piroska Nagy, IMR 24 (Turnhout: Brepols, 2018), pp. 131–164 BREPOLS PUBLISHERS 10.1484/M.IMR-EB.5.113465

To guard against this kind of error requires more than a casual commitment to cultural relativism.

Of course, the constructed nature of 'pleasure' of any kind — sensual, aesthetic, spiritual — is something that medieval historians now take for granted. Few today subscribe openly to the older views of scholars such as Johan Huizinga, Norbert Elias, Marc Bloch, and Lucien Febvre, that medieval people were impetuous, childlike, turbulent, and violent, and that historical change has been all in the direction of increased control of impulse and appetite.[5] Recent attempts to understand the gender identities and sexual orientations of medieval people have encouraged heightened awareness of the perils of imposing contemporary conceptual grids on the past.[6]

But there is one respect in which historians might nonetheless do well to inform themselves of these developments. Until recently Western moralists and social scientists understood pleasure in a unidimensional fashion. A tendency to think this way about pleasure is still widespread in Western countries today. While there is no place here to go into the complex history of thinking about pleasure between the Middle Ages and the twentieth century, it is worth noting the 'family resemblances' that link the analytical apparatus of a Peter Damian or a Peter Lombard with twentieth-century theories such as Freudian psychoanalysis or, until very recently, theories used in neuroscience. Such resemblances can easily be taken as reflecting a straightforward universal physiological truth. But present-day neuroscience undercuts such a view.

According to twelfth-century theologians, the pursuit of pleasure resulted from powerful bodily cravings, strengthened by original sin, so powerful that they could overwhelm reason and the will, if they were not kept in check by constant self-discipline. These ideas had been accepted for centuries, but twelfth-century reformers were beginning to apply them, with unprecedented vigour, to social life, via attempts to reform marriage, enforce incest taboos, deny inheritance rights to 'illegitimate' children, and, in general, to penalize sexual pleasure, and thereby reduce or eliminate it because it was considered almost always sinful. The Gregorian reformers of the period saw most aristocrats

[5] Reddy, 'Historical Research on the Self and Emotions'. Norbert Elias's notion of the 'process of civilization', however, continues to influence many researchers; see, for example, certain articles in the special issue on Elias of *Vingtième Siècle: Revue d'histoire*, no. 106, including Wouters, 'Comment les processus de civilisations se sont-ils prolongés?'.

[6] Kuefler, 'Male Friendship and the Suspicion of Sodomy in Twelfth-Century France'; McLaughlin, *Sex, Gender, and Episcopal Authority in an Age of Reform*; Schultz, *Courtly Love, Love of Courtliness, and the History of Sexuality*.

as vice-ridden and 'turbulent'. The latter charge, especially, that they were personally 'turbulent' (rather than conforming to an aristocratic common sense about lordship), continues to find supporters among present-day historians.[7] Thus, aristocrats' most refined skills and most cultivated performances were often taken to be signs of a *breakdown* of inhibition, a *lack* of self-discipline. This clerical tendency still leaves its traces in the historiography of the present, as Michel Zink's verdict on William IX suggests.[8]

The historian must be able to appreciate clerical discourse without granting it more authority than it actually enjoyed in the twelfth century. But this task of achieving a proper appreciation is complicated by the fact that, today, commonsense concepts such as the 'sex drive', the 'pleasure principle', or the brain's 'pleasure center' continue to encourage a reductionistic attitude towards persons such as courtiers and ladies, even though it is obvious they were pursuing complex life plans when they sang a song or flirted with a handsome companion.

It is worth noting that the sexual revolution of the late twentieth century did little to discourage reductionistic thinking about sex, aiming, as it did, to liberate a 'natural' and therefore innocent hankering for sexual pleasures. Destigmatization of sexual desires, if pursued by 'consenting adults', has made substantial progress. But until recently, scholars did not challenge the Freudian or Lacanian idea that desire enjoyed a covert hegemony over other emotions such as shame or longing. Only in the last few years has attention turned to the role of other emotions such as shame or longing in the shaping of sexual identity.[9]

Popular culture is still awash in messages about the sharp sting of sexual cravings. One longs for sexual release in the same impersonal way one longs for food, it is supposed; any partner of the appropriate type will do, just as any café can satisfy a craving for a sandwich. Some recent examples from among scores of films built around the assumed reality of impersonal lust are *The Other Woman* (2014), *Amour et turbulences* (2013), *No Strings Attached* (2011), and *L'Amour dure trois ans* (2011). Sexual cravings are now considered potentially good, or at least morally indifferent in themselves, but they are still closely associated with bodily 'appetites' such as hunger or thirst.

Michel Zink's verdict about William IX is an example of a kind of slippage that can easily occur in historical research on pleasure. Zink appears to agree

[7] See my discussion of this matter in Reddy, *The Making of Romantic Love*, pp. 61–67.

[8] White makes a similar point in his essay 'The Politics of Anger'.

[9] Marcus, 'Queer Theory for Everyone'; Cvetkovich, *An Archive of Feeling*; Sedgwick and Frank, *Touching Feeling*.

with Bishop Hildebrand of Tours who claimed that William IX 'burned with secret fires'.[10] But one must remember to ask: Can anyone 'burn with secret fires' unless a complex process of historical change has shaped an array of practices that can embody, and doctrines that can explain, such a state? Present-day neuroscience says this is impossible.

William IX was the first, or the first we know about, to produce literature about sexual relationships of an entirely new kind. Whether he was innovating himself or imitating others — and most likely he was doing both — he was doing something of very recent vintage; and this requires the historian's careful attention. A change occurred. Medievalists concerned with pleasure must be more than routinely vigilant if they wish to avoid misapplying their own era's common sense to a moment when a crucial feature of that common sense first became current and, perhaps, inspired opposition and satire.

With respect to pleasure, as with respect to some other issues, maintaining the necessary vigilance may be easier to do if one is aware of some of the profound transformations in our understanding of human nature that are being suggested by the latest advances in neuroscience. The idea of a sex drive, along with the idea of any purely physiological understanding of pleasure, is under attack.

In this paper, therefore, I first attempt a summary review of developments in neuroscience and their impact on the neuroscientific understanding of pleasure. The importance of presenting this summary stems from two considerations. First, new understandings of pleasure are part of a much larger shift, one that, as it turns out, provides substantial support for the cultural historian's methodological commitments. Just as these commitments require her to mistrust her own era's common sense, so neuroscience is currently undermining many features of that common sense. Second, as Daniel Gross and Stephanie Preston have argued in an important recent essay, the funding methods that prevail in neuroscience research discourage synthesis and overview, while encouraging researchers to dramatize the findings of their own laboratories, even to exaggerate their importance.[11] Journalists who attempt to explain these findings to a larger public tend to repeat the simple, dramatic claims that frame specific reports. Thus, larger trends that characterize the field, which may be well known to many specialists, are seldom discussed in print and are difficult for outsiders to appreciate.

[10] Quoted in William IX of Aquitaine, *The Poetry*, ed. and trans. by Bond, pp. 130–33.

[11] Gross and Preston, 'Emotion Science and the Heart of a Two-Cultures Problem'.

Following this overview of the neuroscience of pleasure in its larger context, I examine the role of pleasures in twelfth-century courts, as an example of an important topic in medieval history that is readily susceptible to anachronistic misreading. Finally, I offer a reading of the songs of William IX of Aquitaine as expressions of the complex interweaving of pleasures, loyalties, and favour in twelfth-century courts.

Pleasure and Present-Day Neuroscience

Once thought of as a straightforward physiological response, pleasure is now understood as a complex array of response patterns in which learning and 'high levels' of cognition play a central role. There is increasingly clear structural evidence that the brain is a kind of operating system, a kind of staging platform for cultural variation and historical change.[12] Of course, translating these research results into terms that are useful for historians is no easy task. Some regard it as an impossible one, but that is too pessimistic.

Translation is complicated by the tendency of neuroscientists and experimental psychologists to kidnap normal English words such as *emotion* or *perception* and to apply them unproblematically to certain response patterns or certain imaging results. Initially aware that the correspondence of the word and the evidence is approximate at best, they soon fall into a lazy habit of equating the two. Thus, in 1956, when James Olds announced the existence of 'pleasure centers in the brain',[13] he borrowed the everyday English word *pleasure* to refer to whatever it was that made rats, when implanted with electrodes, 'work to deliver repeated electrical stimulation to the ventral tegmentum in the midbrain up through the ventral pallidum, ventral thalamus and nucleus accumbens'.[14] But soon, abetted by the popular press, experts were talking about the brain's 'pleasure center' as if it were settled science that a one-to-one correspondence existed between these brain structures and all experienced pleasure. Surreptitiously, some experts then began to think that a response not involving the nucleus accumbens and associated structures could not be 'pleasure'. This is the step that accomplishes the 'kidnapping' of the word; it is not always

[12] For further discussion, see Reddy, 'Humanists and the Experimental Study of Emotions'; Reddy, 'Neuroscience and the Fallacies of Functionalism'.

[13] Olds, 'Pleasure Centers in the Brain'; Olds and Milner, 'Positive Reinforcement Produced by Electrical Stimulation of Septal Area and Other Regions of Rat Brain'.

[14] Berridge, 'Pleasures of the Brain', p. 115.

acknowledged, and humanists and others must exercise caution when reading the kind of jargon-laden prose that results.

In the study of emotions, this kidnapping has been both open and persistent in the 'basic emotions theory' of Paul Ekman and his followers; Ekman insists that the term 'emotions' can only apply to the responses that generate seven specific facial expressions which he regards as universal and hard-wired.[15] Not emotions, according to Ekman, are such things as love, pride, ambition, admiration, avarice, hope, resignation, nostalgia. These and all other affects must be explained as blends of the seven basic emotions. Thanks to advanced imaging research of recent years, reductionistic theories of this kind are gradually being set aside.[16] But the tendency of brain researchers to kidnap and redefine the vocabulary of the self and of experience in order to magnify the significance of their laboratory findings — regrettable but understandable, given the difficulties they often face — is still very much alive.

Historians and other humanist scholars must read experimental psychology and neuroscience with a critical eye, therefore. For example, when research on speech recognition suggests that a semantic level of processing is located upstream from auditory, morphological, and syntactic processing regions, it is a good idea to place mental quotation marks around the terms 'semantic', 'auditory', 'morphological', and 'syntactic'. These terms are borrowed words that are in danger of being kidnapped.[17] At the same time, it is necessary to recognize that the evidence strongly supports both regional specializations of this sort as well as intensive and subtle interactions among regions of the brain that defy the most sophisticated model building. Neuroscientists need the borrowed words, but also need to exercise great caution in their deployment of them.

Keeping the need for quotation marks constantly in mind, one can nonetheless appreciate, via a brief review of major trends of the last forty years, how understandings of 'pleasure' have been transformed in ways similar to understandings of perception, pain, movement, and emotion. In all these areas of research, a new conception of 'top-down' processing has developed to take into account the profound impact of the 'higher levels' of cognitive processing — which are themselves shaped by learning and habituation, that is, by historically situated cultural common sense. These higher levels mediate the seem-

[15] Ekman, 'Basic Emotions'.

[16] See Reddy, 'Humanists and the Experimental Study of Emotions', for a full discussion of this trend.

[17] An intriguing starting point is Batterink and others, 'The Role of Awareness in Semantic and Syntactic Processing'.

ingly concrete world we live in and inform the simplest responses we have to it. The concept of 'top-down' processing rules out any notion of pleasure as an unlearned, uninhibited 'natural' bodily response.

The Role of 'Top-Down' Processing in Perception

Study of visual perception is one of the most developed fields in neuroscience, and the appreciation of the role of top-down processing got an early start in that field, playing a paradigmatic role for investigations in other areas. Beginning in 1973, in a series of experiments, neuroscientist Stephen M. Kosslyn asked participants to remember a previously viewed picture. He then asked them questions about the object in the picture and measured how long it took them to answer. Reaction times were similar to those of other participants who were actually looking at pictures. For example, participants who were remembering a picture of a boat were asked to press a button if they could 'see' the motor at the back; then they were asked if they could 'see' the anchor at the front. Kosslyn found that participants who were *remembering* a picture took just as long to scan from the back of the boat to the front (to check for the anchor) as participants who were actually *looking at* the picture.

Kosslyn explained this kind of result as follows. It was already known that there are as many efferent pathways in the visual system of the brain as there are afferent ones. That is, there are as many nerve fibers sending information down or outward to the 'visual cortex' at the back of the brain as there are sending information up or inward. At the lowest levels, including the so-called V1, V2, and V3 areas of the visual cortex, there are arrays of 'retinotopically' organized neurons. The firing of these neurons corresponds spatially to the firing of cells in the retina, just as pixels on a screen light up to reproduce an image. Kosslyn hypothesized that these areas of cortex constituted a 'visual buffer'. When directed by executive centres higher up (in the prefrontal cortex), information from visual memory of objects, apparently stored in the inferior temporal gyrus, is projected downward to this visual buffer to generate a detailed image; one can then 'inspect' this image generated by memory just as if it were something currently perceived. Likewise, Kosslyn argued that perception of an object involved the projection downward into the visual buffer of information stored in memory, until an adequate 'match' was achieved between incoming information and remembered information.[18]

[18] Kosslyn, *Image and Brain*; the 1973 study is discussed on p. 7; see also pp. 14, 170.

Fast forward forty years, after the revolution in brain imaging made possible by PET, fMRI, and other scanning technologies, and one finds that the basic features of Kosslyn's theory have held up very well. Not all experts are agreed that V1, V2, V3, and V4 are used for visually remembering or imagining an object. But there is a general consensus that visual object recognition involves the projection downward or outward of remembered information in the search for a match with incoming visual data, and that a similar process is involved in remembering or imagining objects. Evidence suggests that this two-way process of object recognition is carried out with astonishing speed.[19] According to Moshe Bar and associates, a low-resolution sample of incoming visual information is rushed forward to the prefrontal cortex, which somehow makes a selection of a range of possible objects, in turn rushing these guesses to the inferior temporal fusiform gyrus, where object memory traces are stored.[20] This memory bank, in turn, starts sending richer information on a limited number of likely candidates downward to regions of the visual cortex, until a match is found. We do not 'know' what we are 'seeing' until we make this match. This whole process is unconscious and can take as little as 200 milliseconds.

Subsequent research has confirmed, in fact, that Kosslyn's general approach is valid not just for visual perception, but for a host of other perceptual processes. In speech recognition, incoming auditory information is being compared not only with memories of lexical items (words) but also with possible meanings, as well as with objects in the visual field, within 200 milliseconds of the initiation of an utterance. Long before the first syllable of a phrase is complete, the language recognition system is already guessing at the likely lexical, syntactical, and *semantic* structure of the utterance under way. These guesses are sent back down to the auditory cortex in search of a match. All of this occurs outside of awareness.[21]

Movement, Mirror Neurons, Embodied Cognition, Pain

The discovery of so-called 'mirror neurons' has stimulated a lot of new research and been much discussed in the popular media. These neurons lie in areas of the

[19] Kosslyn and others, 'Brain rCBF and Performance in Visual Imagery Tasks'.

[20] Gilbert and Li, 'Top-Down Influences on Visual Processing'; Bar and others, 'Top-Down Facilitation of Visual Recognition'.

[21] For example, Yee and Sedivy, 'Eye Movements to Pictures Reveal Transient Semantic Activation during Spoken Word Recognition'; Batterink and others, 'The Role of Awareness in Semantic and Syntactic Processing'; Vigliocca and others, 'Nouns and Verbs in the Brain'.

motor cortex that control muscular movements. Brain-imaging studies show that they are activated when one is perceiving the movements of other people's bodies, as well as when one perceives others' facial expressions. It appears that they are used to run 'simulations' of what one sees. (In mirror-neuron studies, a concept of 'simulation' is in fact in the process of being kidnapped — transformed from an intentional and imaginative activity into a structurally hard-wired 'processing' strategy.) These simulations involve the passing of visual information to the prefrontal cortex and from there back out to motor neurons. In one study published in 2010, participants read emotional passages from novels before and after treatment with Botox. Previous studies had shown that reading emotional passages was associated with very slight contractions of facial muscles reflecting the activation of 'mirror' neurons as part of the process of emotional comprehension. But researchers found that Botox, which temporarily paralyses muscle tissue near the skin, 'selectively slowed the reading of sentences that described [emotional] situations that normally require the paralyzed muscle for expressing the emotions evoked by the sentences'.[22]

This kind of discovery has given rise to theories of 'embodied cognition', according to which cognition is aided at every step by the running of such simulations, which entail reactions not just of motor neurons but of the body itself. The hypothesized architecture of such simulations is similar to that of visual perception and speech recognition. Sketchy information is rushed to centres in the prefrontal cortex, which centres send directions back downward — to memory areas and to the visual, auditory, and motor cortices. Somehow, very high-level executive areas of the prefrontal cortex are able to provide sketchy candidates that speed the search for a match. In doing so, they often trigger simulations. In the prefrontal cortex are those crucial zones that provide the so-called cross-modal links that enable the brain to compare visual, auditory, tactile, and motor input; nearby prefrontal regions handle 'emotional' processing as well as 'executive control' of many other systems.[23]

Research on pain has undergone a similar, perhaps even more dramatic transformation. The old idea of a one-to-one relationship between tissue

[22] Havas and others, 'Cosmetic Use of Botulinum Toxin-A Affects Processing of Emotional Language', p. 895. See also, e.g., Iacoboni and Dapretto, 'The Mirror Neuron System and the Consequences of its Dysfunction'.

[23] On 'executive control' by the dorsal lateral prefrontal cortex, see, e.g., Decety, 'Dissecting the Neural Mechanisms Mediating Empathy'; Gilbert and Li, 'Top-Down Influences on Visual Processing'; Craig, 'How Do You Feel — Now?'; Littrell, 'Perspectives Emerging from Neuroscience on How People Become Addicted and What to Do About It'.

damage and perceived pain has been set aside, as researchers have found that neurons projecting from the midbrain and brainstem into the spinal cord can inhibit pain neurons and produce analgesia; pain neurons can also be sensitized by inflammation and repeated stimulation. Higher up, pain perception is highly malleable through deployment of attentional resources, pursuit of goals, and the influence of social contexts.[24]

Emotions

And so with emotions. An early neurophysiological theory of emotions associated them with certain subcortical centres such as the amygdala or the hypothalamus. These structures were imagined to be a kind of primitive interrupt system that could produce affective responses of aversion or attraction independent of cognition.[25] But here, too, the rich two-way pathways between the amygdala and certain regions of the prefrontal cortex have been shown to activate with great rapidity, permitting the 'executive' or 'regulatory' functions of the prefrontal cortex to modulate amygdala reactions almost as quickly as they arise. Not only is the amygdala constantly and massively modulated by input from the prefrontal cortex, but it also influences perception through its own set of direct pathways to sensory regions of the cortex, for example, to the retinotopically organized visual cortex. An emotionally significant object will literally leap out of the visual field, as V1 neurons activate more intensely in response to amygdala input, which is in turn modulated by the prefrontal cortex.[26]

The currently emerging wisdom is that emotions are associated with widely distributed networks of activation involving cortical and subcortical regions in nearly simultaneous responses. As Luis Pessoa has recently remarked,

> the architectural features of the brain are such that they provide massive opportunity for cognitive-emotional interactions [...] given inter-region interactivity, and the fact that networks intermingle signals of diverse origin, although a characterization of brain function in terms of networks is needed, the networks themselves are best conceptualized as neither 'cognitive' nor 'emotional'.[27]

[24] Larivière and others, 'Changes in Pain Perception and Descending Inhibitory Controls Start at Middle Age in Healthy Adults'; Sullivan, 'Finding Pain between Minds and Bodies'.

[25] Duncan and Feldman Barrett, 'Affect Is a Form of Cognition'.

[26] Damaraju and others, 'Affective Learning Enhances Activity and Functional Connectivity in Early Visual Cortex'.

[27] Pessoa, 'Beyond Brain Regions', p. 159.

Recent review articles suggest that the amygdala, even though it is located beneath the neocortex, far from being some kind of mediator of primitive reflexes, is in fact a hub that handles strategic deployment of attentional resources in various cortical regions.[28] Hence its involvement in startle and fear responses is just a function of its larger role in the shifting of attention to whatever is currently important. Amygdala response is, in turn, highly sensitive to inhibitory signals from the prefrontal cortex. Emotion, like vision, pain, speech recognition, or the perception of others' bodies, is as much a 'top-down' as a 'bottom-up' process.[29]

Research on desire has seen a similar change. Understanding of sexual desire, arousal, and satisfaction has undergone a complete reversal among clinical researchers on sexuality. Where Alfred C. Kinsey measured sexual satisfaction by counting orgasms in the 1940s and 1950s, recent research suggests that most people do not consider penile tumescence or vaginal lubrication as always pleasant, or even as a reliable indication that one has become sexually aroused. Brain imaging studies have failed to locate any one brain region that specializes in sexual arousal, indicating it is mediated by broadly distributed networks, just like emotional states. Instead, sexual desire and gratification are found to be heavily influenced by social context and emotional state — that is, sexual desire is associated with the kind of executive control or emotional regulation that brain imaging associates consistently with the prefrontal cortex.[30]

Pleasure

It should come as no surprise, then, that research on pleasure in general has followed a similar trajectory. As noted above, in 1956, James Olds announced the existence of 'pleasure centers in the brain'.[31] Since the onset of brain imaging, however, the experience of pleasure has been shown to be much more complex. In the last fifteen years, Kent Berridge and associates have developed a theory that distinguishes a 'liking' system from a 'wanting' system. This theory

[28] Pessoa, 'Emotion and Cognition and the Amygdala'; Salzman and Fusi, 'Emotion, Cognition, and Mental State Representation in Amygdala and Prefrontal Cortex'; Pessoa, 'On the Relationship Between Emotion and Cognition'.

[29] Pessoa and Adolphs, 'Emotion Processing and the Amygdala'.

[30] This research is reviewed in Reddy, *The Making of Romantic Love*, pp. 9–15.

[31] Olds, 'Pleasure Centers in the Brain'; Olds and Milner, 'Positive Reinforcement Produced by Electrical Stimulation of Septal Area and Other Regions of Rat Brain'.

has attracted wide attention. Berridge has noted that the mere fact that a rat will repeatedly self-stimulate when electrodes are placed in certain parts of the brain does not prove that the self-stimulation is actually pleasurable.

Berridge argues in addition that the human research on what Olds called the 'pleasure center' confirms that 'pleasure' is the wrong term. In the 1970s, some psychiatrists began using electrodes implanted in the so-called pleasure centres in humans to treat certain chronic conditions such as intractable pain or severe depression. Some patients repeated the self-stimulation as many as 1200 to 1500 times in a row on a single day. Improvement in their conditions was obvious. After repeated stimulation, these patients reported that the world became 'motivationally brighter and more attractive'.[32] But, notes Berridge, patients also often reported strong thirst, hunger, or sexual arousal. In addition, they did not report feelings of pleasure. Reviewing the research, Berridge argues that these electrodes were stimulating a 'wanting' system, not a 'liking' system. The wanting system, he argues, is set in motion when neurons in the ventral tegmental area release dopamine. Far from being the key to pleasure as was long believed, dopamine is now seen as a source of general arousal that prepares the organism for goal-seeking activity.

Berridge and associates distinguish genuine pleasure from mere wanting, in part, by means of mouth movements in animals and human infants. In human infants, Berridge and a co-author remark, sweet foods 'elicit a contented licking of the lips, but bitter tastes instead elicit disgust gapes and headshakes. Homologous "liking" orofacial expressions are elicited also in apes and monkeys, and even in rats and mice'.[33] Berridge has identified two linked 'hotspots' in rats, one in the nucleus accumbens, one in the ventral pallidum, that reliably induce these pleasure responses when stimulated via microinjections of opioids. But slight movements of the injection location can result in very different responses, including disgust.

To clarify the wanting versus liking distinction, Berridge and associates note that one continues to find the taste of chocolate pleasant even after one has eaten one's fill. In effect, while the responses of the liking system are constant, the wanting system will track the intake of chocolate and turn itself off.[34] Liking versus wanting is also regarded as helpful in explaining addiction. Exposure to addictive drugs at first brings both pleasure and wanting. But

[32] Berridge, 'Pleasures of the Brain', p. 117.

[33] Berridge and Kringelbach, 'Neuroscience of Affect', p. 298.

[34] Berridge and Kringelbach, 'Neuroscience of Affect', p. 296.

experimental evidence suggests that the wanting system can become sensitized by repeated exposure so that it is set off merely by the sight, for example, of drug paraphernalia, whereas the liking system is hypothesized to become less sensitive to the drug with repeated exposure.[35]

Neuroscience is thus giving the word *pleasure* back to the humanists — to speak allegorically — but threatening to kidnap *wanting* and *liking* in return for *pleasure*'s release. Doubtless the usefulness of Berridge's model will run its course, and we will eventually get *wanting* and *liking* back as well. In the meantime, the model, suitably equipped with quotation marks, remains suggestive.

Still another set of studies has uncovered a keyboard-like array of neurons in the medial shell of the nucleus accumbens in rats. Each 'microdomain' of the medial shell, if given a microinjection of a GABA (gamma-Aminobutyric acid) agonist (which blocks the inhibitory effect of GABA) or glutamate antagonist (which blocks the excitatory effect of glutamate), elicits a different mixture of desire or dread. At the caudal (that is, posterior) end of the nucleus accumbens, intense desire, that is, the wanting system, is set in motion when these injections inhibit the action of nearby neurons. At the rostral or anterior end, intense fear or dread results. But the precise response of the microdomains in between changes according to context; many microdomains that elicit desire when the rat is in a peaceful context will elicit dread if the rat is over-stimulated with bright lights and loud music.[36]

Although the amygdala was long associated more closely with negative emotions, just as the nucleus accumbens was associated with pleasure, recent studies suggest the wiring is much more complex. Many different emotional states involve, in various ways, the same set of cortical and subcortical regions, including the ventral medial prefrontal cortex, the orbitofrontal cortex, the anterior cingulate cortex, and the insula, as well as the subcortical (and once thought to be more 'primitive') regions of the nucleus accumbens, ventral pallidum, ventral tegmental area, amygdala, and hypothalamus. In each case, cortical regions are involved both in monitoring the states of subcortical

[35] Littrell, 'Perspectives Emerging from Neuroscience on How People Become Addicted and What to Do About It'.

[36] As Berridge and Kringelbach put it, 'A motivation-releasing drug microinjection inhibits NAc neurons with a local 0.5–1.0 mm diameter micro-domain corresponding to a single "key" of the keyboard (via a GABA agonist or AMPA glutamate antagonist). This drug inhibition of accumbens microdomains prevents the endogenous NAc inhibition of targets, and so releases particular downstream motivation generating circuits into final activation to produce the intense motivations that are observed'. Berridge and Kringelbach, 'Neuroscience of Affect', p. 301.

structures but also in modulating or regulating them through 'massive projections' of efferent pathways. Still other cortical regions are in turn activated or deactivated by these subcortical 'hubs'. Determining which centres 'trigger' or 'inhibit', which 'respond' to or are 'modulated' by others is often a matter of guesswork, because pathways running in both directions link them all.

Using an innovative PET scanning technique, Valorie N. Salimpoor and associates recently found evidence of a close association between moments in a piece of music that participants rated as peak emotional experiences and the moments of peak releases of dopamine in these same participants, demonstrating that response to music is handled, at least in part, by the same processes that are activated by cocaine, methamphetamine, and other addictive stimulants.[37] Neuroscientists studying the pleasure elicited by music, art, and other aesthetic endeavours presume that the complex cognitive work involved in appreciating a work of art occurs in prefrontal cortical regions. These are the same regions that, according to Salimpoor and Robert J. Zatorre, 'underlie advanced thinking and reasoning, abstraction, integration of mental processes with emotional responses, and integration of past and present to create expectations and anticipation'.[38] These areas also integrate sensory modalities and movement, as when sight, hearing, and motion are combined in dance. It is, then, the cognitive response of these 'advanced' or 'executive' areas of the prefrontal cortex (as they are sometimes called) that triggers the pleasure system as well as the wanting system in distinctive ways, when one is pleased by music.

As Amy Arnsten, Kent Berridge, and others have noted, these 'executive' regions of the prefrontal cortex have direct 'massive' links to every structure in the liking and wanting systems; the prefrontal cortex can therefore order up its own dopamine from the ventral tegmental area, Arnsten notes, initiating what Berridge would call the 'wanting' system. And it can do so, to all appearances, based on very abstract processing, such as that required to understand a complex chord progression or melody.[39]

For Berridge and others, then, pleasure must be understood as an emotion, not a mere bodily response. For Berridge, a pleasant sensation generates no pleasure unless a positive affect is elicited by it, which affect reflects either the person's approval of the sensation's effect, or else the person's inclination to

[37] Salimpoor and others, 'Anatomically Distinct Dopamine Release during Anticipation and Experience of Peak Emotion to Music'.

[38] Salimpoor and Zatorre, 'Neural Interactions that Give Rise to Musical Pleasure', p. 62.

[39] Arnsten, 'Stress Signalling Pathways that Impair Prefrontal Cortex Structure and Function'.

approve of it (which includes knowing what it is and knowing the implications of approving it).[40] Like fear, anger, sadness, or happiness, pleasure involves a network of activations within the same affect-related set of subcortical and nearby cortical areas; like them, it can be initiated by a wide variety of contexts, whose evaluation involves the most 'advanced' regions of the cortex. Each 'emotion's' network may be different, as may each 'pleasure's' network, but all are supported by overlapping sets of regions which are positioned to mediate among the various senses, muscular movements, motivation, memory, and decision making. Therefore, in terms of the neural structures involved, pleasure, pain, hunger, or thirst are just as much 'emotional' as fear, joy, anger, or love.

According to Berridge and Kringelbach, in a review article of 2013, the triggering of the liking system is the common feature of all states that have a positive valence, that is, all states that are inherently rewarding, from the tasting of sweets to the appreciation of a painting by Picasso or a symphony by Mozart.[41] Appreciation of sweet taste appears to be, in some sense, inborn, but learning soon intervenes. Overall, there is plenty of room in this organization of response patterns for learning — that is, plenty of room for culture and history to have their say. It should be hardly surprising, in the end, that neuroscience should confirm the crucial role of the cultural in human affairs.

The Neuroscience of Pleasure and the Historian

Thus the cultural historian may comfort herself that, the more carefully the empirical dimension is examined, the more stiffly it resists reductionistic accounts of human experience. At first neuroscientists used imaging technology to move beyond a *presumed* reductionism, to look for concrete evidence that *demonstrated* the existence of a hidden mechanism governing human feeling. But they have found that scans of brain activity fail to offer any support. If anything, the brain's architecture appears designed to *prevent* the direct application of an unfiltered response pattern to any context. Even though it is obviously designed to provide extremely rapid responses, it turns out that even the fastest responses rely on learning and are subject to 'executive control'.

[40] Berridge, 'Pleasures of the Brain'; see, for example, p. 106, where he characterizes 'liking' as 'the core process that underlies sensory pleasure and causes positive affective reactions'.

[41] 'Affect, the hedonic quality of pleasure or displeasure, is what distinguishes emotion from other psychological processes', according to Berridge and Kringelbach, 'Neuroscience of Affect', p. 294.

Part of the problem in conceptualizing pleasure is metaphysical rather than physical. Once the world is divided between mental (or spiritual) phenomena and material phenomena, it becomes difficult to explain how one dimension can ever come into contact with the other. This is true whether the division is drawn along Platonic lines, Aristotelian lines, or Cartesian lines. Terms such as 'passion', 'affect', 'emotion', 'desire', and 'appetite' have been used for centuries to name an intermediate range of things that bridge the gap. 'Emotions' and their correlates are imagined to exist on both sides. They are at once bodily and meaningful. But conceptualizing how they accomplish this intermediation then becomes, in turn, very difficult. The philosopher Michel Meyer has briefly sketched out the various ways, inspired but always unsatisfactory, that philosophers since Plato have attempted to solve the riddle.[42]

Just as present-day neuroscientists have a tendency to 'kidnap' everyday terms of experience and use them as labels for patterns identified in the laboratory, so, for instance, Augustine struggled to establish a language that could consistently relate experience with bodily existence. As Peter Brown has noted, 'Unlike the hasty Jerome, and even unlike Ambrose, Augustine was exceptionally careful to point out, in frequent, patient expositions of the Letters of Paul, that the flesh was not simply the body: it was all that led the self to prefer its own will to that of God'. This resulted from 'a lasting distortion of the soul itself. With Adam's Fall, *the soul lost the ability to summon up all of itself, in an undivided act of will*, to love and praise God in all created things. Concupiscence was a dark drive to control, to appropriate, and to turn to one's private ends, all the good things that had been created by God to be accepted with gratitude and shared with others. It lay at the root of the inescapable misery that afflicted mankind'.[43] This is how concupiscence became something more than a bodily condition and gained its spiritual meaning: it was virtually a detached fragment of the will that could drag the rest of the will into sin.

Damien Boquet has explored the difficulties which Cistercian theologians faced explaining the relation between body and soul in the twelfth century. Boquet notes 'a certain fluidity in the terminology used by Aelred of Rievaulx'[44] which permitted him to speak of love, in some instances, as something separate from affect, as a separate capacity instilled by God which free will uses either

[42] Meyer, *Le Philosophe et les passions*; see also Deluermoz and others, 'Écrire l'histoire des émotions'; Changeux and Ricoeur, *Ce qui nous fait penser*.

[43] Brown, *The Body and Society*, p. 418; emphasis added.

[44] Boquet, *L'Ordre de l'affect au Moyen Âge*, p. 198.

for good or for evil. Each impulse to love is initiated by reason, by affect, or by both. Rare is that orderly act of love in which reason reins in affect's energy and affect softens reason's commands — this is the reward of a long effort of self-discipline. Love inspired solely by affect, in contrast, becomes too sensual, giving rise to what Aelred called a 'perverted love that strips man of his humanity and makes him bestial, which stifles, so to speak, and erases what there is in him of reason, of nobility, and finally of utility'. In this analysis, Aelred used the concept of love to give spiritual meaning to affect, where affect was understood as a disturbance deriving from bodily existence.[45]

Thus the experts of the period offered various explanations of the number and definition of the soul's faculties, and of the precise character of their complex interactions. But they followed Augustine in considering, in a general way, that pleasure became 'bestial' when it involved enjoyment of the things of this world without appreciation of them as God's gifts, to be employed only as part of a life of devotion and obedience. Even the highly politicized pleasures of earthly courts, therefore, were inevitably seen as entailing a failure of self-discipline, a giving in to a lower nature, rather than as requiring a particular kind of self-discipline.

Pleasure in Twelfth-Century Courts

Twelfth-century courts, whether of local lords or of sovereign princes, were places where one could expect to find a variety of pleasures: the pleasures of food and drink, to be sure, and also those of music, news, storytelling, humour, gambling, pageantry and luxury, and amorous intrigue. The game of chess, tight-fitting dresses, pointed shoes, and new hairstyles came into fashion in the late eleventh century, as travel and long-distance trade awakened new tastes.[46] But courts were also central sites in a ceaseless and highly involving game of manoeuvre for favour, honours, legitimacy, and authority. Outward displays of affection and loyalty were paired with behind-the-scenes gossip and plotting. Hardly anyone who entered such a court, from the lowliest clerk to the sovereign her- or himself, could afford to ignore this game, or to neglect the current state of play. Courtly pleasures were just one feature of the game. Court pastimes permitted one to parade the excess resources that flowed from well-regulated holdings with obedient subjects and, at the same time, to display

[45] Boquet, *L'Ordre de l'affect au Moyen Âge*, pp. 203–07.

[46] Reddy, *The Making of Romantic Love*, p. 74.

one's finesse, one's ease, one's long experience with lordly status, and thus one's aptitude for additional favours, offices, authority.[47] The pleasures of court were business, pursued sometimes with a grim determination.

In the Occitan verse *Ensenhamen* of Arnaut-Guilhem de Marsan, a Gascon lord in the Angevin orbit, written in the 1170s or 1180s, an old hand instructs a young man how to get on at court.[48] A thousand persons, we are told, were playing chess and backgammon, singing, or telling stories, as the old hand told the young man of the great lovers Paris, Tristan, Aeneas, Linaura, Yvain, Apollonius of Tyre. These figures were presented, not as pleasant fictions, but as models one must strive to emulate. The old hand gave detailed instructions on how a young man could avoid appearing stupid or flat-footed at court: what to wear; how to trim one's beard; how to avoid appearing stingy in providing food or drink (if hosting a dinner), or stung if one lost a bet; how to equip one's horse for a tournament; how to conduct oneself in the mêlée. The payoff for mastery of literature, gaming, dress, and horsemanship, according to the old hand, was the favour of ladies. A lady wants nothing to do with a lover who is quickly done with court or war, and who must depend on fate. She wants a man who 'every day can increase his worth' ('a totz jorns pus | fassa son pretz en sus', lines 521–22).

At the end of the *Ensenhamen*, the old hand brags of the high-status ladies who have granted him their favour and alludes to others whose names he dare not mention. The pleasures of court are, from the point of view of the *Ensenhamen*, complex problems to be solved, problems crucial to one's identity and status. How one enjoys them displays one's true rank, which is only partially a matter of family and status, and is more like an aura or charisma one broadcasts via subtle cues only insiders understand. Enjoying the pleasures of court in the right way gives access to favour, including the favour of great ladies, and thus to still other pleasures whose superiority has as much to do with self-esteem as with mere sensory perception. Arnaut-Guilhem de Marsan's work attracted at least some attention, launching a new genre of advice literature.

Arnaut-Guilhem may have made visits to the court of Richard Coeur-de-Lion in Poitiers in the 1170s, or paid his respects to Richard's sister Joanna,

[47] Crouch, *The Birth of Nobility*, pp. 24–44; Jaeger, *The Origins of Courtliness*, pp. 116–17. Barlow's biography of Thomas Becket describes the rise of this consummate 'courtier' in a revealing way; see Barlow, *Thomas Becket*, pp. 41–63.

[48] Arnaut-Guilhem de Marsan, *L'Ensenhamen*, ed. by de Cauna, French trans. by Gouiran; on this *Ensenhamen*, see de Cauna, Introduction'; see also Monson, *Les Ensenhamens occitans*; Lejeune, *Littérature et société occitane au Moyen Âge*, pp. 261–70.

when she travelled south for her wedding with William II of Sicily in 1176.[49] When Joanna crossed the Channel, her father Henry II paid over 17 pounds for the fitting out of eight ships to carry her, her party, and her furnishings and clothing, including robes for the wedding ceremony that cost 'a staggering' 115 pounds, 5 shillings, 5 pence, according to Colette Marie Bowie.[50] Joanna's party was led by Richard of Dover, who had replaced the murdered Thomas Becket as Archbishop of Canterbury three years before. The party included, among five other bishops, the Archbishop of Rouen, who had presided over Henry the Young King's submission to his father the year before, at the close of the failed rebellion of Henry II's sons of 1173–74. Doubtless some of these courtiers, including Arnaut-Guilhem, as they smiled in celebration or congratulations for Joanna, were acutely aware of the many people who were not present, including former associates of Thomas Becket (whose new status as martyr-saint was deftly appropriated by Henry II beginning in 1172) and the many barons whose support of the rebellious sons in 1173–74 had earned ruthless retribution.[51]

Better known today than Arnaut-Guilhem de Marsan are the northern critics of the Angevin court, clerical authors writing in Latin, including John of Salisbury and Walter Map, who provide glimpses of the underside of courtly splendours.[52] Walter Map's extended comparison of the court to hell, at the beginning of his satirical *De nugis curialium* (*c.* 1189), indicates his familiarity with the pitfalls of combining so much apparent pleasure with so much serious business.[53] Every courtier was prey to tedium, anxiety, discouragement, humiliation. Waiting for an audience, for the right moment to speak, one watched one's purse empty out or, worse, one's debts mount up, as weeks turned into months. Loss of favour usually brought loss of access. Reinstatement depended on the intercession of friends, such as those who soothed Henry II's

[49] De Cauna, relying on charter evidence, places him in the entourage of Eleanor of Aquitaine's daughter, on her way to marry Alphonse VIII of Castille in 1170; see de Cauna, 'Introduction', p. 11. See also Chauvenet, 'L'Entourage de Richard Coeur de Lion en Poitou et en Aquitaine'.

[50] Bowie, 'The Daughters of Henry II and Eleanor of Aquitaine', p. 91.

[51] Bowie, 'The Daughters of Henry II and Eleanor of Aquitaine', p. 161. On the rebellion of 1173–74, see Flori, *Aliénor d'Aquitaine*, pp. 120–47; Strickland, 'Arms and the Men'. On Henry II's court, see also Türk, *Nugae curialium*; Vincent, 'The Court of Henry II'.

[52] Türk, '*Curialis Nugator — Il perfetto cortegiano*'.

[53] Map, *De Nugis Curialium, Courtiers' Trifles*, ed. and trans. by James, rev. by Brooke and Mynors.

anger at John of Salisbury in 1156–57.[54] Thus anyone at court was bound to cultivate friendships as vigorously as she or he pursued lordly favour.

In her or his own court, a lord was prone to suspicion and to anger. The danger of rebellion was constant and often could only be countered by ensuring one had the real loyalty of a majority of one's supposedly loyal barons, that is, of enough of them to overawe the rest. This is how William IX of Aquitaine survived the rebellion that met his accession in 1086; how Stephen of Blois secured the succession to the English crown in 1135. This is how Henry II's father, Geoffrey, Count of Anjou, survived a rebellion inspired by his jealous brother around 1140; how Ermengard of Narbonne survived the attempted takeover of her lands in 1142; how Henry II himself survived the rebellions of 1173–74 and 1183.[55] Thus smiles, deference, enjoyments at court were scrutinized with care; to enjoy its pleasures was implicitly to claim that, at least for the present, one was loyal.

The twelfth century brought a significant increase in the social significance of courtly pleasures. But it also brought a significant, perhaps not unrelated, shift in clerical attitudes towards pleasure. Paradoxically, instead of recognizing the growing significance of refined enjoyments in the pursuit of, and display of, political authority, theologians and preachers of the Gregorian Reform period tended to distinguish pleasures of the flesh more sharply than ever from spiritual pleasures. Peter Damian urged men, when they saw a beautiful woman, to think of what she would look like as her flesh rotted after death. Bernard of Clairvaux also viewed physical beauty with disgust; one of his followers called a beautiful woman a 'sack of excrement'. In his sermons on the Song of Songs, Bernard transformed the erotic splendour of that text into an allegory about the relation between the soul and God.[56] The line between fleshly and spiritual pleasures was drawn in such a way that it was virtually impossible for theologians

[54] Constable, 'The Alleged Disgrace of John of Salisbury in 1159'.

[55] On William IX's accession in 1086, see Richard, *Histoire des Comtes de Poitou*, II, 119–30. On Ermengard of Narbonne, see Cheyette, *Ermengard of Narbonne and the World of the Troubadours*, pp. 14–21; on Stephen of Blois, see Bradbury, *Stephen and Matilda*, pp. 14–22. On Geoffrey Plantagenêt, Count of Anjou, and his rebellious brother Helie, see Lemesle, 'Le Comte d'Anjou face aux rébellions (1129–1151)'.

[56] Reddy, *The Making of Romantic Love*, pp. 77–89, and works cited there, suggesting that Bernard's sermons may have been inflected by awareness of contemporary troubadour love songs. Bernard was not the first to offer this sort of allegorical interpretation of the Song of Songs, although the usual approach was to treat it as an allegory about the relation between Christ and his Church (Piroska Nagy, personal communication). See Matter, *The Voice of my Beloved*.

to grasp, in their abstract schemas, a fundamental fact of the courts. This fact was that young men and women were obliged to perfect their skills in singing, in fashion, in conversation, in horsemanship, or in games of chance as a means of fulfilling their duty to self and family.[57]

When Philip I of France dismissed his wife and married Bertrada of Montfort in 1092, Bishop Ivo of Chartres did not congratulate Bertrada for her remarkable charms but sent Philip a long letter explaining the dangers of lust.[58] Orderic Vitalis reserved his 'fiercest denunciations', according to Mathew Kuefler, for the court of William Rufus of England (ruled 1087–1100). 'They devoted their nights to feasts and drinking-bouts, idle chatter, dice, games of chance, and other sports, and they slept all day', Orderic complained. Male same-sex liaisons abounded there: 'the effeminates [*effeminati*] throughout the realm ruled supreme, and carried on their debaucheries without restraint, and loathsome Ganymedes [*catamitae*], who ought to be consumed by flames, abused themselves with foul sodomite-things [*sodomitica*]'.[59] In the aftermath of William Rufus's death, bishops gathered in 1102 and issued a condemnation of sodomy, threatening offenders with anathema. But Bishop Anselm of Canterbury urged that the anathema threat not be published, 'considering that this sin had been so prevalent up to now that almost no one blushed at it; and that as a result many, not realizing its gravity, had thrown themselves into it'.[60]

Only at the end of the twelfth century and in the early years of the thirteenth were concessions made on singing and storytelling; Pierre the Chanter and Thomas of Chobham allowed that singing about the deeds of princes or the lives of the saints, if one avoided lechery and turpitude, might be done without sin.[61] Earlier, controversy had arisen over the question whether sexual pleasure was sinful, and whether it was a venial or a mortal sin, even when enjoyed within legitimate marriage. Here, too, Pierre the Chanter and Thomas of Chobham took a conciliatory stance; sexual pleasure within marriage was still sinful, to be sure, but only '*venialissime*', only very slightly.[62]

[57] Türk, *Nugae curialium*, pp. 68–94, discusses John of Salisbury's inability to grasp the political stakes of courtly behaviour.

[58] Duby, *The Knight, the Lady and the Priest*, pp. 7–14.

[59] Kuefler, 'Male Friendship and the Suspicion of Sodomy in Twelfth-Century France', pp. 194–95.

[60] Poly, *Le Chemin des amours barbares*, pp. 392–93.

[61] Baldwin, 'The Image of the Jongleur in Northern France around 1200', pp. 643–44.

[62] Boquet, 'L'Amour en Occident … et ailleurs'.

Clerical understanding of the 'flesh' simply did not make sense in the context of the serious business of courtly enjoyments. Clerical condemnation tended to leave courtiers and visitors at court without any guide to their behaviour. Perhaps this helps to explain the transformation that Thomas Becket underwent, when he changed from the most successful of Angevin courtiers, trusted chancellor of Henry II, and tutor to his son, into the intransigent Archbishop of Canterbury in 1162.[63] Named to the see of Canterbury, Thomas, perhaps because he was a perfectionist in all he did, found himself pushed across the temporal-spiritual divide and suddenly recognized he had entirely new rules to guide his behaviour. He also had a new and very strong incentive to deploy clerical rigidity and reductionism; after all, the theology of the day endowed primates such as Thomas with ultimate authority over the doings of temporal government. Prelates such as Thomas or Bernard of Clairvaux were not interested in describing courts. They sought the best means to translate their spiritual claims into real influence. The harsh rhetoric of condemnation and anathema was for many an irresistible tool.

Into the Breach: William IX and his Songs

William IX's 'obscene' or 'ribald' songs belong to the context of the twelfth-century court as much as do his ardent love songs, as well as all the love songs of the troubadours who followed him. This claim is worth underscoring because, not surprisingly, contemporary clerical chroniclers seemed unaware of this crucial feature of his lyrics when they harshly condemned both his songwriting and his behaviour.

It is now widely recognized that Merovingian and Frankish elite males often took secondary wives as much to ensure they would have heirs as in pursuit of 'pleasure'. These practices were still very much alive in the eleventh century. William IX's father dismissed two childless wives before marrying his mother, and some scholars suggest that William IX himself dismissed a first wife when she was unable to bear him children.[64] If these scholars are right, it was only

[63] Barlow, *Thomas Becket*, pp. 64–87.

[64] Richard, *Histoire des Comtes de Poitou*, II, 8–13, 44–67; Bezzola, 'Guillaume IX et les origines de l'amour courtois'. Ruth Harvey disputes this view, however, in a very careful and persuasive rereading of the original sources. In her view there was no first marriage to a certain Ermengard of Anjou, and William's marriage to Philippa of Toulouse was his only marriage. She also doubts that William ever repudiated her, given his very serious interest in claiming the title of Count of Toulouse, which she had a strong claim to as the previous count's only

when he wished to stray from the bed of his second marriage that he fell afoul of the reforming spirit, because of the appointment of a reform-minded bishop in Poitiers.

Gradually across the twelfth century, Church reformers succeeded in establishing the exclusive legitimacy of monogamous marriage, in outlawing divorce, in reducing the incidence of 'incestuous' liaisons, and in labeling male same-sex ties as 'unmanly'. Nonetheless, as David Crouch has pointed out, aristocrats continued to value 'bastard' sons for their loyal service and their value in marital alliances with lesser lords.[65] Courtly pleasures and political advancement continued to be intricately intertwined.

But for clerical chroniclers, William IX was a seeker of pleasure and nothing else. He burned so ardently for the wife of one of his viscounts, claimed William of Malmesbury, that he dismissed his own wife, carried off the viscountess, and installed her in the ducal palace, braving clerical condemnation and an interdict on his lands to keep her nearby. He was 'poisoned by the viperish hiss of this whore', concluded William of Malmesbury.[66] As noted above, Bishop Hildebrand of Tours also charged that he 'burned with secret fires'. Much later in the century, Geoffrey of Vigeois dismissed William as a 'vehement lover of women'.[67]

The analogy between sexual appetite and fire can be traced back to Ovid.[68] For Ovid, this fire distracted the dutiful Roman citizen — whose proper concern was the virtuous conduct of politics and war — and led him to fritter his life away on seductions and secret meetings. For clerical chroniclers, William IX's burning desires drew him away from Christian chastity and alienated him from clerical authority. In his frenzy, he drew his sword on Bishop Pierre II of Poitiers,

surviving child. But it is worth pointing out that William may have installed Maubergeonne in his palace in Poitiers without formally repudiating Philippa. Clerical observers would have regarded this as a blatant violation of marital fidelity, but it was, after all, a long-standing aristocratic tradition to have secondary wives, and it cannot be ruled out that William and Philippa both regarded Maubergeonne in this light. Harvey's interpretation notably fails to deal with the fact that William married his son to Maubergeonne's daughter, thus establishing an enduring tie between the ducal and the vicecomital families. See Harvey, 'The Wives of the "First Troubadour", Duke William IX of Aquitaine'.

[65] Crouch, *William Marshal*, p. 69.

[66] Quoted in William IX of Aquitaine, *The Poetry*, ed. and trans. by Bond, pp. 128–31.

[67] Quoted in Bezzola, *Les Origines et la formation de la littérature courtoise en occident*, pp. 270–71. For further discussion of these verdicts, see Reddy, *The Making of Romantic Love*, p. 103.

[68] Edwards, *The Flight from Desire*, p. 66.

while that reforming bishop was in the act of pronouncing excommunication against him.[69]

A twelfth-century comital court such as William IX's was part of the institutional realization of lordship; it was dominated by, and existed to serve the authority of, a single local lord. Of those under her or his authority, some were attached to her or his service as household knights, as female companions to the lord (if she were female) or to the lord's wife, as stewards, or as young nobles seeking training and hoping to be 'knighted'. Of those under her or his (often only nominal) authority, some were lesser lords (male or female) in their own right, viscounts or untitled castellans within the count's orbit; they and their spouses could be drawn to court (on those occasions when the lord 'held court') for a variety of reasons: to build or maintain relationships with the lord and with one's fellows, to seek marriage partners for self or offspring, to bring a complaint against a person or institution within the lord's territory, to plot rebellion in the shadows.

Given the variety of motives for coming to such a court, in which the advance of one's own status was often paramount, court interactions and courtly expression were highly susceptible to irony, in the strict sense that one often had to say something while meaning something else.[70] Much of the humour of the court derived from bringing this irony gracefully to the attention of the group. Irony in the troubadour love song could take a variety of forms. The songwriter might actually feel love for no one, despite the poignancy of her or his song. Or, in refusing to name the beloved, or using only a nickname for the beloved, one might suggest an identity different from the real one. In claiming that she has refused the songwriter's advances, a troubadour might seek to protect his beloved's honour. Or the troubadour might offer the song as praise to the lord's lady (or the lord herself), in which case the longing to make love to her, expressed in the poem, was supposed to be taken as ironic exaggeration of one's admiration and dutiful submission. Troubadour songs echoed the elaborate posturing that was a survival skill at any court of the period.

[69] Pierre II's interdiction involved William IX's despoiling of certain Church property, according to Alfred Richard; it was renewed, in his view, by a papal legate in view of William's dismissal of his legitimate wife; see Richard, *Histoire des Comtes de Poitou*, II, 200–206. Gerald A. Bond, however, believes Pierre II's refusal to annul William IX's marriage to Philippa of Toulouse was the real bone of contention between them; see Bond, 'Introduction', pp. xxix–xxxiii; Reddy, *The Making of Romantic Love*, p. 76.

[70] A useful discussion of the meaning of 'irony' can be found in Gaunt, *Troubadours and Irony*, pp. 5–18.

William IX's ribald songs were written from the position of the lord who dominated the court. Only a few twelfth-century songwriters wrote from this position; for example, Raimbaut d'Orange or the Comtessa de Dia. Raimbaut also employed sarcasm and ribald innuendo. But no one did so with the hauteur displayed by William IX, one of the most powerful European lords of his day. In his ribald songs, his status as ruler is on display.

In Song 1, for example, he complains that he has two excellent lovers, Agnes and Arsen, who are jealous of each other, and who are thus forcing him to make a choice.[71] He would like to keep them both. But he formulates his complaint as a comment about two horses. It was a matter of course at the time for a knight to have more than one mount; if one horse were killed or wounded, then his page could quickly bring forward another, already well-trained and familiar. The availability of extra mounts could easily be a matter of life and death. William IX complains his two excellent mounts are jealous of each other. The idea of two horses being jealous of each other is absurd, and obviously not in accord with the military needs of a knight. William's joke is to treat the women as comparable to horses: greatly appreciated, utterly necessary, they ought to be properly submissive to the owner's will.

But within this joke there is a buried assumption about desire and pleasure. Horses can be replaced. One's relationship to a horse is not entirely personal; quite the opposite, it is instrumental. The horse's purpose is that one be carried boldly into battle. In similar fashion, William prefers to keep his current mounts.

> Si.ls pogues adomesgar a mon talen,
> Ja no volgr'aillors mudar mon garnimen
> Que meils for'encavalguatz de negun home viven.
>
> [If I could tame them to my liking,
> I would never want to take my equipment elsewhere,
> Because I would be better mounted than any man alive.] (lines 10–12)[72]

The clear implication, however, is that he could get other mounts if he had to. William IX's other ribald songs tell a similar story. Sexual pleasure, a necessary

[71] The Bond edition of William IX's songs is used here: William IX of Aquitaine, *The Poetry*, Song 1, pp. 2–5.

[72] William IX of Aquitaine, *The Poetry*, ed. and trans. by Bond, pp. 2–3. In addition, if William IX was attempting to treat both Philippa and Maubergeonne as his legitimate wives, as suggested in note 69 above, this song could be read as a comment on his difficulties with the Church in the mid-1110s.

element of noble life for both men and women, can only be obtained from an appropriately noble partner; some are better than others, but they are all of a kind. This is the language of a lord who has been surrounded his whole life by aspirants, eager for his favour. William wrote as if he could make as many jokes about it as he liked. Belittling his subordinates in this way (whether they were male or female) might alienate some of them some of the time, but any who were alienated could be replaced. William's humour was, therefore, itself an act of lordship or domination. As his subordinates laughed at his ribald songs, they must have realized at the same time that William was drawing a sharp line between himself and them.[73]

But William is also making a link between domination and sexual desire that was quite consonant with theological views of desire being promoted by the Gregorian Reform. It was the Church that now insisted, more stridently than before, that sexual desire was the manifestation of a bodily appetite like hunger or thirst. As such, it could be satisfied by any object of the appropriate type. It was not personal. As a great lord, William could replace a lover easily. And he associates this power with his desire — most crudely when he complains of those who guard 'cunt' in Song 3.[74] But he also insists on noblewomen's right to an appropriate partner in Song 2. Those who guard a noblewoman too closely, he insists, only force her to look for satisfaction with an underling or servant.[75] But if she is free to make love with a noble partner of her choice, all gain by it. 'Si com autra res en merma, | qui.n pana, e cons en creis' ('Although any other thing decreases, | if someone steals from it, the cunt increases').[76]

William is proposing that noble men and women both have an interest in relative freedom in the choice of lovers, an interest deriving from an impulse or craving to which they must respond, and which might threaten their honour if not properly satisfied. William was thus a pioneer in imagining a social context and social practices that would give life to the theologians' rather abstract idea of sexual desire as appetite. He saw a way to integrate desire-as-appetite

[73] Such jocular line-drawing is implicit in the story told by Geoffrey of Vigeois of William IX and Ebles of Ventadorn's friendly rivalry over who could make the most worthy dinner preparations for unexpected guests; see Geoffrey of Vigeois, *Chronica*, ch. 69, excerpted in William IX of Aquitaine, *The Poetry*, ed. and trans. by Bond, pp. 126–29.

[74] William IX of Aquitaine, *The Poetry*, ed. and trans. by Bond, pp. 10–13.

[75] On noblewomen's sexual needs, see Song 2, William IX of Aquitaine, *The Poetry*, ed. and trans. by Bond, pp. 6–9.

[76] Song 3, lines 11–12, in William IX of Aquitaine, *The Poetry*, ed. and trans. by Bond, pp. 10–11.

into the life of the court. A lord could not dominate her or his subordinates unless they were, to some extent, interchangeable; if one or a few rebelled, there must be enough who remained faithful to overwhelm the rebels. A lord could not afford to rely too much on any one person. Thus, in a period when a system of informal aristocratic polygamy was being attacked vigorously by clerical reformers, William IX's ribald songs reformulated the lord's politically shrewd granting of sexual favours as the honourable indulgence of a sexual appetite, as a kind of brazen aristocratic debauchery.

In William IX's love songs we find a sharply different perspective. William now writes as a subordinate, an aspirant, who begs a noble lady of great power to accord him her favour. Like a lesser lord whose political options were dominated by the presence of a nearby count, William now offers fealty that is utterly personal. There is no question of replacing the lady with another. (Even if one considered such a thing, a subordinate knew that all thought of changing sides must be carefully hidden at court.) The pleasure that William anticipates in his love songs is that of political protection that is expressed through, or sealed by, sexual caresses. The protection of lordship is explicitly (and ironically) associated with lovemaking in Song 9.

> Enquer me menbra d'un mati
> Que nos fezem de guera fi
> E que.m donet un don tan gran:
> Sa drudari'e son anel;
> Enquer me lais Dieus viure tan
> C'aia mas mans soz so mantel!
>
> [I still remember one morning
> When we put an end to war
> And when she gave me a gift so great:
> Her intimacy and her ring;
> God let me yet live long enough
> That I might have my hands beneath her cloak!] (lines 19–24)[77]

According to Rita Lejeune's convincing reading of this stanza, William jokingly sexualizes the ritual of submission of vassal to lord, which involved the giving of a ring and the joining of hands (the vassal's in prayer, the lord's around the vassal's). A vassal might well find himself with his hands beneath the lord's cloak. Thus, in this song, fealty is equated with sexual caress.[78]

[77] Song 10, in William IX of Aquitaine, *The Poetry*, ed. and trans. by Bond, pp. 36–39.

[78] Lejeune, *Littérature et société occitane au Moyen Âge*, pp. 141–50.

From these considerations, and others, it is evident that the idea of sexual pleasure, and the practices which that idea inspired, were undergoing a transformation in the twelfth century.[79] This transformation is all the more difficult for present-day historians to evaluate in that the change, on a practical level, was driven in part by an idea of sexual desire as an appetite, a notion already old, now being put to new uses, and which is still, eight centuries later, very close to the present-day commonsense notion of the sex drive.

What few scholars have recognized is that William IX's ribald songs are as innovative as his love songs. The idea that sexual craving was powerful and dangerous was put into dramatic sermons preached through the Loire valley, as well as William IX's own lands, by Robert of Arbrissel, among others between 1095 and 1115. Three women linked to William IX, his first two wives and a daughter, became nuns in Robert's monastery of Fontevrault after 1101.[80] William seemed to be protesting that, if we aristocrats are to remain outside the cloister, then we must be provided with appropriate 'mounts' lest we turn to ignoble sexual partners. But he also protested, in his love songs, that a sexual partnership was something more than an alliance to satisfy an appetite, that the theology was somehow implausible, in the end. From this latter insight grew the ideal of courtly love.

The idea of sexual desire as an appetite survived in various forms into recent times. As recent research has shown, when Christian theology lost its hegemony over thinking about human nature, beginning in the seventeenth century, aspiring social scientists were anxious to build secularized 'scientific' theories based on commonsense Western ideas about the human body. These commonsense ideas were, for the most part, of Christian origin.[81]

The idea of the 'pleasure center' of the brain, and the powerful cravings it could unleash, was believed to be settled science in the late twentieth century. It is an idea quite consonant with Christian doctrine about original sin and the reductionist style of thinking about sexuality associated with this doctrine. It is only in the last few years that the very lessons of brain architecture have begun to offer support for what every cultural historian must recognize, that is, that human experiences tend to be shaped holistically.[82] Before a 'desire' can

[79] An array of further evidence is examined in Reddy, *The Making of Romantic Love*.

[80] Zink, *Les Troubadours*, pp. 71–76; Reddy, *The Making of Romantic Love*, pp. 77–78.

[81] Especially revealing on this transition are Laqueur, *Solitary Sex*; Davidson, *The Emergence of Sexuality*.

[82] Compare the old and the new models of brain processes, for example, in Duncan and Feldman Barrett, 'Affect Is a Form of Cognition'.

be experienced as appetitive, a very substantial amount of learning must take place. This cultural learning intervenes between perception and action. Should anyone doubt the validity of this idea (as something more than just a methodological rule of thumb for cultural historians), the complex networks of response patterns recently mapped out by neuroscience show that higher levels of 'executive control' are deeply involved, from the very first few milliseconds, in any experience of 'pleasure'.

Works Cited

Primary Sources

Arnaut-Guilhem de Marsan, *L'Ensenhamen d'Arnaut-Guilhem de Marsan*, ed. by Jacques de Cauna, with a French trans. by Gerard Gouiran (Monein: Pyremond, 2007)

Map, Walter, *De Nugis Curialium, Courtiers' Trifles*, ed. and trans. by M. R. James, rev. by C. N. L. Brooke and R. A. B. Mynors (Oxford: Clarendon Press, 1983)

William IX of Aquitaine, *The Poetry of William VII, Count of Poitiers, IX Duke of Aquitaine*, ed. and trans. by Gerald A. Bond (New York: Garland, 1982)

Secondary Works

Arnsten, Amy F. T., 'Stress Signalling Pathways that Impair Prefrontal Cortex Structure and Function', *Nature Reviews Neuroscience*, 10 (2009), 410–22

Baldwin, John W., 'The Image of the Jongleur in Northern France around 1200', *Speculum*, 72 (1997), 635–63

Bar, Moshe, and others, 'Top-Down Facilitation of Visual Recognition', *Proceedings of the National Acadamy of Science*, 103 (2006), 449–54

Barlow, Frank, *Thomas Becket* (Berkeley: University of California Press, 1986)

Batterink, Laura, and others, 'The Role of Awareness in Semantic and Syntactic Processing: An ERP Attentional Blink Study', *Journal of Cognitive Neuroscience*, 22 (2009), 2514–29

Berridge, Kent C., 'Pleasures of the Brain', *Brain and Cognition*, 52 (2003), 106–28

Berridge, Kent C., and Morten L. Kringelbach, 'Neuroscience of Affect: Brain Mechanisms of Pleasure and Displeasure', *Current Opinion in Neurobiology*, 23 (2013), 294–303; <http://dx.doi.org/10.1016/j.conb.2013.01.017>

Bezzola Reto, 'Guillaume IX et les origines de l'amour courtois', *Romania*, 66 (1940), 145–237

——, *Les Origines et la formation de la littérature courtoise en occident (500–1200). Part II: La Société féodale et la transformation de la littérature de cour*, 2 vols (Paris: Champion, 1960)

Bloch, R. Howard, *Medieval Misogyny and the Invention of Western Romantic Love* (Chicago: University of Chicago Press, 1991)

Bond, Gerald A., 'Introduction', in William IX of Aquitaine, *The Poetry of William VII, Count of Poitiers, IX Duke of Aquitaine*, ed. and trans. by Gerald A. Bond (New York: Garland, 1982), pp. x–lxxxvii

Boquet, Damien, 'L'Amour en Occident … et ailleurs', *Les Émotions au Moyen Âge, carnet d'EMMA* (blog), 31 December 2012, <http://emma.hypotheses.org/1844> [accessed 20 November 2014]

——, *L'Ordre de l'affect au Moyen Âge: Autour de l'anthropologie affective d'Aelred de Rievaulx* (Caen: CRAHM, 2005)

Bowie, Colette Marie, 'The Daughters of Henry II and Eleanor of Aquitaine: A Comparative Study of Twelfth-Century Royal Women' (unpublished doctoral thesis, University of Glascow, 2011)

Bradbury, Jim, *Stephen and Matilda: The Civil War of 1139–53* (Stroud: Sutton, 1996)

Brown, Peter, *The Body and Society: Men, Women, and Sexual Renunciation in Early Christianity* (New York: Columbia University Press, 1988)

Cauna, Jacques de, 'Introduction', in Arnaut-Guilhem de Marsan, *L'Ensenhamen d'Arnaut-Guilhem de Marsan*, ed. by Jacques de Cauna, with a French trans. by Gerard Gouiran (Monein: Pyremond, 2007), pp. 5–61

Changeux, Jean-Pierre, and Paul Ricoeur, *Ce qui nous fait penser: La Nature et la règle* (Paris: Odile Jacob, 1998)

Chauvenet, Frédérique, 'L'Entourage de Richard Coeur de Lion en Poitou et en Aquitaine', in *La Cour Plantagenêt (1154–1204): Actes du Colloque tenu à Thouars du 30 avril au 2 mai 1999*, ed. by Martin Aurell (Poitiers: Université de Poitiers, Centre d'études supérieures de civilisation médiévale, 2000), pp. 137–49

Cheyette, Frederick L., *Ermengard of Narbonne and the World of the Troubadours* (Ithaca, NY: Cornell University Press, 2001)

Constable, Giles, 'The Alleged Disgrace of John of Salisbury in 1159', *English Historical Review*, 69 (1954), 67–76

Craig, A. D., 'How Do You Feel — Now? The Anterior Insula and Human Awareness', *Nature Reviews Neuroscience*, 10 (2009), 59–70

Crouch, David, *The Birth of Nobility: Constructing Aristocracy in England and France 900–1300* (Harlow: Pearson, 2005)

——, *William Marshal: Knighthood, War, and Chivalry, 1147–1219*, 2nd edn (London: Longman, 2002)

Cvetkovich, Ann, *An Archive of Feeling: Trauma, Sexuality, and Lesbian Public Cultures* (Durham, NC: Duke University Press, 2003)

Damaraju, Eswar, and others, 'Affective Learning Enhances Activity and Functional Connectivity in Early Visual Cortex', *Neuropsychologia*, 47 (2009), 2480–87

Davidson, Arnold I., *The Emergence of Sexuality: Historical Epistemology and the Formation of Concepts* (Cambridge, MA: Harvard University Press, 2001)

Decety, Jean, 'Dissecting the Neural Mechanisms Mediating Empathy', *Emotion Review*, 3 (2011), 92–108

Deluermoz, Quentin, and others, 'Écrire l'histoire des émotions: De l'objet à la catégorie d'analyse', *Revue d'histoire du XIXe siècle*, 47 (2013), 155–89

Duby, Georges, *The Knight, the Lady and the Priest: The Making of Modern Marriage in Medieval France*, trans. by Barbara Bray (New York: Pantheon, 1983)

Duncan, Seth, and Lisa Feldman Barrett, 'Affect Is a Form of Cognition: A Neurobiological Analysis', *Cognition and Emotion*, 21 (2007), 1184–1211

Edwards, Robert R., *The Flight from Desire: Augustine and Ovid to Chaucer* (New York: Palgrave Macmillan, 2006)

Ekman, Paul, 'Basic Emotions', in *Handbook of Cognition and Emotion*, ed. by T. Dalgleish and M. J. Powers (New York: Wiley, 1999), pp. 45–60

Flori, Jean, *Aliénor d'Aquitaine: La Reine insoumise* (Paris: Payot, 2004)
Gaunt, Simon, *Troubadours and Irony* (Cambridge: Cambridge University Press, 1989)
Gilbert, Charles D., and Wu Li, 'Top-Down Influences on Visual Processing', *Nature Reviews Neuroscience*, 14 (2013), 350–63
Gross, Daniel M., and Stephanie D. Preston, 'Emotion Science and the Heart of a Two-Cultures Problem', in *Science and Emotions after 1945: A Translatlantic Perspective*, ed. by Frank Biess and Daniel M. Gross (Chicago: University of Chicago Press, 2014), pp. 96–117
Havas, David A., and others, 'Cosmetic Use of Botulinum Toxin-A Affects Processing of Emotional Language', *Psychological Science*, 21 (2010), 895–900
Harvey, Ruth, 'The Wives of the "First Troubadour", Duke William IX of Aquitaine', *Journal of Medieval History*, 19 (1993), 307–25
Iacoboni, Marco, and Mirella Dapretto, 'The Mirror Neuron System and the Consequences of its Dysfunction', *Nature Reviews Neuroscience*, 7 (2006), 942–51
Jaeger, C. Stephen, *The Origins of Courtliness: Civilizing Trends and the Formation of Courtly Ideals, 939–1210* (Philadelphia: University of Pennsylvania Press, 1985)
Kosslyn, Stephen M., *Image and Brain: The Resolution of the Imagery Debate* (Cambridge, MA: MIT Press, 1994)
Kosslyn, Stephen M., and others, 'Brain rCBF and Performance in Visual Imagery Tasks: Common and Distinct Processes', *European Journal of Cognitive Psychology*, 16 (2004), 696–716
Kuefler, Mathew, 'Male Friendship and the Suspicion of Sodomy in Twelfth-Century France', in *The Boswell Thesis: Essays on Christianity, Social Tolerance, and Homosexuality*, ed. by Mathew Kuefler (Chicago: University of Chicago Press, 2006), pp. 179–212
Laqueur, Thomas W., *Solitary Sex: A Cultural History of Masturbation* (New York: Zone, 2003)
Larivière, Marianne, and others, 'Changes in Pain Perception and Descending Inhibitory Controls Start at Middle Age in Healthy Adults', *Clinical Journal of Pain*, 23 (2007), 506–10
Lejeune, Rita, *Littérature et société occitane au Moyen Âge* (Liège: Marche Romane, 1979)
Lemesle, Bruno, 'Le Comte d'Anjou face aux rébellions (1129–1151)', in *La Vengeance, 400–1200*, ed. by Dominique Barthélemy, François Bougard, and Régine Le Jan (Roma: École française de Rome, 2006), pp. 199–236
Littrell, Jill, 'Perspectives Emerging from Neuroscience on How People Become Addicted and What to Do About It', *Journal of Social Work Practice in the Addictions*, 10 (2010), 229–56
Marcus, Sharon, 'Queer Theory for Everyone: A Review Essay', *Signs*, 31 (2005), 191–218
Matter, E. Ann, *The Voice of my Beloved: The Song of Songs in Western Medieval Christianity* (Philadelphia: University of Pennsylvania Press, 1990)
McLaughlin, Megan, *Sex, Gender, and Episcopal Authority in an Age of Reform, 1000–1122* (Cambridge: Cambridge University Press, 2010)
Meyer, Michel, *Le Philosophe et les passions: Esquisse d'une histoire de la nature humaine* (Paris: Librairie générale française, 1991)

Monson, Don A., *Les Ensenhamens occitans: Essai de définition et de délimitation du genre* (Paris: Klinksieck, 1981)
Olds, James, 'Pleasure Centers in the Brain', *Scientific American*, 195 (1956), 105–16
Olds, James, and P. Milner, 'Positive Reinforcement Produced by Electrical Stimulation of Septal Area and Other Regions of Rat Brain', *Journal of Comparative and Physiological Psychology*, 47 (1954), 419–27
Pessoa, Luiz, 'Beyond Brain Regions: Network Perspective of Cognition–Emotion Interactions', *Behavioral and Brain Sciences*, 35 (2012), 158–59
——, 'Emotion and Cognition and the Amygdala: From "What Is It?" to "What's to Be Done?"', *Neuropsychologia*, 48 (2010), 3416–29
——, 'On the Relationship Between Emotion and Cognition', *Nature Reviews Neuroscience*, 9 (2008), 148–58
Pessoa, Luiz, and Ralph Adolphs, 'Emotion Processing and the Amygdala: From a "Low Road" to "Many Roads" of Evaluating Biological Significance', *Nature Reviews Neuroscience*, 11 (2010), 773–82
Poly, Jean-Pierre, *Le Chemin des amours barbares: Genèse médiévale de la sexualité européenne* (Paris: Perrin, 2003)
Reddy, William M. 'Historical Research on the Self and Emotions', *Emotion Review*, 1 (2009), 302–15
——, 'Humanists and the Experimental Study of Emotions', in *Science and Emotions after 1945: A Transnational Perspective*, ed. by Frank Biess and Daniel M. Gross (Chicago: University of Chicago Press, 2014), pp. 41–66
——, *The Making of Romantic Love: Longing and Sexuality in Europe, South Asia, and Japan (900–1200)* (Chicago: University of Chicago Press, 2012)
——, 'Neuroscience and the Fallacies of Functionalism', *History and Theory*, 49 (2010), 412–25
Richard, Alfred, *Histoire des Comtes de Poitou*, 3 vols (1903; repr. Monein: Pyremonde, 2005–08), II, 119–30
Salimpoor, Valorie N., and Robert J. Zatorre, 'Neural Interactions that Give Rise to Musical Pleasure', *Psychology of Esthetics, Creativity, and the Arts*, 7 (2013), 62–75
Salimpoor, Valorie N., and others, 'Anatomically Distinct Dopamine Release during Anticipation and Experience of Peak Emotion to Music', *Nature Neuroscience*, 14 (2011), 257–64
Salzman, C. Daniel, and Stefano Fusi, 'Emotion, Cognition, and Mental State Representation in Amygdala and Prefrontal Cortex', *Annual Review of Neuroscience*, 33 (2010), 173–202
Schultz, James A., *Courtly Love, Love of Courtliness, and the History of Sexuality* (Chicago: University of Chicago Press, 2006)
Sedgwick, Eve Kosofsky, and Adam Frank, *Touching Feeling: Affect, Pedagogy, Performativity* (Durham, NC: Duke University Press, 2003)
Strickland, Matthew, 'Arms and the Men: War, Loyalty and Lordship in Jordan Fantosme's Chronicle', in *Medieval Knighthood*, vol. IV, *Papers from the Fifth Strawberry Hill Conference 1990*, ed. by Christopher Harper-Bill and Ruth Harvey (Woodbridge: Boydell, 1992), pp. 187–220

Sullivan, Mark D., 'Finding Pain between Minds and Bodies', *Clinical Journal of Pain*, 17 (2001), 146–56

Türk, Egbert, '*Curialis Nugator — Il perfetto cortegiano*: Deux manières d'appréhender une même réalité sociale', in *La Cour Plantagenêt (1154–1204): Actes du Colloque tenu à Thouars du 30 avril au 2 mai 1999*, ed. by Martin Aurell (Poitiers: Université de Poitiers, Centre d'études supérieures de civilisation médiévale, 2000), pp. 217–28

——, *Nugae curialium: Le Regne d'Henri II Plantegenêt (1145–1189) et l'éthique politique* (Geneva: Droz, 1977)

Vigliocca, Valerie, and others, 'Nouns and Verbs in the Brain: A Review of Behavioural, Electrophysiological, Neuropsychological and Imaging Studies', *Neuroscience and Biobehavioral Reviews*, 35 (2011), 407–26

Vincent, Nicholas, 'The Court of Henry II', in *Henry II: New Interpretations*, ed. by Christopher Harper-Bill and Nicholas Vincent (Woodbridge: Boydell, 2007), pp. 278–334

White, Stephen D., 'The Politics of Anger', in *Anger's Past: The Social Uses of an Emotion in the Middle Ages*, ed. Barbara H. Rosenwein (Ithaca, NY: Cornell University Press, 1998), pp. 127–52

Wouters, Cas, 'Comment les processus de civilisations se sont-ils prolongés?', *Vingtième Siècle: Revue d'histoire*, no. 106 (2010), 161–75

Yee, Eiling, and Julie C. Sedivy, 'Eye Movements to Pictures Reveal Transient Semantic Activation during Spoken Word Recognition', *Journal of Experimental Psychology: Learning, Memory, and Cognition*, 32 (2006), 1–14

Zink, Michel, *Les Troubadours: Une histoire poétique* (Paris: Perrin, 2013)

Didactic Pleasures

Taking Pleasure in Virtues and Vices: Alcuin's Manual for Count Wido

Barbara H. Rosenwein*

For Mayke de Jong, Carolingianist extraordinaire

The Carolingian scholar and courtier Alcuin (d. 804) wrote a treatise on the virtues and vices that hardly mentioned pleasure. And yet I shall argue here that Alcuin meant his treatise as a whole to bring pleasure, that is, to be a source of pleasure to its initial reader, Wido (a powerful Carolingian layman), and to those who came after him. Further, I shall argue that although Alcuin wrote about what he called virtues and vices, we may think of them as emotions. This is because, by the time Alcuin was writing, the pagan classical tradition regarding the emotions (variously called *pathe*, *perturbationes*, *passiones*, *motus animi*, and so on) had been largely assimilated into Christian schemes of the virtues and vices. Alcuin's treatise was a forerunner of the emotional self-help books that we see today. These, too, rarely talk directly about pleasure. But they mean to bring tranquility and peace to their modern readers. Those are the pleasures that this paper is about.

My neighbourhood public library devotes many shelves to books on emotions written by experts to help laypeople cope with the challenges of their private and public lives. Some of these books have grand pretensions. Edmund Bourne and Lorna Garano, for example, want to help everyone deal with anxiety. They provide what they describe as 'an array of simple tools to help you find

* I reuse here parts of my article 'Rereading *Askese und Laster*: The Case of Alcuin', by kind permission of Andreas Schwarcz. I thank Riccardo Cristiani for helping me think through Alcuin's work in general and for his many interventions on this paper in particular.

Barbara H. Rosenwein (brosenw@gmail.com) is professor emerita of Loyola University, Chicago.

Pleasure in the Middle Ages, ed. by Naama Cohen-Hanegbi and Piroska Nagy, IMR 24 (Turnhout: Brepols, 2018), pp. 167–179 BREPOLS PUBLISHERS 10.1484/M.IMR-EB.5.113466

greater calm and stability in the midst of complex, even chaotic times'.[1] Mark Epstein asserts that all lives are filled with traumas. Therefore, with Buddhism as his guide, he hopes to show his readers how traumas can be 'bearable, even illuminating'.[2] Mihály Csíkszentmihályi asks what in human life generates 'happiness' and 'enjoyment'. He arrives at the notion of 'flow' — the feeling of 'being carried away by a current' as we pursue a task that absorbs our attention.[3] He hopes that by showing how 'flow' is a natural outcome of human evolution, he will help 'build a stable, meaningful future'.[4]

Other emotions self-help books are directed to a specific readership. Self-help author Barbara Sher, for example, anxious to make a middle-aged audience happier, assures them that 'you're about to embark on an amazing new beginning'.[5] Likewise, Jungian analyst James Hillman speaks to the aging, finding uplifting potential despite the ailments of old age: memory loss, heart attacks, and so on. For example, he reminds readers that the heart that loves never fails no matter what happens to the physical heart. In this way, he intends his book to offer 'the promise of refreshing the reader's mind'.[6] Again addressing a specific readership, Elisabeth Kübler-Ross and David Kessler offer solace to the bereaved by outlining the 'five stages of loss'. They hope that their insights may make 'us better equipped to cope with life and loss'.[7] With an even narrower audience in mind, Ellen Mohr Catalano and Nina Sonenberg offer methods to cure compulsive shoppers. They promise the reader the ability 'to master your problem'. Ultimately, they hope, their step-by-step method will 'help you reach your own will, wisdom, and desire for change. With these forces, there is no problem you cannot resolve'.[8]

These are strong claims. They seem particularly modern. In fact, however, they have a deep ancestry. That is the case with the treatise written at some point between 801 and 804 by Alcuin.[9] Like modern 'self-help' books, his *On*

[1] Bourne and Garano, *Coping with Anxiety*, p. ix.

[2] Epstein, *The Trauma of Everyday Life*, p. 3.

[3] Csíkszentmihályi, *The Evolving Self*, p. xiii.

[4] Csíkszentmihályi, *The Evolving Self*, p. xvi.

[5] Sher, *It's Only Too Late If You Don't Start Now*, p. xiii. See her website: <http://barbarasher.com/index.htm>.

[6] Hillman, *The Force of Character and the Lasting Life*, p. xiii.

[7] Kübler-Ross and Kessler, *On Grief and Grieving*, p. 7.

[8] Catalano and Sonenberg, *Consuming Passions*, pp. 4, 7.

[9] Alcuin, *De virtutibus et vitiis*, ed. by Migne [henceforth *DVV*]. Alcuin was at Tours in

the Virtues and Vices was directed to a layman, in this case the powerful warrior and aristocrat Wido, count of the Breton march. Like Barbara Sher, Alcuin provided his reader with short chapters, which he termed *sermones* (sermons) and provided with short titles. He did so, Alcuin said, in order that 'my words may inhere more easily in the memory of your devotion, knowing that you are busy in many reflections on secular matters'.[10] The idea was, apparently, for Wido to hurry home to read one chapter or another as his worldly cares allowed. Finally, like the authors of modern self-help books, Alcuin meant his treatise to make his reader happier. In his dedicatory epistle, he noted that Wido, who was involved 'in warlike matters', had asked him for guidance. Alcuin wanted to give him solace (*solatium*) via his little book, 'so that your *animus*' (mind? soul? spirit? we shall have to return to this word), 'fatigued by external troubles (*molestiis*), may make a reversion to itself in which it may rejoice (*in quo gaudeat*)'.[11] Compare this to Bourne and Garano's purposes in their book on anxiety, or Hillman's hope to refresh his reader's mind. All of these authors wished to bring a kind of pleasure to their readership by implementing an emotional transformation. In the case of Alcuin, it was from an *animus* weighed down by troubles to one joyously returned to itself. Why did he think his moral treatise would have this effect? I argue in this paper that his treatise was as much about emotions as it was about morality, and, like the modern authors, Alcuin assumed that understanding and mastering emotions was the key to happiness.

* * *

It was not just Wido who constituted Alcuin's readership. His treatise *On the Virtues and Vices* was enormously popular throughout the Middle Ages, with over 140 manuscripts extant and translations into a number of vernacular languages.[12] The solace that it offered was general and long-lasting.

801 and died there in 804. For the date of the treatise, see Dubreucq, 'Autour du *De virtutibus et vitiis* d'Alcuin', pp. 269–70, and Sedlmeier, *Die laienparänetischen Schriften der Karolingerzeit*, pp. 120–21. For Wido, see Smith, *Province and Empire*, pp. 52–53, 67–68.

[10] The opening letter and the final *peroratio* of the treatise were edited separately as Alcuin, *Epistola* 305, ed. by Dümmler, here p. 464: 'Quatenus facilius vestrae devotionis memoriae haec mea dicta inhaerere potuissent, sciens te in multis saecularium rerum cogitationibus occupatum'.

[11] Alcuin, *Epistola* 305, ed. by Dümmler, p. 464: 'ut animus exterioribus fatigatus molestiis, ad se ipsum reversus habeat, in quo gaudeat'. To be sure, it was a topos of the time to claim that one wrote on request. See Wallach, *Alcuin and Charlemagne*, pp. 232–33, and Dubreucq, 'Autour du *De virtutibus et vitiis* d'Alcuin', p. 271.

[12] Szarmach, 'A Preliminary Handlist of Manuscripts'.

What sort of treatise was it? Alcuin himself did not call it *On the Virtues and Vices*. That title came from Alcuin's anonymous biographer.[13] Rather, Alcuin called it *Sentences of Paternal Admonition*.[14] Mayke de Jong has explored the meaning of the admonitory tradition in the Carolingian period.[15] It harked back to Gregory the Great's *Pastoral Care*. Gregory saw the pastor as a kind of therapist: he should 'enter into' the emotional lives of his flock in order to lead them to better thoughts, feelings, and behaviours.[16] Writing for clerics, he advised them, for example, 'how to admonish in one way those who are happy and in another way those who are sad'.[17] His method was to remind the happy about the tortures awaiting them while telling the sad about the joys of heaven. With a lay audience, Alcuin's task was a bit different: it was to give Wido a basic guide to dealing with all his emotional and moral states.

Composed of thirty-five chapters, Alcuin's treatise began with a short discussion of wisdom. Thereafter came three chapters on the theological virtues (faith, charity, and hope), followed by one on the importance of reading. Chapters 6–26 covered various virtues alongside what Donald Bullough has called 'spiritual exercises': such activities as confession and penance and such feelings as compunction of heart.[18] Chapters 27–34 covered the eight principal vices (listed by Alcuin as pride, gluttony, fornication, avarice, anger, acedia, sadness, and vainglory) while chapter 35 summarized what Alcuin had said about the four cardinal virtues (prudence, justice, fortitude, and temperance) in an earlier treatise, his *Disputatio de rhetorica*.[19] Finally, the treatise was bookended by letters: the dedication, already mentioned, and a final epistle in which Alcuin assured Wido that even the habits of a layman and his secular way of life did not close the door to celestial beatitude.[20]

Although its purpose — a moral guide for a layman — was quite cutting edge for the Carolingian period, the contents of *On the Virtues and Vices* were not.[21]

[13] *Vita Alcuini*, ed. by Arndt, p. 195.

[14] He did so in his dedicatory letter to the treatise: see Alcuin, *Epistola* 305, ed. by Dümmler, p. 464: 'paternae ammonitionis sententias'.

[15] De Jong, *The Penitential State*, pp. 118–22.

[16] See Rosenwein, *Emotional Communities in the Early Middle Ages*, ch. 3.

[17] Gregory the Great, *Pastoral Care* III.3, ed. by Rommel, trans. by Morel, p. 272: 'Quod aliter ammonendi sunt laeti atque aliter tristes'.

[18] Bullough, 'Alcuin and Lay Virtue', pp. 85–87, quote at p. 85 n. 53.

[19] Alcuin, *Disputatio de rhetorica*, ed. and trans. by Howell, pp. 146–52.

[20] Alcuin, *Epistola* 305, ed. by Dümmler, pp. 464–65.

[21] Sedlmeier, *Die laienparänetischen Schriften der Karolingerzeit*, p. 7, points out that mir-

Indeed, the entire treatise is a pastiche of commonplaces drawn from earlier authors such as Cassian, Defensor of Ligugé, Gregory the Great, and Isidore of Seville. Not long ago pseudo-Augustine would have been added to the list, but Donald Bullough has argued convincingly that passages that used to be attributed to pseudo-Augustine were probably written by Alcuin himself.[22]

There is indeed some solace to be derived from reading and rereading well-known pieties. But what made the treatise most useful, I submit, was Alcuin's handy and succinct presentation of the emotions that Wido might feel and how he should deal with them. How is it possible to say that a compendium of 'virtues and vices' (as his ninth-century biographer put it) or 'admonitions' (as Alcuin termed it) was in fact a popularization of thought about emotions? There is really nothing very remarkable in doing so. The emotions and the virtues-vices tradition had always been two sides of the same coin. When Aristotle

rors for laymen began at the end of the eighth century and continued only for about fifty years thereafter. His own study, designed as an 'umfassende Untersuchung' of the genre, takes up only five texts.

[22] Rochais, 'Le *Liber de virtutibus et vitiis* d'Alcuin', argued that most of Alcuin's treatise depended on Defensor of Ligugé. This was roundly disputed by Wallach, *Alcuin and Charlemagne*, pp. 236–37, who asserted that Alcuin's sources were, rather, Isidore of Seville, *Sententiae* and pseudo-Augustine, *Sermones* 98, 108, 254, 291, 297, 302, and 304. Much more recently, Bullough, 'Alcuin and Lay Virtue', pp. 85–87, pointed out that some of the Latin flourishes in pseudo-Augustine, *Sermo* 302 were characteristic of Alcuin and, further, that there is no independent manuscript tradition for the sermon until its transmission by Hrabanus Maurus, a student of Alcuin (see *Clavis patristica pseudepigraphorum medii aevi*, ed. by Machielsen, IA, no. 1087). Bullough concluded that 'it is surely far more probable that Hrabanus's homily-text is one of a series in which he has combined extracts from one or more chapters of the *De virtutibus et vitiis* with prefatory and concluding passages of his own. It would therefore be Alcuin who originally drew on the *Sententiae* [of Isidore of Seville]'. The *Clavis patristica* suggests that the same manuscript tradition was the case with pseudo-Augustine, *Sermones* 98 (no. 883), 108 (no. 893), 291 (no. 1076), and 304 (no. 1089), i.e. there is no independent source for them until Hrabanus's homilary. That leaves pseudo-Augustine's *Sermo* 254 unaccounted for, but Bullough, *Alcuin*, pp. 354–55, argues that this too is Alcuin's, albeit heavily dependent on 'two or three different works of Isidore', namely the *Sententiae*, the *Synonyma*, and the pseudo-Isidorian *Testimoniae divinae scripturae et patrum*. The sermons of pseudo-Augustine used by Hrabanus are listed in Étaix, 'Le Recueil de sermons composé par Raban Maur pour Haistulfe de Mayence'. Wallach, *Alcuin and Charlemagne*, pp. 242–46, 252–54, adduces other sources for Alcuin, including Peter Chrysologus, *Sermo* 53, Caesarius of Arles, *Sermo* 18, Gregory the Great, *Moralia in Iob*, and Cassian, *Collationes*. Dubreucq, 'Autour du *De virtutibus et vitiis* d'Alcuin', p. 274, adds Julian Pomerius, *De vita contemplativa*. Sedlmeier, *Die laienparänetischen Schriften der Karolingerzeit*, p. 130, suggests a different way to think about source use: not *which* source but how closely (or loosely) Alcuin quoted them.

argued that virtue was the mean between vicious extremes, he specified that feeling fear, desire, anger, or pity 'at the right time, on the right occasion, towards the right people, for the right purpose and in the right manner, is to feel the best amount of them, which is the mean amount — and the best amount is of course the mark of virtue'.[23] The Stoics, who elaborated influential theories of the emotions, considered almost all of them to be bad, hence vicious. But they did admit a few emotions, *eupatheiai*, to be good, hence virtuous.[24] The early Christian ascetic tradition as practiced, for example, by Evagrius Ponticus in the fourth century theorized that the emotions were 'bad thoughts' sent by the demons. They should be countered by other 'bad thoughts' in a psychomachia, literally psychological warfare.[25] In the fifth century, John Cassian considered the emotions (he called them *commotiones* and *passiones*) to be vices (*vitia*), and he suggested countering them by withdrawal from the material world.[26] But Augustine, writing around the same time as Cassian, had a more positive take. He thought that emotions were connected to the will. When the will was right (*voluntas recta*) — when, that is, it was directed towards God — the emotions were virtues; when the will was turned away from God, they were vices.[27]

Gregory the Great (d. 604) grafted this more positive view onto the ascetic's distrust of emotions. In general, Gregory condemned emotions as 'cogitations (*cogitationes*)' that tended to overwhelm the mind if not kept in check. In a famous passage on those cogitations, he named the seven capital vices (*inanis gloria*, *invidia*, *ira*, *tristitia*, *avaritia*, *ventris ingluvies*, and *luxuria*), visualizing them organically as a sort of tree with pride (*superbia*) as its root. Gregory aimed to extirpate all of them, root and branch. However, sometimes, as when the pastor needed to reach out to his flock, a few emotions had to be enlisted to help weaker men rise to their salvific potential. In this way, even by the time of Gregory, virtues and vices had become more or less equivalent to emotions. And Gregory, like Augustine, thought that, if rightly used, emotions could be praiseworthy.[28]

[23] Aristotle, *Nicomachean Ethics*, II.3, trans. by Rackham, p. 93.

[24] For a convenient review of Stoic theory, see Sorabji, *Emotion and Peace of Mind*, esp. pp. 29–54.

[25] Rosenwein, *Emotional Communities in the Early Middle Ages*, pp. 46–47.

[26] See Rosenwein, *Emotional Communities in the Early Middle Ages*, ch. 1.

[27] See Rosenwein, 'Christianizing Cicero's *Perturbationes*', esp. pp. 36–40.

[28] See Rosenwein, *Emotional Communities in the Early Middle Ages*, ch. 3.

Most modern studies of medieval emotion theories stop around the time of Augustine and pick up only with twelfth-century monks like Saint Bernard and scholastics like Abelard.[29] But recently, Edward Peters has suggested that the period in between also had its psychological theorists. They wrote what Peters called 'moral theology', not doctrine or theory. They were 'therapists' rather than philosophers or theologians. Peters dubbed their writings 'paleopsychology'.[30] Alcuin's treatise is a good example of the genre.[31]

Because it was meant to be therapeutic, Alcuin's treatise had two salient features that I will take up in this paper. First, emotions did not come from an external source, but rather from within the individual. Second, emotions were not stable but followed various steps as they developed.

* * *

Alcuin associated emotions (which, as we have seen, were largely the same as virtues and vices) with a variety of sites pertaining either to the body or to the soul. In this he was eclectic, simply allowing his sources to assign the site. The important point for him was to make clear that, in the words of Edward Peters, men and women were 'autonomous human actors' moved 'to think, feel, and act as they did' by their own 'physiology, spirit, and intellect'.[32] From Cicero, whose *De inventione* Alcuin knew well, he learned that the *animus* was the home of both reason (*ratio*) and the unreasonable *affectiones* (feelings).[33] (The word *animus* had had a variety of meanings even in Cicero's day: it was the rational soul, the mind, the will, memory, consciousness, the heart, and so on.[34] That is why I do not translate it here.) When Alcuin gave the purpose of his treatise, he said it was for the *animus* to make a joyful return to itself. He also connected the *animus* to compassion for, as he wrote, 'we merit the mercy (*misericordiam*) of God and forgiveness of our sins by [our] compassion (*miseratione*) and alms to the poor, since he who does not turn his *animus* away from

[29] For example Casagrande and Vecchio, 'Les Théories des passions dans la culture médiévale'; Knuuttila, *Emotions in Ancient and Medieval Philosophy*, chs 2 and 3.

[30] Peters, '*Vir inconstans*'.

[31] Indeed, Peters, '*Vir inconstans*', p. 69, cites this work.

[32] Peters, '*Vir inconstans*', p. 59.

[33] Cicero, *De inventione*, I.2, trans. by Hubbell, p. 4, for *ratio animi* and I.41 (p. 80) for *affectio animi*. Alcuin used the *De inventione* in his *Disputatio de rhetorica*.

[34] Lewis and Short, *A Latin Dictionary*, *s.v.*

the poor quickly turns the Lord's ear to himself'.[35] Sometimes he connected the *animus* to envy as well: 'Nothing can be more evil than envy', and 'every envious man is tormented in his *animus*'.[36]

But for Alcuin the *animus* was just one site of the emotions. Envy, which tormented the *animus* (as we have just seen), also 'vexes the sense (*sensum*), burns the breast (*pectus*), and afflicts the mind (*mentem*)'.[37] In short it was a global infection, and to understand and describe it, Alcuin gladly drew on a large panoply of notions about the human faculties involved in motivation and action. The biblical injunction to 'love God with all your heart (*cor*), soul (*anima*), and mind (*mens*)' allowed him to link the emotions to all of them.

Consider compunction. Typically, Alcuin — drawing from the *conpunctum corde* of Psalm 108. 17 and other sources — paired it with the heart in the phrase *compunctio cordis*.[38] An offspring of humility, compunction was the key emotion involved in confession, penitence, and pardon. Alcuin, drawing on traditional formulations, put the heart effectively within the mind when he said that 'compunction of heart is the humility of the mind (*humilitas mentis*)'.[39] Nor were heart and mind enough; the soul/spirit (*anima*) was involved as well: 'The *anima* of a person, which is pricked (*compungitur*) in prayer, is extremely effective for salvation. When compunction is poured forth through prayer, without doubt the presence of the Holy Spirit is there in our hearts'.[40]

[35] *DVV*, col. 625: 'Ita misericordiam Dei et indulgentiam peccatorum nostrorum, pauperum miseratione et eleemosynis meremur: quoniam qui suum ab inope non avertit animum, cito ad se Domini convertit auditum'.

[36] *DVV*, col. 630: 'Nihil nequius potest esse invidia [...]. Omnis enim invidus animo torquetur'.

[37] *DVV*, col. 630: 'Invidia sensum mordet, pectus urit, mentem affligit'. Lockett, *Anglo-Saxon Psychologies in the Vernacular and Latin Traditions*, pp. 284–99, discusses Alcuin's approach to the nature of the soul in his *De anima*: he tended to 'whitewash over pertinent controversies' (p. 296) such as the materiality or non-materiality of the soul. Alcuin presumably knew Augustine's work on the soul; Augustine (see p. 186) at times specified the relationships among the *anima*, *animus*, and *mens*. But at other times, as in his *Soliloquia*, he left the question hanging.

[38] *DVV*, cols 620–21, includes an entire chapter 'de compunctione cordis' (on compunction of the heart). For the affective import of this term, see Nagy, *Le Don des larmes au Moyen Âge*, pp. 425–30.

[39] *DVV*, col. 620: 'Compunctio cordis est humilitas mentis'.

[40] *DVV*, col. 621: 'Anima hominis quae in oratione compungitur, valde illi proficit ad salutem. Cum per orationem compunctio effunditur, Spiritus sancti praesentiam adesse cordibus nostris non dubium est'.

Not every chapter of Alcuin's treatise was about an emotion. Wisdom (*sapientia*), the subject of his first chapter, for example, was about a changeless goal. Unlike the virtues and vices, wisdom was not (at least in Alcuin's treatment of it) 'perfectible', mutable, or subject to human control. But the virtues and vices were different. Alcuin accepted Augustine's dictum: if rightly directed, emotions led to God; if wrongly directed, they led to perdition. He made clear, for example, that anger (*ira*, *iracundia*) might be both virtuous and vicious: 'Anger is just and necessary when a person gets angry against his own sins and is indignant against himself when he does evil'.[41] But 'anger is wicked when it disturbs the mind such that it loses its proper capacity of judgement'.[42]

If, as I am arguing here, the virtues and vices were indeed equivalent to the emotions for Alcuin, then we may say that he named some thirty-seven emotions in this treatise. That's not a bad haul. To be sure, it does not match the multiple terms that may be found in ancient theoretical discussions, as, for example, in Cicero's *Tusculan Disputations*.[43] But even more important than quantity is content. Cicero never mentioned *acedia*, *avaritia*, or *compunctio*. Alcuin's list did not include Cicero's many words of distress and anxiety, such as *aegritudo* (distress), *adflictatio* (misery), and *lamentatio* (lamentation). The differences point up the fact that emotions — how they are defined and which ones are emphasized — change over time. Nevertheless, the differences should not blot out the similarities: *both* lists have *desiderium* (desire), *desperatio* (despair), *gaudium* (joy), *invidia* (envy), *ira* (anger), *laetitia* (happiness), and many other terms.

* * *

Along with the shift from pure theory, as exemplified by Cicero's *Tusculan Disputations*, to the works of moral theology, such as Alcuin's treatise, came a new interest in how the emotions worked together. This is the second feature of his therapeutic approach I wish to stress. Because, unlike the Stoics, Alcuin was not interested in extirpating all emotions but rather was, like Augustine of Hippo and Gregory the Great, interested in how emotions might aid the salvific process, he spent time on how one emotion led to another or, indeed, might be transformed into something else.

[41] *DVV*, col. 631: 'Illa ira est justa et necessaria, quando homo contra propria irascitur peccata, et contra seipsum indignatur, dum male agit'.

[42] *DVV*, col. 631: 'Illa ira mala est, quae mentem turbat, ut rectum consilium perdat'.

[43] See Rosenwein, 'Christianizing Cicero's *Perturbationes*', pp. 34–35.

Consider Alcuin's discussion of sadness, *De tristitia*. It comes in the middle of his discussion of the eight principal vices, largely but by no means entirely borrowed from Gregory the Great. Alcuin's account of sadness is short enough to present in full:

> Tristitiae duo sunt genera: unum salutiferum, alterum pestiferum. Tristitia salutaris est, quando de peccatis suis animus contristatur peccatoris, et ita contristatur, ut confessionem et poenitentiam agere quaerat, et converti se ad Deum desideret. Alia est tristitia hujus saeculi, quae mortem operatur animae, quae nihil in bono opere proficere valet, quae animum perturbat, et saepe in desperationem mittit, ut futurorum spem abstollat bonorum. Ex ipsa nascitur malitia, rancor, animi pusillanimitas, amaritudo, desperatio. Saepe etiam et praesentis vitae nulla delectatio. Quae vincitur per laetitiam spiritualem, et spem futurorum, et consolationem Scripturarum, et fraternum [in spirituali jucunditate] colloquium.[44]
>
> [There are two sorts of sadness, one salvific, the other destructive. Sadness is salvific when the mind (*animus*) of the sinner is made sad (*contristatur*) by its own sins; and it is so saddened (*contristatur*) that it seeks to do confession and penance and desires itself to be turned (*converti se […] desideret*) to God. The other is the sadness of this world, which brings about the death of the soul (*animae*), which does not manage to produce anything good, which perturbs (*perturbat*) the mind and often drives it to despair (*desperationem*), so that it takes away the hope (*spem*) of future good things. From [this sort of sadness] are born malice, rancor, weakness of mind, bitterness, and despair. Often there is even no delight (*delectatio*) in the present life. [This sadness] is conquered by spiritual happiness (*laetitiam spiritualem*) and hope (*spem*) of future things, the consolation (*consolationem*) of Scripture, and fraternal talk in spiritual jocularity (*jucunditate*).]

Let us unpack this chapter. There is movement and change at every moment. Salvific sadness starts with sin. Then, conscious of his (or her) sinfulness, the sinner moves to confess and do penance and thence desires to be 'converted (*converti*)' to God. Worldly sadness, on the other hand, leads ultimately to the death of the soul by first 'perturbing' the mind, that is, stirring it up with the sorts of anxieties that led Cicero to call *all* emotions *perturbationes*.[45] Then worldly sadness leads to despair. But there are specific antidotes. While Gregory the Great had told the pastor simply to tell the sad members of his flock about the joys of heaven, Alcuin named two abstract ideas — spiritual happiness and

[44] *DVV*, col. 635.

[45] In the *Tusculan Disputations*, Cicero translated the Stoic *pathe* by the Latin *perturbationes animi*. See Rosenwein, 'Christianizing Cicero's *Perturbationes*', pp. 31–36.

hope — but also two specific salves: the Bible and a certain kind of conversation, perhaps of the sort that Alcuin 'recorded' in his dialogue on rhetoric.[46]

* * *

What pleasure did Alcuin expect Wido to get out of his therapy? While Alcuin had a very different view of the human condition than do the writers of modern self-help manuals, nevertheless there are also some continuities. Just as Catalano and Sonenberg hoped that compulsive shoppers would master their impulses by better understanding them, so Alcuin meant Wido to gain better control over his feelings and acts. Just as Bourne and Garano provided 'simple tools' for anxieties, Alcuin gave specific antidotes for unwelcome and immoral feelings. And just as Kübler-Ross and Kessler told the bereaved what stages of grief they should expect, so Alcuin listed the steps by which sadness would ascend to godliness or descend to suicide. Like modern self-help books, Alcuin's treatise offered a kind of wisdom. It is no accident that the first chapter of his treatise was *de sapientia*, which, as he said, was the key to the *vita beata*. Is not the *vita beata* the goal of every life, even today?

[46] Alcuin, *Disputatio de rhetorica*, is presented as a pleasing and enlightening dialogue between a 'wise pupil' and a 'revered master'.

Works Cited

Primary Sources

Alcuin, *De virtutibus et vitiis liber ad Widonem comitem*, in *PL*, CI, cols 613–38

——, *Disputatio de rhetorica et de virtutibus sapientissimi Regis Caroli et Albini magistri*, in *The Rhetoric of Alcuin and Charlemagne: A Translation, with an Introduction, the Latin Text, and Notes*, ed. and trans. by Wilbur Samuel Howell (Princeton, NJ: Princeton University Press, 1941)

——, *Epistola* 305, ed. by Ernst Dümmler, in *Epistolae Karolini aevi*, II, MGH Epistolae, 4 (Berlin: Monumenta Germaniae Historica, 1895; repr. 1994), pp. 464–65

Aristotle, *Nicomachean Ethics*, trans. by Harris Rackham, Loeb Classical Library, 73 (Cambridge, MA: Harvard University Press, 1932)

Cicero, *De inventione*, in Cicero, *On Invention*, trans. by Harry M. Hubbell, Loeb Classical Library, 386 (Cambridge, MA: Harvard University Press, 1960)

Clavis patristica pseudepigraphorum medii aevi, IA–B, ed. by John J. Machielsen (Turnhout: Brepols, 1990)

Gregory the Great, *Pastoral Care*, in Grégoire le Grand, *Règle pastorale II*, ed. by Floribert Rommel, trans. by Charles Morel, Sources chrétiennes, 382 (Paris: Editions du Cerf, 1992)

Vita Alcuini, ed. by Wilhelm Arndt, MGH Scriptores, 15.1 (Hannover: Monumenta Germaniae Historica, 1887), pp. 185–97

Secondary Works

Bourne, Edmund J., and Lorna Garano, *Coping with Anxiety: 10 Simple Ways to Relieve Anxiety, Fear & Worry* (Oakland, CA: New Harbinger, 2003)

Bullough, Donald A., *Alcuin: Achievement and Reputation* (Leiden: Brill, 2004)

——, 'Alcuin and Lay Virtue', in *Predicazione e società nel medioevo: riflessione etica, valori e modelli di comportamento* (*Preaching and Society in the Middle Ages. Ethics, Values and Social Behaviour*), ed. by Laura Gaffuri and Riccardo Quinto (Padova: Centro Studi Antoniani, 2002), pp. 71–92

Casagrande, Carla, and Silvana Vecchio, 'Les Théories des passions dans la culture médiévale', in *Le Sujet des émotions au Moyen Âge*, ed. by Piroska Nagy and Damien Boquet (Paris: Beauchesne, 2008), pp. 107–22

Catalano, Ellen Mohr, and Nina Sonenberg, *Consuming Passions: Help for Compulsive Shoppers* (Oakland, CA: New Harbinger, 1993)

Csíkszentmihályi, Mihály, *The Evolving Self: A Psychology for the Third Millennium* (New York: Harper, 1994)

Dubreucq, Alain, 'Autour du *De virtutibus et vitiis* d'Alcuin', in *Alcuin, de York à Tours: Écriture, pouvoir et réseaux dans l'Europe du haut Moyen Âge*, ed. by Philippe Depreux and Bruno Judic (Rennes: Presses Universitaires de Rennes, 2004), pp. 269–88

Epstein, Mark, *The Trauma of Everyday Life* (New York: Penguin, 2013)
Étaix, Raymond, 'Le Recueil de sermons composé par Raban Maur pour Haistulfe de Mayence', *Revue des Études Augustiniennes*, 32 (1986), 124–37
Hillman, James, *The Force of Character and the Lasting Life* (New York: Random House, 1999)
Jong, Mayke de, *The Penitential State: Authority and Atonement in the Age of Louis the Pious, 814–840* (Cambridge: Cambridge University Press, 2009)
Knuuttila, Simo, *Emotions in Ancient and Medieval Philosophy* (Oxford: Clarendon Press, 2004)
Kübler-Ross, Elisabeth, and David Kessler, *On Grief and Grieving: Finding the Meaning of Grief through the Five Stages of Loss* (New York: Scribner, 2005)
Lewis, Charlton T., and Charles Short, eds, *A Latin Dictionary* (Oxford: Clarendon Press, 1879)
Lockett, Leslie, *Anglo-Saxon Psychologies in the Vernacular and Latin Traditions* (Toronto: University of Toronto Press, 2011)
Nagy, Piroska, *Le Don des larmes au Moyen Âge: Un instrument spirituel en quête d'institution, v^e^–xiiie siècle* (Paris: Albin Michel, 2000)
Peters, Edward, '*Vir inconstans*: Moral Theology as Palaeopsychology', in *In the Garden of Evil: The Vices and Culture in the Middle Ages*, ed. by Richard Newhauser, Papers in Mediaeval Studies, 18 (Toronto: Pontifical Institute of Mediaeval Studies, 2005), pp. 59–73
Rochais, Henri, 'Le *Liber de virtutibus et vitiis* d'Alcuin', *Revue Mabillon*, 41 (1951), 77–86
Rosenwein, Barbara H., 'Christianizing Cicero's *Perturbationes*', *Quaestiones Medii Aevi Novae*, 17 (2012), 29–45
——, *Emotional Communities in the Early Middle Ages* (Ithaca, NY: Cornell University Press, 2006)
——, 'Rereading *Askese und Laster*: The Case of Alcuin', in *Urkunden — Schriften — Lebensordnungen: Neue Beiträge zur Mediävistik*, ed. by Andreas Schwarcz (Wien: Böhlau, 2014), pp. 77–89
Sedlmeier, Franz, *Die laienparänetischen Schriften der Karolingerzeit: Untersuchungen zu ausgewählten Texten des Paulinus von Aquileia, Alkuins, Jonas' von Orleans, Dhuodas und Hinkmars von Reims* (Neuried: Ars Una, 2000)
Sher, Barbara, *It's Only Too Late If You Don't Start Now: How to Create Your Second Life at Any Age* (New York: Dell, 1999)
Smith, Julia M. H., *Province and Empire: Brittany and the Carolingians* (Cambridge: Cambridge University Press, 1992)
Sorabji, Richard, *Emotion and Peace of Mind: From Stoic Agitation to Christian Temptation. The Gifford Lectures* (Oxford: Oxford University Press, 2000)
Szarmach, Paul E., 'A Preliminary Handlist of Manuscripts containing Alcuin's *Liber de virtutibus et vitiis*', *Manuscripta*, 25 (1981), 131–40
Wallach, Liutpold, *Alcuin and Charlemagne: Studies in Carolingian History and Literature* (Ithaca, NY: Cornell University Press, 1959)

Sin, the Business of Pleasure, and the Pleasure of Reading: Exemplary Narratives and Other Forms of Sinful Pleasure in William Peraldus's *Summa de vitiis*

Richard Newhauser

Sin and Pleasure

As recent scholarship on the emotions and the passions in the Middle Ages has amply demonstrated, the relationship between sin and pleasure is more complex than it might seem to be at first sight.[1] The multifaceted signification that pleasure could have for medieval authors in the moral tradition may be indicated, for example, by the ways in which scholastic theologians differentiated between the *dis*pleasures of sins such as sloth, envy, and despair, or on the other hand the way the specific pleasures associated with each sin were distinguished from those of other sins. Differentiating between wrath and envy, for example, the influential Dominican moral theologian William Peraldus (*c.* 1200 – *c.* 1271) noted in his *Summa de vitiis* (composed in the early thirteenth century) that each of these vices demonstrated a different, but related, form of disordered love:

[1] Among many other studies, see for example Cohen, *The Modulated Scream*; Casagrande and Vecchio, *Piacere e dolore*; Barton, 'Gendering Anger'; Rosenwein, *Anger's Past*.

Richard Newhauser (Richard.Newhauser@asu.edu) is professor of English and Medieval Studies at Arizona State University, Tempe. His research concentrates on the moral tradition and sensory studies; he is editor of *A Cultural History of the Senses in the Middle Ages* (London: Bloomsbury, 2014) and is currently directing a project to edit and translate into English William Peraldus's *Summa de vitiis*.

Pleasure in the Middle Ages, ed. by Naama Cohen-Hanegbi and Piroska Nagy, IMR 24 (Turnhout: Brepols, 2018), pp. 181–202 BREPOLS PUBLISHERS 10.1484/M.IMR-EB.5.113467

> In peccato uero ire et inuidie est amor alieni mali pure. Sed in hoc uidentur differre illa duo uicia, quia in peccato ire amor alieni mali ortum uidetur habere a malo alterius. Iste enim qui irascitur alicui ideo uult ei malum quia malum ab eo recipit. Ira enim appetitus est uindicte. In peccato inuidie amor alieni mali ortum habet a propria malicia, scilicet a superbia. Inuidus enim ideo uult malum alterius, ne ille sibi preficeretur. Vnde peccatum inuidie in materia communicat cum peccato ire, sed finem recipit a peccato superbie.[2]

> [Now, in the vices of wrath and envy the love of someone else's evil appears in its purity. But these two vices seem to be differentiated in that in the vice of wrath one's love of someone else's evil apparently arises out of an evil in that other person. For a person who is angry with someone desires that person's evil because he receives some evil from him. For wrath is the desire for vengeance. But in the vice of envy, the love of someone else's evil arises out of one's own malice, namely out of pride. For the envious person desires another person's evil so that he will not be made his superior. Whence, the sin of envy shares its substance with the sin of wrath, but adopts its goal from the sin of pride.]

Medieval theologians also conceived of the possibility of the simultaneity and interconnection of pain and pleasure within the soul: thus, the pain of disease, and the suspicion that it might be a divine visitation for past sinful acts, was understood to coexist with a certain measure of joy at the extraordinary opportunity afforded to the soul by a disease of the body in the process of achieving salvation; despair occasioned by the loss of earthly goods was conceived of as coinciding with the pleasure of gaining spiritual goods through material loss. Moreover, theologians developed a conception of not only actively seeking the pain that arises from the guilt of pleasure in sin, but also — as Carla Casagrande and Silvana Vecchio have reminded us — of registering a state of 'dis-pleasure' (*displicentia*) in the midst of legitimate and virtuous pleasure, as William of Auxerre did when writing of conjugal sex in the *Summa aurea* (composed between 1215 and 1229).[3]

And, ultimately, while moral theologians were aware that pleasure was a key element in hamartiological analysis, they also knew that it was only one among many other factors in both the commission and the effect of sin. As Peter of Limoges, the author of an important pastoral text of the late thirteenth century, noted, to understand sin merely as a matter of delegitimized pleasure is

[2] Peraldus, *Summa de vitiis*, Tract. de Superbia, Lyon, Bibl. mun., MS 678, fol. 84va (Paris, Bibl. Maz., MS 794, fol. 113rb).

[3] Casagrande and Vecchio, 'Introduzione', p. 7.

to espouse the limited perspective of the as yet uneducated sinner. Peter, whose *Moral Treatise on the Eye* was a bestselling sermon aid (composed between 1275–76 and 1289), adopted the scientific principles of optics for ethical examination in this work, observing in Chapter 6, for example, that

> Peccatum potest certitudinaliter apprehendi secundum gradum proprie quantitatis ab eo qui peccatum directe respicit oculo racionis. Hoc autem modo doctor aliquis uel quicumque alius studiosus peccatum respicit, qui ueritatem in singulis speculando de peccatorum gradibus agnoscendis considerat uel inquirit. Et hec quidem noticia potissime prelatis est necessaria qui tenentur habere scienciam discernendi inter lepram et lepram, ut dicitur Leuitici xiii. Peccator autem quando peccatum committit, ipsam culpam non directe sed quasi per fractam lineam respicit seu oblique. Non enim aspicit ad ipsam peccati deformitatem siue maliciam sed pocius ad delectacionem annexam, quia secundum Dyonisium nullus ad malum aspiciens facit quod facit.[4]

> [A sin can be comprehended with certainty according to the degree of its own proper magnitude by someone who looks at the sin directly with the eye of reason. And this is the way a professor or anyone else who is studious looks at sin: by reflecting on and inquiring into the truth through an examination of each and every thing that ought to be known about the degrees of sins. And indeed this concept is necessary above all for prelates, who are required to have the knowledge to differentiate between different kinds of lepers, as it is said in Leviticus 13. Now, when a sinner commits a sin, he does not see this fault directly, but rather through a refracted line or obliquely, for he does not perceive the sin's deformity or evil, but rather the pleasure connected with it, since according to Dionysius no one does what he does with an eye to evil.]

Sin, thus, as the quotation from Dionysius makes clear, obfuscates from the eye of the sinner the many factors that motivate his/her sinful action: due to the nature of sin, sinners are self-deceptive, perceiving only the immediately obvious factor of pleasure in their actions. Beyond this, the point Peter emphasizes is that to understand all the factors involved in sinning — the full breadth and implications of an act of evil — is a matter of moral education, and that all Christians should be engaged in this educational project. But it is also clear from this passage that pleasure is merely one of the factors involved in the pro-

[4] Peter of Limoges, *Tractatus moralis de oculo*, 6.11, BnF, MS lat. 16396, fol. 9^{r-v}. See also *Johannis Pithsani archiepiscopi Canthuariensis ordinis fratrum minorum liber de oculo morali foeliciter incipit*. For a translation based on the early printed edition, with emendations from the best manuscripts, see Peter of Limoges, *The Moral Treatise on the Eye*, 6.11, trans. by Newhauser, p. 37.

cess of edification, the only one perceivable to the uneducated sinner before the process of his/her moral enlightenment has been achieved. Peter's observation is, finally, a statement of moral optimism, for he assumes that this enlightenment is not only within everyone's grasp, but that once it has been accomplished — once the sinner can perceive through direct lines of sight — the temptation to sin will be vanquished.

In fact, one can go a step further than the observation that pleasure is only one factor among many in the examination of sin. Given a teleological perspective, some moral analyses posit that pleasure might not even be the most important element involved in the commission of every sin. William Peraldus's *Summa de virtutibus* (*c.* 1249) shares in common with the *Summa fratris Alexandri* (also of the mid-thirteenth century, and perhaps one of the sources of Peraldus's work on the virtues) a statement that leads precisely in this direction, attributed in both works to Gregory the Great. In the initial treatise of the compendium on the virtues, Peraldus affirms that 'Gregorius: "Absit ut tanta sit delectatio in uiciis, quanta est in uirtutibus"' (Gregory [says]: 'As much pleasure as might be absent from the vices, just that much pleasure is present in the virtues').[5] In this assertion, and perhaps influenced by Albert the Great, Peraldus reflects a distinction used by some moral theologians between a pleasure that is a passion, and thus is a phenomenon that has the potential to be morally compromised, and a pleasure that results from virtue, and thus is one that belongs to the wide range of non-sensory pleasures available to human beings.[6]

The Complexity of Medieval Pleasure

The sensitivity to questions of pleasure and the important distinctions in the relationship between pleasure and pain, as well as between different types of pleasure, are characteristic of the analysis of these issues by medieval moral theologians, but they have hardly been foregrounded in some contemporary presentations of the Middle Ages intended for the mass market. They are, for example, completely occluded in claims of the sort made recently by Stephen Greenblatt about medieval pain and pleasure. Concerning monastic theology

[5] Peraldus, *Summa de virtutibus*, 1.7, Lyon, Bibl. mun., MS 678, fol. 177rb. For a printed edition, see Peraldus, *Summa virtutum ac vitiorum*, I, fol. 8rb. The exact sentence can also be found in Alexander of Hales (attrib.), *Summa theologica*, liber 2, pars 2, inq. 1, tract. 3, quaest. 1, cap. 4, num. 43, ed. by PP. Collegii S. Bonaventurae, III, 61.

[6] See Vecchio, 'Il piacere da Abelardo a Tommaso', p. 80.

and its imagined general applicability to a broader ideology before the Italian Renaissance, Greenblatt asserts that in the Middle Ages 'in one of the great cultural transformations in the history of the West, the pursuit of pain triumphed over the pursuit of pleasure', or that in medieval thought for the next millennium following Lactantius (*c.* 240 – *c.* 320 CE) 'pleasure is a code name for vice'.[7] These are, of course, little more than caricatures of the variety of ways of thinking about sin, pleasure, and pleasure's opposite that have been found to be indicative of a number of medieval theological texts. But then, so is Greenblatt's depiction of the opposite of asceticism as it had developed over the centuries in the atmosphere of the Roman Curia and, by the 1430s, was satirized in Lapo da Castiglionchio the Younger's *De curiae commodis dialogus*.[8] Here, Greenblatt identifies the practice of hedonistic pleasure seeking and moral depravity that fills out a caricature of the contrast to an ascetic medieval period, namely that other popular notion of a 'bawdy' Middle Ages. It is made palpable for Greenblatt in the lurid details of Lapo's satire of curial festivities with their

> witty gossip, along with fantastic food and drink served by beautiful, young, hairless boys. And for those whose tastes do not run in the direction of Ganymede, there are the abundant pleasures of Venus. Mistresses, adulterous matrons, courtesans of all descriptions occupy a central place in the curia, and appropriately so, since the delights they offer have such a central place in human happiness. Lewd songs, naked breasts, kissing, fondling, with small white lap-dogs trained to lick around your groin to excite pleasure — and all for remarkably low prices.[9]

As John Parker has noted, Greenblatt's narrow materialism flattens out the notion of pleasure to mean essentially a physical immoderation — either rejected wholesale or embraced lasciviously — but the same Tertullian (*fl.* *c.* 200 CE) cited often by Greenblatt as decisive for the development of a medieval ascetical rejection of pleasure already understood, as did Peraldus a thousand years later, that one of the greatest of virtuous pleasures is an aversion to the passion of pleasure in its worldly immediacy.[10] Many critics of *The Swerve* have taken the book to task especially for the failures of its historiography — in the field of

[7] Greenblatt, *The Swerve*, pp. 102–03.

[8] For the text and translation, see Lapo da Castiglionchio the Younger, *De curiae commodis*, ed. and trans. by Celenza.

[9] Greenblatt, *The Swerve*, p. 140.

[10] Parker, 'The Epicurean Middle Ages', p. 326. See Tertullian, *De spectaculis*, 29.2, ed. by Dekkers, p. 251: 'Quae maior uoluptas quam fastidium ipsius uoluptatis…?'.

science, or the phenomenon of manuscript production and transmission, or its brand of New Historicism, or its practice of periodization altogether[11] — and along with all of these blemishes one can add the work's startling oversimplification of the complex reality of pleasure, in particular medieval pleasure and its relationship to sin. But Greenblatt's dualistic and exaggerated view of pleasure performs important cultural work for him in defining — one could say paying homage to — the modern. Unlike schemes of established eras of history current in the Middle Ages, for example — such as the pattern of time before the law, during the law, and during grace — the Renaissance established a model of three ages (Antiquity, the Middle Ages, and the Renaissance) that culminated in itself. Greenblatt's entire approach in *The Swerve*, and his devaluation of medieval pleasure in particular, recapitulates this procedure. As Lee Patterson pointed out some time ago, defining periods of history that result in the self-understanding of the present characterizes the practice of history from a modern perspective, for this procedure of periodization helps define modernity in particular: 'Because its central move is to establish a sharp divide between the before of tradition and the after of modernity, it serves not only to define the modern but to enact it'.[12]

Recent investigations by psychologists and others working in the social sciences on human pleasure have agreed with the analysis of many theologians by underscoring how multifaceted the phenomenon is. The distinction between pleasures of the senses and those that are non-sensory is basic to these contemporary studies. As one psychologist specializing in the investigation of emotions has put it:

> Sensory pleasures often lead to the assumption that neural sensitivities exist that, when activated by stimuli, directly lead on to pleasure. Evolution proposes a rationale for this assumption: recognizing objects (foods, mates) as pleasant promotes reproductive fitness, just as recognition of harmful objects as aversive does [...]. However, there exist other kinds of pleasure for which the link to particular sensory stimuli is not so clear.[13]

[11] Parker's article is part of a forum in *Exemplaria* 25.4 (2013) presenting a number of reviews of *The Swerve*. I have cited Parker's article as being of particular importance for my own reading of the book, but all of the reviews in the forum are essential reading for understanding *The Swerve*.

[12] Patterson, 'The Place of the Modern in the Late Middle Ages', p. 54.

[13] Frijda, 'On the Nature and Function of Pleasure', p. 103.

Among the categories of pleasures enumerated here that are not grounded in sensory experience one finds a number already familiar from the analysis of medieval thinkers: diffuse likings of objects such as possessions or money, pleasures of relief caused by the removal of what is unpleasant rather than by pleasant sensory stimuli themselves, achievement pleasures caused by reaching desired goals. And beyond these can be added aesthetic pleasures derived from hearing, seeing, or reading works of art. Whether one understands pleasures as factors in the evolutionary biology of human beings, or as a set of cultural constructions built on a biological foundation, or as part of a fixed list of essential elements in human psychology that are often 'by-products of mental systems that have evolved for other purposes',[14] the expansive view of these phenomena in the social sciences regularly includes not just the pleasure of food and sex, but also such things as the pleasure resulting from religious practice. Moral theologians obviously started from very different assumptions about pleasure than social scientists do, seeing in pleasure both a divine gift and the potential incitement to vice; nevertheless, as has been seen already and as will be expanded in more detail in what follows, medieval moral theologians such as William Peraldus were likewise expansive and nuanced in their understanding of pleasure, in particular in its relationship to sin.

William Peraldus on Pleasure

When a moral thinker like Peraldus speaks on matters of vice and virtue, it makes sense for us to listen. Certainly three centuries and more of medieval and Counter-Reformation readers did, making Peraldus's double *Summae* — the *Summa de vitiis* and the *Summa de virtutibus* — the most influential pastoral treatments of ethics produced in the late Middle Ages. Peraldus probably studied at the university in Paris before entering the Dominican Order there and eventually becoming the prior of the Dominicans in Lyon.[15] He wrote with such authority, and was accepted as such in his own time, that he is often referred to in contemporary manuscripts as the archbishop (or suffragan) of that city, though he never held this office. His *Summa de vitiis* contains an introduction to sin in general, seven treatises on the deadly sins, and a final one

[14] Bloom, *How Pleasure Works*, p. 8.

[15] On the author's life, still essential is Dondaine, 'Guillaume Peyraut, vie et œuvres'. On the treatment of the seven deadly sins among early Scholastic authors in Paris, see Young, *Scholarly Community at the Early University of Paris*, pp. 168–207.

on the sin of the tongue. It was completed about 1236 and circulated together with its companion volume on the virtues shortly after the latter was completed around 1249. The work on the vices is still extant in over six hundred manuscripts, and the treatment of the virtues in something well over half that many.[16] As Leonard Boyle pointed out, Peraldus's texts had a secure place in all Dominican libraries: after he had retired from being general of the Dominicans in 1263, Humbert of Romans noted that every priory should have good copies of basic texts used by the lectors for teaching, and among them he named specifically Peraldus's *Summa de vitiis* and his *Summa de virtutibus*.[17] They served as the major inspiration for a very large number of Latin and vernacular compendia of ethics. Peraldus's treatment of the vices also extended far beyond the boundaries of the Order of Preachers; it determined the form and content not only of many Latin treatises on the seven deadly sins and contrary virtues for confessors and preachers,[18] but also of just as many vernacular texts on the vices, including the *Fiore di virtù*, the *Somme le roi*, the *Spiegel der Sonden*, Michel Beheim's *Büchlein von den sieben Todsünden*, *The Book of Vices and Virtues*,[19] and many others. Its influence extended to a number of other genres, as well: encyclopedias (such as Brunetto Latini's *Li livres dou tresor*), or penitential manuals such as Heinrich von Langenstein's *Erchantnuzz der sund*, or the work of poets like Dante Alighieri and Geoffrey Chaucer.[20] It was, in fact, so essential

[16] On the transmission of the work on the vices, see Dondaine, 'Guillaume Peyraut, vie et œuvres'; Kaeppeli, *Scriptores Ordinis Praedicatorum Medii Aevi*, no. 1622; Bloomfield and others, *Incipits of Latin Works on the Virtues and Vices*, no. 1628. The latter text is now emended in Newhauser and Bejczy, *A Supplement to Morton W. Bloomfield et al.* For the work on the virtues, see Verweij, 'The Manuscript Transmission of the *Summa de Virtutibus* by Guillielmus Peraldus'.

[17] Boyle, 'Notes on the Education of the *fratres communes*', p. 257.

[18] For the concept of the contrary virtues, formerly known as 'remedial virtues', see Newhauser, 'Preaching the "Contrary Virtues"'.

[19] For editions of the *Fiore di virtù*, see Newhauser, *The Treatise on Vices and Virtues in Latin and the Vernacular*, p. 38. Frère Laurent, *La Somme le roi*, ed. by Brayer and Leurquin-Labie. *Die Spiegel der Sonden*, ed. by Verdam. For Beheim's *Büchlein*, see McDonald, 'Singing Sin'. *The Book of Vices and Virtues*, ed. by Francis.

[20] Latini, *Li livres dou tresor*, ed. by Carmody. Wolf, '*Propter utilitatem populi*'; Newhauser, 'The Parson's Tale and its Generic Affiliations'. Wenzel, 'Dante's Rationale for the Seven Deadly Sins'. Newhauser, 'The Parson's Tale'; Wenzel, 'The Source of Chaucer's Seven Deadly Sins'; Wenzel, 'The Source for the *Remedia* of the Parson's Tale'. On the reception of Peraldus's *summae*, see Newhauser, *The Treatise on Vices and Virtues in Latin and the Vernacular*, pp. 127–30; Wenzel, 'The Continuing Life of William Peraldus's *Summa vitiorum*'.

that by the fifteenth century, when Jean Gerson was chancellor of the University of Paris, he observed that the loss of all the books in the world could be tolerated if only Peraldus's *Summa de vitiis* (and his treatment of the virtues) would survive.[21] All of this qualifies Peraldus's texts as being among the most successful of Dominican works on moral instruction and the preparation of sermons to emerge from the reimagining of the bonds between the Church and the Christian community codified in Lateran IV (1215–16).

The *Summa de vitiis* in particular furthered the call to introspective examination of the conscience that forms the core of many sermons and preparation for confession, but it also emphasizes the socially embedded identity of the individual. The order of sins in the *Summa* moves from the corporeal to the spiritual, but also from the individual to the communal. As Peraldus notes at the beginning of the treatment of pride:

> De facili potest uideri quare de superbia, ira, et inuidia posterius tractetur, quia hec tria uicia amorem nostrum inordinatum reddunt ad proximum; quatuor uero precedentia inordinatum reddunt ad nos ipsos. Inordinatio uero alicuius in se prior est quam inordinatio ipsius ad alium. Preterea prius est quod animale, deinde quod spirituale. Vnde cum quatuor prima uitia humana sint et ita quodammodo carnalia, in ordine doctrine priora sunt. Tria uero que secuntur, que diabolica sunt et spiritualia, posteriora sunt.[22]

> [It can easily be seen why pride, wrath, and envy should be discussed later [in the *Summa*] since these three vices refer our disordered love to a fellow human being; the four preceding ones refer this disordered [love] to ourselves. Indeed, disorder occurs in a person's own self before that person's disorder is directed towards another person. Moreover, what is worldly comes first, then what is spiritual. For this reason, since the first four vices [namely, in the order: gluttony, lust, avarice, sloth] are human, and thus in a certain sense fleshly, in the order of teaching they come earlier. The three which follow, however, which are diabolical and spiritual, come afterwards.]

It was within this larger Augustinian context of sin understood as disordered love and in which individual identity emerges as above all ethically contoured and bound to a nexus of social groupings by obligations of the love of one's fellow human being (*caritas*) that Peraldus's reflections on pleasure and sin are located.

[21] See Arnould, *Le 'Manuel des Péchés'*, p. 29, n. 3.

[22] Peraldus, *Summa de vitiis*, Tract. de Superbia, Lyon, Bibl. mun., MS 678, fol. 84^{va-vb} (Paris, Bibl. Maz., MS 794, fol. 113rb).

In its Augustinian framework, the pleasure of sex was identified with concupiscence of the flesh,[23] one of an all-encompassing triad of evils Augustine developed on the basis of I John 2. 16. And it is against this background that we can understand Peraldus's exegesis in his treatment of the sin of lust that connects the deceitful woman of Proverbs 5, whose end is said to be bitter as wormwood, with carnal pleasure itself.[24] Peraldus also cites Augustine's words in the *Confessions*, often repeated in the moral tradition, concerning the other sin besides lust in Gregory the Great's category of corporeal vices, namely gluttony. Here, the point is that some pleasure may come along with eating, like a travelling companion, and that while eating food is necessary for the health of the body, sometimes the miserable soul in the grips of gluttony will rejoice in hiding under the cloak of health its real aim, namely an increase of gustatory pleasure.[25] But for Peraldus, fully attuned to the needs of preaching and penance in a complex social situation, the matter of pleasure did not remain simply an acknowledgement of humanity's proclivity to sinfulness, or at best the weak first precarious step over the slippery slope leading to the culmination of a sinful act. Pleasure in itself is not culpable; only when it moves beyond the bounds of temperance or involves a specifically illicit object does it become sinful. His treatment of gluttony contains warnings against seeking delicacies of food, but it also recognizes that the desire in appetite can hardly or not at all achieve its aim of keeping human beings alive *except* by way of some pleasure, an appreciation of the essential utility of pleasure at the moment of satisfying hunger, not just its presence alongside the act of eating:

> Quia si delectabilia tibi dantur in adiutorium carni aduersus spiritum concupiscenti, erunt duo contra unum, et uincitur spiritus; unde Bernardus: 'De condimentis sufficiat ut comestibilia fiant, non concupiscibilia. Sufficit enim concupiscencie malicia sua. Que cum uix aut nullo modo pertransire possit ad finem explendum

[23] See Vecchio, 'Il piacere da Abelardo a Tommaso', p. 68.

[24] Peraldus, *Summa de vitiis*, Tract. de Luxuria, Lyon, Bibl. mun., MS 678, fol. 19[vb] (Paris, Bibl. Maz., MS 794, fol. 12[rb]): 'Ad penitentiam pertinet quod legitur Prouerbiorum v de muliere fallaci, per quam uoluptas intelligitur: *Nouissima autem illius amara quasi absinthium*'. The biblical reference is Proverbs 5. 4.

[25] Peraldus, *Summa de vitiis*, Tract. de Gula, Lyon, Bibl. mun., MS 678, fol. 17[ra] (Paris, Bibl. Maz., MS 794, fol. 8[ra]): 'Frequenter enim dum hoc fit quod salus esse debeat edendi, adiungit se pedisseca periculosa iocunditas, et plerumque precurrit, ut eius causa fiat quod causa salutis fieri debuit, et gaudet infelix anima ut obtentu salutis obumbret negocium uoluptatis'. The passage is adopted from Augustine, *Confessionum libri XIII*, 10.31.44, ed. by Verheijen, p. 178.

> necessitatis nisi per uiam quantamcumque delectationis, si ceperit habere irritamenta, fiunt duo contra unum, et periclitatur consciencia'.[26]

> [Since delicious things assist your flesh that lusts against your spirit, there are two against one, and your spirit is overcome; whence Bernard says: 'Concerning spices, let it suffice that [your food] becomes edible, not [excessively] desirable. For the evil in desire is sufficient by itself. As desire can hardly or not at all reach its aim of filling its need except by way of some pleasure, if it then has some [additional] stimulus, there are two against one, and conscience loses out'.]

In acknowledging that pleasure is an essential part of appetite, not just ancillary to it, Peraldus takes a first step towards the analysis of gustatory pleasure as more than simply something to be avoided.[27] As will be seen, for him the sense of taste has an important role to play in judgement.

Moreover, Peraldus can conceive of an act of lust in which corporeal pleasure is not the primary factor for the sinner, who is more interested in engaging in adulterous behaviour precisely because it is said to be annoying to God:

> Potest ostendi quam contumeliosum sit istud peccatum Deo ex hoc quod luxuriosus illud dulcius reputat quod Deo est contumeliosius. Magis enim amat interdum coniugatam turpem quam solutam pulchram. Vnde non uidetur querere in peccato suo uoluptatem suam sed Dei contumeliam; unde Ieronimus: 'Libidinosa mens inhonesta ardentius prosequitur et quod non licet dulcius suspicatur'.[28]

> [How great an insult this sin [of lust] is to God can be shown by the fact that a lustful person considers sweeter what to God is more insulting. For sometimes he loves an ugly married woman more than a beautiful unmarried one. In this he does not seem to seek in his sin his own pleasure so much as an insult to God; whence Jerome: 'A lustful mind pursues dishonourable things more fiercely and believes to be sweeter what is not allowed'.]

The range of *delectatio* (pleasure) in particular among the rest of the vices often stays relatively close to its usage in the context of the corporeal sins in implicating creaturely comforts. In line with the goals of Lateran IV, Peraldus is writing

[26] Peraldus, *Summa de vitiis*, Tract. de Gula, Lyon, Bibl. mun., MS 678, fol. 18vb (Paris, Bibl. Maz., MS 794, fol. 10vb–11ra). For the quotation attributed to Bernard, see William of Saint-Thierry, *Epistola ad Fratres de Monte Dei*, 134, ed. by Verdeyen, CCCM, 88, p. 256.

[27] Cf. the interesting analysis of the long process of a 'revolution of taste' in Italy in Giannetti, 'Of Eels and Pears'.

[28] Peraldus, *Summa de vitiis*, Tract. de Luxuria, Lyon, Bibl. mun., MS 678, fol. 20va (Paris, Bibl. Maz., MS 794, fol. 13va). For the quotation from Jerome, see *Epistulae*, 117.7, ed. by Hilberg, II, 430.

to ensure the unity of the entire Christian community. The degree to which he conceived of this task as a matter of insisting on orthodox positions stands out clearly in his *Tractatus de fide* in the *Summa de virtutibus*, less a philosophical analysis of faith than a detailed presentation of doctrinal mistakes and the errors of heretics, such as those he preached against in the south of France and in the adjacent Alpine regions.[29] In the *Treatise on Faith* he again insists, in fact, on the necessary utility of pleasure when he argues that the modern dualist heretics of his day demonstrated their lack of faith by their faulty senses, perceiving only pure evil in corruptible matter, which they said was the product of the principle of evil. On the other hand, Peraldus notes, the senses are needed to distinguish what is good from what is bad; all matter has the potential for goodness and for giving pleasure, being the creation of a single, good God:

> Item quilibet sensus dicit aliquid bonum in eis [i.e. corruptibilibus], ut gustus dicit aliquod uinum bonum; Iohannis ii: *Tu autem seruasti uinum bonum usque adhuc* [John 2. 10]. Dicit auditus uocem aliquam bonam. Dicit uisus formam aliquam bonam. Dicit tactus uestem aliquam bonam et suauem. Dicit odoratus aliquem odorem bonum. Ergo sicut ille qui negat niuem esse albam sensu indiget, sic Manichei omni sensu uidentur indigere. Ipsi uidentur esse ceci et surdi et aliis sensibus indigentes, nec digni sunt ut contra errorem eorum disputetur.[30]

> [Likewise, every sense proclaims something good in [corruptible matter], as the sense of taste declares that some wine is good; John 2: *But you have kept the good wine until now*. The sense of hearing declares that a certain tone is good. The sense of sight proclaims that a certain shape is good. The sense of touch declares that some article of clothing is good and pleasing. The sense of smell proclaims that an odor is good. Thus, just as someone who denies that snow is white lacks sense, so the Manichaeans appear to lack all their senses. They appear to be blind and dumb and lacking their other senses, nor is it worth disputing with them about their error.]

The Business of Pleasure

But within the community of the Church, *delectatio* (pleasure) was also differentiated by the social position of those engaged in pleasurable activity in Peraldus's view of sin. In discussing the prideful pleasures of clothing, for example, Peraldus notes that belts adorned with gold and silver are especially repre-

[29] Newhauser, 'Unerring Faith in the Pulpit'.

[30] Peraldus, *Summa de virtutibus*, 3.8, Lyon, Bibl. mun., MS 678, fol. 197$^{\text{bis va–vb}}$. See also Peraldus, *Summa virtutum ac vitiorum*, I, fol. 40ra.

hensible because they are worn demonstratively over one's stomach, which in his view is the most humbling part of the body. But in an aside he also likens the morally tenuous situation of wearing an adorned belt over one's stomach to the greater displeasure God takes in pride when it is exhibited by a poor person: being indigent gives one all the more reason to be humble, which should suppress pride and its attendant pleasures of fashion.[31] In their ability to access pleasure, the marked gap between the poor and the well-to-do is perhaps most apparent in this realm of fashion, and Peraldus spends a good deal of time detailing and arguing against the pleasure one might take in displays of women's long trailing gowns, decorated belts, saffron-coloured headbands, cosmetics, wigs, clothing with slashes cut into it, and perforated shoes.[32]

Elsewhere, he draws on the power of commercial activity in the imagination of the urban populations in the earlier thirteenth century, where buying and selling had already become appropriate and often utilized metaphors by preachers and confessors to express moral action. The Dominican tradition of penitential handbooks developed during this period to minister, among others, to merchants assumes 'that commercial activity can, in principle, be useful and honourable',[33] something which Peraldus affirms in his treatment of avarice in the *Summa de vitiis*.[34] Though the focus on greed as the chief factor of immorality in the High Middle Ages was not the first time moralists had viewed this vice as the catalyst of all that was wrong with human society,[35] social changes in connection with the spread of the profit economy in the eleventh century made it even more likely that moralists could use the corrosive sin of avarice as

[31] Peraldus, *Summa de vitiis*, Tract. de Superbia, Lyon, Bibl. mun., MS 678, fol. 101$^{ra–rb}$ (Paris, Bibl. Maz., MS 794, fol. 142ra): '<Inter> [MSS: Item] ornatus uero qui propter materiam reprehensibiles sunt specialiter uidentur esse reprehensibiles corrigie serice deaurate uel deargentate, et hoc multiplici ratione. Primo, quia superbia talium corrigiarum in loco humiliationis est; unde Michee vi: *Humiliatio tua in medio tui* [Micah 6. 14]. Vnde sicut superbia in paupere amplius displicet Deo quam in diuite (quia pauper habet materiam humilitatis et quoddam repressiuum superbie), sic potius displicet Deo superbia circa uentrem, ubi tanta materia humilitatis est, quam displiceat in alia parte hominis'.

[32] Peraldus, *Summa de vitiis*, Tract. de Superbia, Lyon, Bibl. mun., MS 678, fols 101ra–102va (Paris, Bibl. Maz., MS 794, fols 141va–144rb).

[33] Langholm, *The Merchant in the Confessional*, p. 47.

[34] Peraldus, *Summa de vitiis*, Tract. de Avaritia, Lyon, Bibl. mun., MS 678, fol. 46va (Paris, Bibl. Maz., MS 794, fol. 52rb): 'Quarto loco inter species auaricie dicendum est de fraudibus negociatorum. Et notandum quod negociatio in se bona est et hominibus necessaria'.

[35] Newhauser, *The Early History of Greed*.

a model to explain the evils of the times. As Lester Little and Alexander Murray have argued, because the use of cash as an agent of exchange allowed more people to manifest the signs of wealth, and to desire to be wealthy altogether, than the limited number of the aristocracy which had had access to the immovable wealth in land in the early Middle Ages, the complaints of moralists from the late tenth century onwards contain descriptions which once again emphasized the trope of the entire world falling prey to greed.[36] In the rhetorical ammunition Peraldus assembles on numerous occasions in his treatment of the vices to persuade those accustomed to the merchant trade against illicit *delectatio*, the business of pleasure is configured as an especially bad market transaction, the kind which leaves one looking unwise or, worse, dehumanized. Among those whom prideful clothing harms, he observes with characteristic misogyny, is the woman who wears such clothing herself because this clothing causes her to be treated like a horse:

> Ex quo equus habet signum uenalitatis in fronte, iam non queritur utrum sit uenalis sed pro constanti habetur et de precio queritur. Sic ex quo aliqua mulier ornatum meretricium habet, ipsa sollicitata nisi fortis ualde sit, labitur de facili. Quia ut ait poeta:
>
> Casta est quam nemo rogauit.[37]
>
> [When a horse has a for-sale sign on its forehead, no one asks whether it is for sale but takes this for granted and asks for its price. In the same way, a woman who wears some meretricious adornment is solicited, and unless she is very strong, she easily slips, for as a poet says:
>
> She is chaste whom no one has asked.]

And among the arguments that can bring people to detest the sin of lust, Peraldus suggests focusing on the shame it can lead to, which he develops with two exempla:

> Et quidam qui sibi abscidit linguam ut uehementia doloris temperaret uehementiam temptationis dixit: 'Absit ut tanti emam unde peniteam!' Insipiens mercator est qui forum facit unde certus est quod penitebit. Exemplum: Quedam uirgo esti-

[36] Little, 'Pride Goes before Avarice'; Little, *Religious Poverty and the Profit Economy in Medieval Europe*, pp. 35–39; Murray, 'Money and Robbers', pp. 89–90; Murray, *Reason and Society in the Middle Ages*, p. 61.

[37] Peraldus, *Summa de vitiis*, Tract. de Superbia, Lyon, Bibl. mun., MS 678, fol. 103va (Paris, Bibl. Maz., MS 794, fol. 145vb). The verse is taken from Ovid, *Amores*, 1.8.43, ed. by Kenney, p. 19. It was quoted with some frequency by later medieval authors.

mans quod delectatio huius peccati esset quoddam magnum desiderio illius uirginitatem sibi auferri permisit; deinde uidens pro qua uili re tantum thesaurum amisisset, adeo penituit quod uoluit se interficere.[38]

[And someone who cut off his tongue so that the fierceness of pain would temper the fierceness of temptation said: 'Far be it from me to buy so expensively what I would regret afterwards!' It is a foolish merchant who carries out a transaction he is sure to regret. For example: A certain virgin, thinking that the pleasure of this sin would be something wonderful, let herself be deprived of her virginity through this desire. Then realizing that for such a shameful thing she had lost such a great treasure, she regretted it so much that she wanted to commit suicide.]

Narrative Pleasure

Exempla like these are a consistent feature of Peraldus's examination of sin and virtue, as they were increasingly in many treatises in the moral tradition from the late twelfth century on. The Cistercians played an important early role as storytellers, but the mendicants were adept in developing, collecting, and organizing exempla collections throughout the later medieval centuries. An appreciable number of the copies of Peraldus's *Summae* contain notations in the margins, sometimes almost the only marginalia in the manuscripts, that indicate where the exempla occur in the text, so one can say that along with its useful (and pleasurable) analysis of sin, Peraldus's text was valued as a storehouse of poetic and narrative material. And he did not shy away from adopting lines of verse from classical poets and stories from secular and vernacular sources for his *Summae*. In skewering the hypocritical pleasure-seeking of prelates, for example, Peraldus notes:

Ypocrita mortuum se simulat mundo — cum in ueritate uiuus sit — donec habeat unam magnam prelationem in qua deliciis possit uacare, tunc aperte ostendit quod uiuus est. Sicut fabulose refertur de uulpe que mortuam se simulauit donec posita fuit super quadrigam in qua erant alectia; tunc comedendo alectia se uiuam ostendit.[39]

[A hypocrite pretends to be dead to the world — while in truth he is alive — until he has gained a rich prelacy where he devotes himself to pleasures, and then it is

[38] Peraldus, *Summa de vitiis*, Tract. de Luxuria, Lyon, Bibl. mun., MS 678, fol. 19vb (Paris, Bibl. Maz., MS 794, fol. 12^{rb-va}). For the quoted statement, see Petrus Cantor, *Verbum abbreviatum (textus prior)*, 123, ed. by Boutry, p. 635.

[39] Peraldus, *Summa de vitiis*, Tract. de Superbia, Lyon, Bibl. mun., MS 678, fol. 127rb (Paris, Bibl. Maz., MS 794, fol. 189ra).

> very clear that he is alive. There is the fable about the fox who pretended to be dead until he was put on a cart in which there were herring; and then he showed he was alive by eating them.]

No matter how unusual a herring-loving fox might sound, Peraldus has the story ultimately, and perhaps directly, from one of the branches of the *Roman de Renart* and has pressed it into service for moral analysis.[40] He certainly was well aware that in composing a text that could be useful for preachers interested in curbing vice, he was focused on a kind of theology aligned with one type of practical philosophy, namely ethics, and that the immediate ends of encouraging moral action made it easier to bring together the goals of moral theology with 'the writings of poets, who were habitually branded as liars',[41] without threatening the position of a more ratiocinative theology as the queen of the sciences.

The increased importance of exempla in the moral tradition in the thirteenth century has much to do with developments in literary theory against the background of the reception of Aristotle in that period and the conception, articulated, for example, by a writer like Roger Bacon (d. *c.* 1292) in the *Moralis philosophia*, that the human *affectus* cannot be led to moral action by logic alone, but rather it is the duty of rhetorical persuasion to move the audience's faculties of imagination and judgement *per delectationem*.[42] In fact, for the reception in the Middle Ages of an author like Ovid, pleasure — no matter how ethically ambiguous it might be in reference to a text like the *Amores* — was conceived of as a central goal of that author.[43] And Dominican writers were among the swelling tide of others who well understood the usefulness, even necessity, of what can be recognized as aesthetic pleasure aroused by narratives that could be employed for an effective sermon.[44] Humbert of Romans, the prior of the Dominicans in Lyon when Peraldus arrived there, observed in his *Liber de dono timoris*:

[40] See *Le Roman de Renart*, III, ed. by Martin, pp. 131–36.

[41] Minnis, 'The Trouble with Theology', pp. 32–33, has called attention to the potential devaluation of theology in reducing it to ethics alone that could occur if it were made the full equivalent of poetry, and the care theologians took to avoid this trouble.

[42] Gillespie, 'The Senses in Literature'.

[43] Gillespie, 'The Study of the Classical Authors from the Twelfth Century to *c.* 1450', p. 190.

[44] Newhauser, 'Jesus as the First Dominican?'.

> <Quonia>m plus exempla quam uerba mouent secundum Gregorium et facilius intellectu capiuntur et alcius memorie infiguntur, necnon et libencius a multis audiuntur suique delectacione quadam plures attrahunt ad sermones, expedit viros predicacionis officio deditos in huiusmodi habundare exemplis.[45]

> [Since, according to Gregory, exempla are more moving than mere words and are more easily grasped by the intellect and are fixed deeper in the memory, and furthermore since they are heard with greater pleasure by many and attract many more to sermons by the delight which they give, it is advantageous for men dedicated to the office of preaching to have an abundance of exempla.]

Peraldus put this advice to good use, creating compendia that analyse, among other matters, the complex relationship between sin, pleasure, and pleasure's opposite — and of course this kind of discursive analysis carried pleasures of its own for medieval readers, as it does for most readers today. But Peraldus also employed the aesthetic pleasure of narrative in composing his works. The wide transmission of his texts testifies to the importance and pleasure of understanding vice and virtue in the late Middle Ages, but also to the importance of adopting forms of pleasure itself as the vehicle for that understanding.

Conclusion

The broad palette of attitudes towards pleasure expressed by medieval authors writing in the moral tradition extended from a utilitarian view of the necessity of gustatory pleasure among human beings for the preservation of life itself to an ascetically oriented denunciation of sexual pleasure, from the aesthetic appreciation of the potential of narrative pleasure in motivating moral choice to a differentiated hamartiological analysis of the potential unimportance of pleasure in the commission of sin. The territory mapped out here is nowhere so influentially expressed as in the works on vice and virtue by William Peraldus. His reflections on the ethics of pleasure were intended initially for the education of novices in the growing Dominican Order, and through them, in particular, the merchant class and an urban aristocracy who swelled their congregations in later medieval cities.[46] But the pragmatism of his approach to the moral status of pleasure, with its emphasis on a spiritual and ethical sense of

[45] Humbert of Romans, *Liber de dono timoris*, BnF, MS lat. 15953, fol. 188^{r}.

[46] On the use of sermon narratives especially for urban elites, see Scanlon, *Narrative, Authority, and Power*, p. 65; Rosenwein and Little, 'Social Meaning in the Monastic and Mendicant Spiritualities'.

community that drew from and was sustained by vibrant commercial activity, proved significantly persuasive well beyond the early thirteenth century. Its practicality can be remarked in Peraldus's adoption of modes of valuation developed in the marketplace as metaphorical expressions of moral value as well. The 'exchange value' of pleasure that emerges here, its potential to be an instrument of ethical amelioration or deterioration, became standard in the analysis of the vices that is so prevalent at the end of the medieval period and that had the effect of equating the individual with his/her internalized moral identity. In the wider context of the *Summa de vitiis*, thus, in the way it encouraged and furthered the call to introspective examination of the conscience that forms the core of many sermons, Peraldus's view of pleasure in relation to sin also has an important place in the development of ideas of the Self in Western culture, a Self conceived of as both a social and an ethical phenomenon obligated by the bonds of love Peraldus articulated at the beginning of his treatment of pride.

Works Cited

Manuscripts

Humbert of Romans, *Liber de dono timoris*, Paris, Bibliothèque nationale de France [BnF], MS lat. 15953

Peter of Limoges, *Tractatus moralis de oculo*, Paris, Bibliothèque nationale de France [BnF], MS lat. 16396

William Peraldus, *Summa de virtutibus*, Lyon, Bibliothèque municipale [Bibl. mun.], MS 678

William Peraldus, *Summa de vitiis*, Lyon, Bibliothèque municipale [Bibl. mun.], MS 678 and Paris, Bibliothèque Mazarine [Bibl. Maz.], MS 794

Primary Sources

Alexander of Hales (attrib.), *Summa theologica (Summa fratris Alexandri)*, ed. by PP. Collegii S. Bonaventurae, 4 vols (Quaracchi: Collegium S. Bonaventurae, 1924–48)

Augustine, *Confessionum libri XIII*, ed. by Luc Verheijen, CCSL, 27 (Turnhout: Brepols, 1981)

The Book of Vices and Virtues: A Fourteenth Century English Translation of the 'Somme le Roi' of Lorens d'Orléans, ed. by W. Nelson Francis, EETS, OS, 217 (London: Oxford University Press, 1942)

Jerome, *Epistulae*, 2nd edn, ed. by Isidor Hilberg, CSEL, 54–56.2, 4 vols (Wien: Tempsky, 1910–18; repr. 1996)

Lapo da Castiglionchio the Younger, *De curiae commodis*, ed. and trans. by Christopher S. Celenza, in *Renaissance Humanism and the Papal Curia: Lapo da Castiglionchio the Younger's 'De curiae commodis'*, Papers and Monographs of the American Academy in Rome, 31 (Ann Arbor: University of Michigan Press, 1999)

Latini, Brunetto, *Li livres dou tresor*, ed. by Francis J. Carmody, University of California Publications in Modern Philology, 22 (Berkeley: University of California Press, 1948)

Laurent (Frère), *La Somme le roi*, ed. by Édith Brayer and Anne-Françoise Leurquin-Labie (Paris: Société des Anciens Textes Français, 2008)

Ovid, *Amores*, ed. by E. J. Kenney, in *P. Ovidi Nasonis Amores, Medicamina faciei femineae, Ars amatoria, Remedia amoris* (Oxford: Clarendon Press, 1961; repr. 1968)

Peraldus, William, *Summa virtutum ac vitiorum Guilhelmi Paraldi Episcopi Lugdunensis de ordine predicatorum*, 2 vols (Paris: Johannes Petit, Johannes Frellon, Franciscus Regnault, 1512)

Peter of Limoges, *The Moral Treatise on the Eye*, trans. by Richard Newhauser, Mediaeval Sources in Translation, 51 (Toronto: Pontifical Institute of Mediaeval Studies, 2012)

——, *Tractatus moralis de oculo*, in *Johannis Pithsani archiepiscopi Canthuariensis ordinis fratrum minorum liber de oculo morali foeliciter incipit* (Augsburg: A. Sorg, 1475 [?])

Petrus Cantor, *Verbum abbreviatum (textus prior)*, ed. by Monique Boutry, CCCM, 196A (Turnout: Brepols, 2012)

Le Roman de Renart, ed. by Ernest Martin, 3 vols (Strassburg: K. J. Trübner, 1882–87)

Die Spiegel der Sonden, ed. by Jacob Verdam, 2 vols (Leiden: Brill, 1900–01)

Tertullian, *De spectaculis*, ed. by E. Dekkers, CCSL, 1 (Turnhout: Brepols, 1954)

William of Saint-Thierry, *Epistola ad Fratres de Monte Dei*, ed. by Paul Verdeyen, in *Opera omnia*, 6 vols, CCCM, 86–89B (Turnhout: Brepols, 1989–2011)

Secondary Works

Arnould, E. J., *Le 'Manuel des Péchés': Étude de littérature religieuse anglo-normande (XIIIe siècle)* (Paris: Droz, 1940)

Barton, Richard E., 'Gendering Anger: *Ira*, *Furor*, and Discourses of Power and Masculinity in the Eleventh and Twelfth Centuries', in *In the Garden of Evil: The Vices and Culture in the Middle Ages*, ed. by Richard Newhauser, Papers in Mediaeval Studies, 18 (Toronto: Pontifical Institute of Mediaeval Studies, 2005), pp. 371–92

Bloom, Paul, *How Pleasure Works: The New Science of Why We Like What We Like* (New York: Norton, 2010)

Bloomfield, Morton W., Bertrand-Georges Guyot, Donald R. Howard, and Thyra B. Kabealo, *Incipits of Latin Works on the Virtues and Vices, 1100–1500 A.D.*, Mediaeval Academy of America, Publication 88 (Cambridge, MA: Mediaeval Academy of America, 1979)

Boyle, Leonard E., 'Notes on the Education of the *fratres communes* in the Dominican Order in the Thirteenth Century', in *Xenia Medii Aevi Historiam Illustrantia oblata*

Thomae Kaeppeli O.P., ed. by Raymund Creytens and Pius Künzle, 2 vols, Storia e Letteratura (Raccolta di Studi e Testi), 141 (Roma: Edizioni di Storia e Letteratura, 1978), I, 249–67; repr. in Leonard E. Boyle, *Pastoral Care, Clerical Education and Canon Law, 1200–1400*, Variorum Collected Studies Series, CS135 (London: Ashgate, 1981), essay VI

Casagrande, Carla, and Silvana Vecchio, 'Introduzione', in *Piacere e dolore: Materiali per una storia delle passioni nel Medioevo*, ed. by Carla Casagrande and Silvana Vecchio, Micrologus' Library, 29 (Firenze: SISMEL/Edizioni del Galluzzo, 2009), pp. 3–11

——, eds, *Piacere e dolore: Materiali per una storia delle passioni nel Medioevo*, Micrologus' Library, 29 (Florence: SISMEL –Galluzzo, 2009)

Cohen, Esther, *The Modulated Scream: Pain in Late Medieval Culture* (Chicago: University of Chicago Press, 2010)

Dondaine, Antoine, 'Guillaume Peyraut, vie et œuvres', *Archivum Fratrum Praedicatorum*, 18 (1948), 162–236

Frijda, Nico H., 'On the Nature and Function of Pleasure', in *Pleasures of the Brain*, ed. by Morten L. Kringelbach and Kent C. Berridge (Oxford: Oxford University Press, 2010), pp. 99–112

Giannetti, Laura, 'Of Eels and Pears: A Sixteenth-Century Debate on Taste, Temperance, and the Pleasures of the Senses', in *Religion and the Senses in Early Modern Europe*, ed. by Wietse de Boer and Christine Göttler, Intersections, 26 (Leiden: Brill, 2012), pp. 289–305

Gillespie, Vincent, 'The Senses in Literature: The Textures of Perception', in *A Cultural History of the Senses*, vol. II, *A Cultural History of the Senses in the Middle Ages*, ed. by Richard G. Newhauser (London: Bloomsbury, 2014), pp. 153–73

——, 'The Study of the Classical Authors from the Twelfth Century to *c.* 1450', in *The Cambridge History of Literary Criticism*, vol. II, *The Middle Ages*, ed. by Alastair J. Minnis and Ian Johnson (Cambridge: Cambridge University Press, 2005), pp. 145–235

Greenblatt, Stephen, *The Swerve: How the World Became Modern* (New York: Norton, 2011)

Kaeppeli, Thomas, *Scriptores Ordinis Praedicatorum Medii Aevi*, 4 vols (Rome: Ad S. Sabinam; Istituto storico Domenicano, 1970–93)

Langholm, Odd, *The Merchant in the Confessional: Trade and Price in the Pre-Reformation Penitential Handbooks*, Studies in Medieval and Reformation Thought, 93 (Leiden: Brill, 2003)

Little, Lester K., 'Pride Goes before Avarice: Social Change and the Vices in Latin Christendom', *American Historical Review*, 76 (1971), 16–49

——, *Religious Poverty and the Profit Economy in Medieval Europe* (London: Paul Elek, 1971)

McDonald, William C., 'Singing Sin: Michel Beheim's "Little Book of the Seven Deadly Sins", a German Pre-Reformation Religious Text for the Laity', in *Sin in Medieval and Early Modern Culture: The Tradition of the Seven Deadly Sins*, ed. by Richard G. Newhauser and Susan J. Ridyard (York: York Medieval Press, in connection with Boydell & Brewer, 2012), pp. 282–303

Minnis, Alastair, 'The Trouble with Theology: Ethical Poetics and the Ends of Scripture', in *Author, Reader, Book: Medieval Authorship in Theory and Practice*, ed. by Stephen Partridge and Erik Kwakkel (Toronto: University of Toronto Press, 2012), pp. 20–37

Murray, Alexander, 'Money and Robbers, 900–1100', *Journal of Medieval History*, 4 (1978), 55–94

——, *Reason and Society in the Middle Ages* (Oxford: Oxford University Press, 1978)

Newhauser, Richard, *The Early History of Greed: The Sin of Avarice in Early Medieval Thought and Literature*, Cambridge Studies in Medieval Literature, 41 (Cambridge: Cambridge University Press, 2000; repr. 2006)

——, 'Jesus as the First Dominican? Reflections on a Sub-theme in the Exemplary Literature of Some Thirteenth-Century Preachers', in *Christ among the Medieval Dominicans: Representations of Christ in the Texts and Images of the Order of Preachers*, ed. by Kent Emery Jr and Joseph Wawrykow, Notre Dame Conferences in Medieval Studies, 7 (Notre Dame: University of Notre Dame Press, 1998), pp. 238–55

——, 'The Parson's Tale', in *Sources and Analogues of 'The Canterbury Tales'*, ed. by Robert M. Correale and Mary Hamel, 2 vols, Chaucer Studies, 28 and 35 (Cambridge: Brewer, 2002–05), I, 529–613

——, 'The Parson's Tale and its Generic Affiliations', in *Closure in 'The Canterbury Tales': The Role of the Parson's Tale*, ed. by David Raybin and Linda T. Holley, Studies in Medieval Culture, 41 (Kalamazoo: Western Michigan University Press, 2000), pp. 45–76; repr. in Richard Newhauser, *Sin: Essays on the Moral Tradition in the Western Middle Ages*, Variorum Collected Studies Series, CS869 (Aldershot: Ashgate, 2007), essay IV

——, 'Preaching the "Contrary Virtues"', *Mediaeval Studies*, 70 (2008), 135–62; repr. in *Classical and Medieval Literature Criticism*, vol. CLIX, ed. by L. J. Trudeau (Detroit: Gale, 2014), pp. 266–81

——, *The Treatise on Vices and Virtues in Latin and the Vernacular*, Typologie des sources du Moyen Âge occidental, 68 (Turnhout: Brepols, 1993)

——, 'Unerring Faith in the Pulpit: William Peraldus' *Tractatus de fide* in the *Summa de uirtutibus*', in *Fides Virtus: The Virtue of Faith from the Twelfth to the Early Sixteenth Century*, ed. by Marco Forlivesi, Riccardo Quinto, and Silvana Vecchio, *Archa Verbi: Yearbook for the Study of Medieval Theology*, Subsidia, 12 (Münster: Aschendorff, 2014), pp. 389–410

Newhauser, Richard, and István Bejczy, *A Supplement to Morton W. Bloomfield et al., 'Incipits of Latin Works on the Virtues and Vices, 1100–1500 A.D.'*, Instrumenta Patristica et Mediaevalia, Research on the Inheritance of Early and Medieval Christianity, 50 (Turnhout: Brepols, 2008)

Parker, John, 'The Epicurean Middle Ages', *Exemplaria*, 25.4 (2013), 324–29

Patterson, Lee, 'The Place of the Modern in the Late Middle Ages', in *The Challenge of Periodization: Old Paradigms and New Perspectives*, ed. by Lawrence Besserman, Garland Library of the Humanities, 1938 (New York: Garland, 1996), pp. 51–66

Rosenwein, Barbara H., ed., *Anger's Past: The Social Uses of an Emotion in the Middle Ages* (Ithaca, NY: Cornell University Press, 1998)

Rosenwein, Barbara H., and Lester K. Little, 'Social Meaning in the Monastic and Mendicant Spiritualities', *Past and Present*, 63 (1974), 18–32

Scanlon, Larry, *Narrative, Authority, and Power: The Medieval Exemplum and the Chaucerian Tradition*, Cambridge Studies in Medieval Literature, 20 (Cambridge: Cambridge University Press, 1994)

Vecchio, Silvana, 'Il piacere da Abelardo a Tommaso', in *Piacere e dolore: Materiali per una storia delle passioni nel Medioevo*, ed. by Carla Casagrande and Silvana Vecchio, Micrologus' Library, 29 (Firenze: SISMEL/Edizioni del Galluzzo, 2009), pp. 67–86

Verweij, Michiel, 'The Manuscript Transmission of the *Summa de Virtutibus* by Guillielmus Peraldus: A Preliminary Survey of the Manuscripts', *Medioevo*, 31 (2006), 103–296

Wenzel, Siegfried, 'The Continuing Life of William Peraldus's *Summa vitiorum*', in *Ad litteram: Authoritative Texts and their Medieval Readers*, ed. by Mark. D. Jordan and Kent Emery Jr, Notre Dame Conferences in Medieval Studies, 3 (Notre Dame: University of Notre Dame Press, 1992), pp. 135–63

——, 'Dante's Rationale for the Seven Deadly Sins (*Purgatorio* XVII)', *Modern Language Review*, 60 (1965), 529–33; reprint in Siegfried Wenzel, *Elucidations*, Synthema, 6 (Louvain: Peeters, 2010), pp. 113–19

——, 'The Source for the *Remedia* of the Parson's Tale', *Traditio*, 27 (1971), 433–53

——, 'The Source of Chaucer's Seven Deadly Sins', *Traditio*, 30 (1974), 351–78

Wolf, Klaus, '*Propter utilitatem populi: Durch nucz willen seines volkes*: Die "staatstragende" Rezeption der "Summa de vitiis" des Guilelmus Peraldus in der spätmittelalterlichen Wiener Schule', in *Laster im Mittelalter / Vices in the Middle Ages*, ed. by Christoph Flüeler and Martin Rohde, Scrinium Friburgense / Veröffentlichungen des Mediävistischen Instituts der Universität Freiburg, 23 (Berlin: de Gruyter, 2009), pp. 187–99

Young, Spencer E., *Scholarly Community at the Early University of Paris: Theologians, Education and Society, 1215–48*, Cambridge Studies in Medieval Life and Thought, 4th ser. (Cambridge: Cambridge University Press, 2014)

The Role of Pleasure in the Acquisition of Good Virtues: Giles of Rome's Idea of Education in his *De regimine principum* (*c.* 1279)

Noëlle-Laetitia Perret

Over the last twenty years a growing number of studies have started to reveal the profound influence of Giles of Rome (1243–1316) on the intellectual and educational culture of later medieval and early Renaissance Europe.[1] The author of a considerable number of Aristotelian commentaries and theological treatises, he was even called *Doctor Fundatissimus* by his contemporaries for his thorough knowledge of Aristotelian philosophy and his intellectual and doctrinal rigour.[2] Around 1279, Giles composed his major political work,[3] entitled *De regimine principum* (*On the Rule of Princes*) and dedicated it to young Philip, the future Philip IV.[4]

[1] The scant attention Giles of Rome has received is explained by the fact that only a few of his works have been edited. Since 1985, a project initiated and directed by Francesco Del Punta and Gianfranco Fioravanti has been undertaken to identify and publish Giles's works. For a biography of Giles, and for a comprehensive list of his works (more than seventy), see Del Punta, Donati, and Concetta, 'Egidio Romano'.

[2] Giles's career as master in theology at the Faculty of Arts was suspended in 1277, when Stephen Tempier, Bishop of Paris, censured Aristotelian and Averroistic heterodoxy. Just before leaving France (he had to wait until 1285 to be rehabilitated) he wrote his 'mirror of princes' (*speculum principis*), entitled *De regimine principum*.

[3] Besides his *De potestate ecclesiastica* (*On Ecclesiastical Power*, trans. by Dyson).

[4] Philip IV (1268–1314) 'the Fair' was King of France from 1285. At the time Giles of Rome dedicated his text to him, he was eleven years old.

Noëlle-Laetitia Perret (noelle-laetitia.perret@unifr.ch) is Maître d'enseignement et de recherche in medieval history at the University of Fribourg (Switzerland) and Membre associée at the École Pratique des Hautes Études (Paris). Her research interests include the social, intellectual, and cultural history of late medieval Europe as well as the history of diplomacy.

Pleasure in the Middle Ages, ed. by Naama Cohen-Hanegbi and Piroska Nagy, IMR 24 (Turnhout: Brepols, 2018), pp. 203–224 BREPOLS PUBLISHERS 10.1484/M.IMR-EB.5.113468

Giles, Friar of the Hermits of St Augustine,[5] divided his treatise on the education of the prince into three books, according to the Aristotelian division of practical philosophy: 'on self government' (ethics); 'on household government' (economics); and 'on civil government' (politics). Until now, this text has been studied first and foremost from the perspective of the history of political thought, with the consequence that Book II, dealing with the role of pleasure in the raising and educating of children, has only been dealt with indirectly.[6]

In this second part of his work, Giles conducts an intense reflection on the role of pleasure in education using notions such as *felicitas*, *bonum perfectum*, and *bonum secundum animam*. As we will see, he follows Aristotle in considering the origins of human nature in a pragmatic manner. He is the first medieval author of a mirror of princes to tackle fundamental questions in philosophical, secular, psychological, and metaphysical terms, outside of any theological conception. Those characteristics and the nearly 'universal' scope of the subjects discussed contributed to the long-lasting success of Giles's treatise, which has been translated into several languages.[7]

Whereas Henri de Gauchi — who first translated *De regimine principum* into French at the request of Philip the Fair in 1282[8] — tried to vulgarize

[5] As a young man, he joined the Hermits of St Augustine before being sent to Paris in 1260 in order to complete his studies at the Faculty of Theology. There, he probably followed Thomas Aquinas's teachings between 1269 and 1272. Giles of Rome was elected general of his order in 1292 and was made Archbishop of Bourges in 1295. He died in 1316.

[6] With a few important exceptions. See in particular Kaufmann, 'Von der Sorge der Eltern für die Erziehung ihrer Kinder von Aegidius Romanus de Colonna' and Schrübbers, 'Regimen und Homo Primitivus'. On children and education in the Middle Ages, see in particular Alexandre-Bidon and Lett, 'Grandeur et renaissance du sentiment de l'enfance au Moyen Âge'; Becchi and Julia, *Histoire de l'enfance en Occident*; and Sigal, 'L'Histoire de l'enfant au Moyen Âge'.

[7] The *De regimine principum* is one of the most copied and translated works of political-advice literature after the pseudo-Aristotelian *Secretum secretorum*. *De regimine principum* immediately resonated and was widely disseminated in Latin and many other languages (French, Italian, Castilian, Catalan, Portuguese, Hebrew, German, Flemish, English, and Swedish).

[8] Seven French versions of the *De regimine principum* have been identified. The text was first translated in 1282 by Henri de Gauchi at the request of Philip the Fair and grew to thirty-six copies. It was followed by six translations (each surviving in a single manuscript) until the end of the fifteenth century: the 'William' version (1330); the anonymous manuscript for Charles V (1372); Gilles Deschamps's translation (1420); the anonymous version by a 'mendicant' (1444); Jean Wauquelin's version for Philip the Good of Burgundy (1452); and the incomplete 'Berlin' version (Staatsbibl., MS Ham. 672), probably executed in northern Italy in the fifteenth century. These French versions of Giles's text take place in the larger process of

Giles's own vulgarization of Aristotle's philosophy through careful abbreviation, most of the other translators took great care to offer their readers translations of the full text. One of them, 'William',[9] who translated the entire work into French in 1330 after being commissioned by a *citoyen* (citizen) in Orléans, added not only examples but also personal opinions and experiences to his translation through interlinear glosses, which occur especially in the passages dealing with pleasure and education.[10]

The following paper therefore aims to highlight how Giles of Rome's examination of the nature of children in his *De regimine principum* brings to light the role of pleasure in their physical and intellectual development. We will observe what kind of pleasure Giles of Rome writes about, how he defines it, and how he draws on Aristotle for this discussion. We will then point out the way in which Giles of Rome's conception of pleasure in education is understood by 'William'. This perspective provides a concrete idea of what Giles of Rome's ideas become when they undergo the process of mediation to a lay public.

A Conception of Pleasure Deeply Influenced by Aristotelian Thinking

Giles of Rome belonged to the first generation of scholars in the West who were exposed to the corpus of Aristotle's moral philosophical works. Latin translations of Aristotle's *Politics* and *Nicomachean Ethics* provided medieval thinkers with a coherent theory of government that offered a substantially different perspective from that of Augustine, whose thinking had previously dominated ideas about human nature in general and about pleasure in particular.

With his widely read *De regimine principum*, Giles was one of the most important transmitters of Aristotle's moral philosophy. The Greek philosopher is Giles's principal authority, whom he usually refers to simply as *Philosophus*. Yet, although there is a significant predominance of Aristotle in his reflec-

French literacy — translations and writing — which evolves precisely from the twelfth century. See Perret, *Les Traductions françaises du 'De regimine principum' de Gilles de Rome*. See also Bérier, 'Traduire en France à la fin du Moyen Age' and Lusignan, *Parler vulgairement*.

[9] As we will see in the text below, we do not have any exact information about William, and we know very little about his activities; maybe he was a teacher in Salins (Burgundy). See Merisalo, 'Guillaume, ou comment traduire Gilles de Rome en 1330' and Merisalo, 'Le *Fidus interpres* et Gilles de Rome'.

[10] When translating Giles, William adds, for example, comments in which he praises the habits of the English when teaching spoken language, and of the Jews when teaching the alphabet to very young children, a process in which the notion of pleasure plays a fundamental role.

tions, Giles was not limited to Aristotelian thought. The influence of Thomas Aquinas's comments on the *Ethics* and *Politics*, as well as his *De regno* and *Summa theologica*, is apparent. Furthermore, Giles drew, mostly implicitly,[11] from many sources, among them classical authors (particularly Cicero and Vegetius), medical sources such as Galen, and many others, such as Dominicus Gundissalinus and Vincent of Beauvais.[12] Moreover, Giles mentions neither his use of the scriptures nor of the Fathers of the Church.

In the second book of *De regimine principum* Giles,[13] following Aristotle, explains the ethical importance of pleasure in the acquisition of virtues. He bases his argumentation in particular on the *Nicomachean Ethics* (Books VII and X), in which Aristotle treats the relationship between happiness and pleasure, and the connection of virtue to pleasure within a reflection on education.[14] The following section shows how Giles, seventeen centuries after Aristotle's death (322 BC), is literally inspired by Aristotle in the way he deals with the notions of pleasure and happiness, and connects them to virtue.

[11] Giles does not often cite the Greek philosopher in an explicit way: in fact, he does not really worry about rendering Aristotle's thoughts with precision. In referring to the Greek philosopher, he is in fact principally concerned with endowing his own writing with a certain authority. This is why he liberally adapts and transposes not only Aristotle's thinking, but also that of Thomas Aquinas and others, usually in an implicit way. So, as Roberto Lambertini shows, Giles of Rome assimilates Aristotle's thinking 'to give the impression to his contemporary readers, and even to future scholars, that he is only reporting Aristotle's thoughts in a simpler way so that even laymen could understand them': Lambertini, 'The Prince in the Mirror of Philosophy', pp. 1524.

[12] Constantino Marmo, Lidia Lanza, and Roberto Lambertini's analyses have contributed substantially to the understanding of Giles's relationship with his sources. See particularly Marmo, '*Hoc autem et si potest tollerari …*'; Lambertini, 'Il filosofo, il principe et la virtù'; Lambertini, '*Philosophus videtur tangere tres rationes*'; Lambertini, 'A proposito della "costruzione" dell' *Oeconomica* in Egidio Romano'; Lanza, 'La *Politica* di Aristotele e il *De regimine principum* di Egidio Romano'.

[13] This second part of Book II is divided into three parts, dealing respectively with marital relations and the proper conduct of women, the upbringing of children, and the management of the household (property, finances, servants, etc). It is therefore dedicated in particular to the problems of education and presents the different periods of childhood and their educational recommendations.

[14] Here, Giles of Rome most probably used Robert Grosseteste's translation of Aristotle's *Ethics*, revised by the Dominican William of Moerbeke around 1260. See Brams, 'The Revised Version of Grosseteste's Translation of the *Nicomachean Ethics*'.

Happiness, Pleasure, and Virtue According to Aristotle and Giles of Rome

Reflection on pleasure lies at the heart of Aristotle's thoughts on ethics. He explores the subject in two main passages: first in the *Nicomachean Ethics*, at the end of Book VII (Chapters 11–14), and then at the beginning of Book X (Chapters 1–5). In his view, pleasure and happiness share common characteristics — but pleasure cannot be reduced to happiness. Aristotle distinguishes between those things such as virtue, intellectual activity, and pleasure which are desirable both for themselves and for the sake of happiness. According to Aristotle, pleasure appears therefore to be a constituent of happiness, along with other good things. Generally, a happy life must therefore include pleasure. In other words, happiness is pleasure, understood to be something intrinsically valuable.[15]

[15] Aristotle, *Nicomachean Ethics*, 1152b, trans. by Rackham: 'Now (1) some people think that no pleasure is a good thing, whether essentially or accidentally. They argue that Good and Pleasure are two distinct things. (2) Others hold that though some pleasures are good, most are bad. (3) There is also a third view, that even if all pleasures are good, nevertheless pleasure cannot be the Supreme Good. [4] (1) To prove that pleasure is not a good at all, it is argued that (a) Every pleasure is a conscious process towards a natural state; but a process can in no case belong to the same order of things as its end; for example, the process of building cannot be a thing of the same sort as the house built. (b) The temperate man avoids pleasures. (c) The prudent man pursues freedom from pain, not pleasure. (d) Pleasures are a hindrance to prudent deliberation, and the more so the more enjoyable they are; for instance, sexual pleasure: no one could think of anything while indulging in it. (e) There is no art of pleasure; yet with every good thing there is an art which produces it. (f) Children and animals pursue pleasures. [5] (2) To prove that not all pleasures are good, it is argued that (a) some pleasures are disgraceful, and discredit the man who indulges in them. (b) Some pleasures are harmful, for certain pleasant things cause disease. (3) To prove that pleasure is not the Supreme Good, it is argued that it is not an end but a process. These then, more or less, are the current views'. In the version used by Giles of Rome — most probably Robert Grosseteste's translation of Aristotle's *Ethics*, revised by the Dominican William of Moerbeke around 1260 — we can read the following passage: 'De delectacione autem et tristicia speculari eius qui politicam philosophatur; iste enim finis architecton ad quem respicientes unumquodque hoc quidem malum, hoc autem bonum simpliciter dicamus. Adhuc autem necessariorum intendere de ipsis; et enim virtutem et maliciam moralem circa tristicias et delectaciones posuimus. Et felicitatem plures cum delectacione esse aiunt; propter quod et beatum nominaverunt a gaudere. Hiis quidem igitur videtur neque una delectacio esse bonum neque secundum se ipsum neque secundum accidens. Non enim esse idem bonum et delectacionem. Hiis autem quedam quidem esse, multe autem prave. Adhuc autem horum tercium, si et omnes bonum, tamen non contingit esse optimum delectacionem. Totaliter quidem igitur non bonum, quoniam omnis delectacio generacio est in naturam sensibilis, neque una autem generacio cognata finibus, puta neque una edificacio domus. Adhuc temperatus fugit delectaniones. Adhuc prudens non triste persequitur, non delectabile. Adhuc impedimentum ei quod est prudentem esse delectationes, et quanto magis

Giles follows closely Aristotle's definition of happiness and pleasure as related to the notion of habit. In *De regimine principum*'s first book, which treats self-control, he presents the first thing to be set out in regard to happiness: 'First it will be shown what his Royal Majesty ought to have as his end and where he should locate his happiness'.[16] He refers to 'the Philosopher' to present what is profitable in moral matters, what is profitable concerning activities, and how they should be carried out in order to enjoy them and to feel pleasure:

> Inde est ergo, quod vult Philosophus 2. Ethic. proficuum esse morali negocio, scrutari ea quae sunt circa operationes, quomodo faciendum sit eas. Operationes autem nostrae ex quatuor (quantum ad praesens spectat) videntur oriri, et diversificari; videlicet, ex finibus, habitibus, passionibus, et moribus. [...] Ad sciendum ergo quae operari debemus, maxime proficuum esse videtur, quem finem nobis praestituere debeamus. Ut dicitur 2. Ethicorum signum generati habitus, est delectationem, et tristitiam fieri in opere, secundum quod alios et alios habitus habemus, in aliis, et aliis actibus delectamur.

> [This is therefore what the Philosopher intends to do when he says in *Ethics* II (2, 1103b29–30) that it is profitable in moral matters to examine thoroughly what concerns activities and how they should be done. Now as regards the present discussion, it would seem that our activities arise from, and are differentiated from another by, four factors, namely, ends, habits, passions, and ways of behaving. [...] Then, in order to know what we ought to do, it seems highly profitable [to know] what end we ought to set ourselves. Moreover, because (as is said in *Ethics* II (3, 1104b3–5)) pleasure or distress in what is done is the sign of an acquired habit — in the sense that we take pleasure in one act or another according as we have one habit or another.][17]

For Aristotle, as for Giles of Rome, the most perfect pleasures are the ones experienced by virtuous people who have the faculty to behave well. In their minds,

gaudet, magis, puta eam que venereorum. Nullum enim utique posse intelligere aliquid in ipsa. Adhuc ars neque una delectacionis, quamvis omne bonus artis opus. Adhuc pueri et bestie persequntur delectationes. Huius autem non omnes studiosas, quoniam sunt et turpes et probrose, et quoniam nocive. Egritudinalia enim quedam delectabilium. Quod autem non optimum delectacio, quoniam non finis, set generacio. Que quidem igitur dicuntur, fere hec sunt'. Aristotle, *Ethica Nicomachea translatio Roberti Grosseteste Lincolniensis*, VII, 13, ed. by Gauthier, pp. 512–13.

[16] Aegidius Romanus, *De regimine principum*, I, I, 2, p. 6; trans. from 'Giles of Rome, On the Rule of Princes (selections)', ed. and trans. by McGrade, Kilcullen, and Kempshall, p. 207.

[17] Aegidius Romanus, *De regimine principum*, I, I, 2, p. 6; trans. from 'Giles of Rome, On the Rule of Princes (selections)', ed. and trans. by McGrade, Kilcullen, and Kempshall, p. 208.

to be a virtuous person means, precisely, to take pleasure in performing virtuous actions. Aristotle, followed by Giles of Rome, considers desire as educable. Thus, the challenge of moral development does not consist of repressing one's desires: the real challenge is to develop these desires properly. Discussing 'The utility of what is to be said' (Book I, Chapter 3), Giles presents his work's ambition:

> Consequitur maiestas regia (quantum ad praesens spectat) quatuor, quae quilibet maxime amare, et desiderare debet. Primo enim lucrabitur maxima bona. Secundo lucrabitur seipsum. Tertio alios. Quarto consequetur, ut habeat ipsum Deum, et felicitatem aeternam
>
> [his Royal Majesty will attain four things for which anyone ought to have the greatest love and desire. First, he will gain (*lucrabitur*) the greatest goods; second, he will gain himself; third, others; and the fourth consequence is that he will have the Lord Himself and eternal happiness.][18]

The notions of human happiness and pleasure represent — as for Aristotle — the fundamental aim of Giles's political and pedagogic theory. Happiness is realized through perfect action, a certain kind of pleasure, and the exercise of virtue. Man — first the Royal Majesty and through him the entire society — arrives at virtue if he has been trained to do so by his education. Ethics and education are one and the same; the happy man is an educated man, having attained virtue through education. Nature reserves particular dispositions for mankind, but only education allows the individual to update or upgrade them in order to fully become a man.

The Fundamental Role of Pleasure in Education

Giles of Rome retains from Aristotle the notion that a human being develops its capacities from birth and that desire for knowledge proceeds from the pleasure of sense perception. From this perspective, he observes that the child experiences pleasure when it breastfeeds: 'from birth we start to experience pleasure: indeed small children take pleasure as soon as they are nursing on their mother's milk'.[19] The child must therefore learn from birth to make good

[18] Aegidius Romanus, *De regimine principum*, I, I, 3, p. 8; trans. from 'Giles of Rome, On the Rule of Princes (selections)', ed. and trans. by McGrade, Kilcullen, and Kempshall, p. 209.

[19] 'Ab ipsa infantia delectari incipimus: nam et pueri statim delectantur, cum incipiunt suggere mammas', Aegidius Romanus, *De regimine principum*, II, II, 6, p. 301 (my translation). Following Giles of Rome, another man of the church, Conrad de Megenberg, is concerned with

use of his or her senses, which are like open doors to the worst temptations related to sensual pleasures. It is an issue of utmost importance that requires everyone's attention. Sound use of reason appears to be the best antidote to unsuitable physical pleasures.

Indeed, Giles of Rome understands reason to be an instrument for the regulation of passions and natural impulses which exist from birth. This view implies that there are two parts to the soul: the irrational, and the part that is endowed with reason. The irrational part is understood as being anterior to the rational part, in the same way that the body is anterior to the soul in its development. This perspective ensues from a representation of human life perceived as successive stages marked by the more or less perfect use of reason. Following Aristotle, Giles of Rome maintains that we must all be led towards finding, from infancy, our pleasures and our pains by means of a good education: 'Hence the importance, as Plato points out, of having been definitely trained from childhood to like and dislike the proper things; this is what good education means'.[20] Thus education proceeds in stages: care of the body must precede that of the soul, and according to this perspective, Giles of Rome prescribes in the second part of Book II specific educational recommendations for each period of childhood.[21]

Giles of Rome divides childhood into three phases (from zero to seven years old, from seven to fourteen, and from fourteen to twenty-one). These periods of human life are perceived, moreover, as key periods that require full attention.[22]

the question and adds some practical suggestions to curb the pleasure that small children experience when breastfeeding: he suggests that women smear their breasts with a mixture of honey and salt to effectively put the child off: 'Sed quoniam difficile est infanti consuetam relinquere mammillam, igitur a principio sue ablactacionis ut plurimum vagit, inquietando vagitu auditores. Refrenandum est desiderium eius hoc modo: sumatur mel sale mixtum et papille mamme inungantur cum illo, et cum puer gustaverit, tanta abhominacione resipiscet, quod amplius non gustabit'. Konrad von Megenberg, *Ökonomik*, I, 2, 10, ed. by Krüger, p. 83.

[20] 'Propter quod oportet duci qualiter confestim ex iuvenibus, ut Plato ait. Quare et gaudere et tristari in quibus oportet; recta enim disciplina hec est': Aristotle, *Ethica Nicomachea translatio Roberti Grosseteste Lincolniensis*, II, 2, ed. by Gauthier, p. 399.

[21] Describing the different periods of childhood, Giles of Rome uses different words such as *infans*, *puer*, *puella*, or *iuvenis* but without being systematic. See Aegidius Romanus, *De regimine principum*, II, II.

[22] Marilyn Nicoud underlined how Bernard de Gordon, in his *Liber conservanda sanitate*, also distinguished different periods of childhood. See Nicoud, *Les Régimes de santé au Moyen Âge*, I, 200. Giles of Rome never refers to medical authors such as Bernard de Gordon or Aldebrandin de Sienne (*The Regimen of the Body*), but he was surely acquainted with them.

The child — the male child — is considered a perfectible being, in constant flux, according to the Aristotelian principle assumed by our writer, who considers that 'nature proceeds from what is imperfect towards that which is perfect'.[23] Here we should mention that Giles of Rome's reflection concerns above all boys, children whose imperfection is considered provisional; girls shows signs of irremediable weakness.

Even if it is care of the body that prevails during the first period of infancy, care afforded to the soul should not, however, be neglected. Giles of Rome advises parents and teachers to encourage children to learn songs, fables, and their own stories in order to exercise their memory, imagination, and moral virtues. Around 1240, Bartholomew the Englishman (1203–1272), like Giles of Rome some years later, advised singing to the child in a gentle voice in order to nurture its senses: 'cantus adhiberi, ut sensus infantuli ex vocis dulcedine delectentur'.[24] Giles refers here indirectly to Aristotle's *De anima*, which affirms that the desire to know proceeds from the pleasure of sensory perception.[25]

Young children, greatly influenced by what they see and hear, need to be kept protected from dishonest displays and licentious remarks. Understood as a being that is easily modelled, the child is particularly exposed to danger merely by its inexperience. It is important to keep an eye on the conversations, gestures, and games that are conveyed to the child, even those to which he would only be taken to observe. It is because he is taught to control his instincts that the child is progressively led to abandon a state close to that of the animal with wild pleasures and to move closer to that of the human being characterized by his rational faculty.

Children's Games: When Pleasure Serves Socialization

Giles also introduces, in the second part of his *De regimine principum*, a discourse on children's games and the appropriate behaviour that he or she should adopt in play activity.[26] Indeed, he observes that children, 'from birth, "natu-

[23] 'Natura enim semper ex imperfecto ad perfectum procedit': Aegidius Romanus, *De regimine principum*, I, 1, 2, p. 5 (my translation).

[24] Bartholomaeus Anglicus, *De genuinis rerum coelestium*, VI, 4, p. 238.

[25] 'Nihil sine phantasmate intelligit anima': Aristotle, *De anima*, III, 7 (431a14).

[26] On children's games in the Middle Ages, see, for example, Mehl, *Des jeux et des hommes dans la société médiévale*; Ortalli, 'Tempo libero e Medioevo'; Orme, 'The Culture of Children in Medieval England'; and Shahar, *Childhood in the Middle Ages*, pp. 104–05 and p. 223.

rally" take pleasure in play'.[27] The image that predominates his thought is that of the child perceived as a small, wild being without limits, always ready to have fun and to play. Play, which characterizes the very nature of the child, is often irrational. However, since it was limited to avoid excess, play appeared to be a useful instrument in the physical and psychic development of the child and even as an effective means for preparing the child to integrate into the society of adults.[28]

Giles appropriates the Aristotelian concept of play, defined as something necessary, a form of relaxation which, however, should not have to be an end in itself. Play allows rest for the soul, and it is not forbidden to give oneself up to it from time to time, on the one condition that it be moderated. Conceived, in contrast to work, as a form of recreation necessary for restoring energies, play is above all an instrument that makes it possible to avoid idleness or laziness. If Giles allows the young child to play, it is to prevent his soul from 'idleness'.[29] While Giles mentions relatively 'classic' games: hoops, archery, chess, etc., Conrad of Megenberg (1309–1374), directly inspired by Giles, adds to the list 'the doll and use of the mirror in order to learn how to talk'.[30] As for adults, Giles advises seeking diversion through play, but only on the condition that their attempts at play be 'moderate and harmless'.[31]

[27] 'Ab ipsa enim infantia connaturale videtur esse pueris delectari iocis': Aegidius Romanus, *De regimine principum*, II, I, 30, p. 138 (my translation).

[28] Later, around 1404–07, Christine de Pizan, in her *Livre du corps de policie*, takes up Giles of Rome's considerations on children's play literally. See Christine de Pizan, *Livre du corps de policie*, I, V, ed. by Lucas, p. 13. More generally, see, for example, Riché and Alexandre-Bidon, *L'Enfance au Moyen Âge*, p. 27; Classen, *Childhood in the Middle Ages and the Renaissance*; Hanawalt, 'Medievalists and the Study of Childhood'.

[29] 'Mens humana nescit ociosa esse': Aegidius Romanus, *De regimine principum*, II, II, 8, p. 307.

[30] 'Decentes vero ludi sunt infantum pupinas tractare, sculptilia volvere et speculis se ipsos intueri': Konrad von Megenberg, *Ökonomik*, I, 2, 14, ed. by Krüger, pp. 89–90. Conrad of Megenberg studied at Erfurt and at the University of Paris, where he taught philosophy and theology. He is one of the most prolific German writers of the fourteenth century and author of, among many texts, the tract *Oeconomia* (*c.* 1350), inspired by Aristotle and Giles of Rome.

[31] 'Aliqua delectabilia quae sunt licitae et innocuae': Aegidius Romanus, *De regimine principum*, II, II, 8, p. 307.

The Right Education and Good Habits in Order to Experience Permitted Pleasure

In his discourse on pleasure and the acquisition of good morals, Giles of Rome principally refers to the tenth book of *Nicomachean Ethics*, in which Aristotle examines the notion of virtue, which he perceives not merely as a form of knowledge, but rather as a form of disposition.[32] It is not enough, Aristotle explains, to know what virtue is; one also has to make an effort to put it into practice. Even if certain people are born with good dispositions, most people acquire them only by means of a good education and good habits. For Aristotle, as for Giles of Rome, moral virtues are acquired in three ways: from nature, which makes people susceptible to them; through habit, which allows people to develop them effectively; and through education, which reveals what they consist of. The acquisition of virtue implies perseverance. The educator must lead the child to imitate an act repeatedly so that the child better integrates it, even if this involves the use of reprimands. Only by proceeding this way will he feel the pleasure of accomplishing it. From this perspective, Giles of Rome agrees with Aristotle's conception of human nature seeking to obtain pleasure.[33]

[32] 'Habitus ex quo bonus homo fit et a quo bene opus suum reddit': Aristotle, *Ethica Nicomachea translatio Roberti Grosseteste Lincolniensis*, II, 5, ed. by Gauthier, p. 402.

[33] Aristotle, *Nicomachean Ethics*, 1175a.1, trans. by Rackham: 'It might be held that all men seek to obtain pleasure, because all men desire life. Life is a form of activity, and each man exercises his activity upon those objects and with those faculties which he likes the most: for example, the musician exercises his sense of hearing upon musical tunes, the student his intellect upon problems of philosophy, and so on. And the pleasure of these activities perfects the activities, and therefore perfects life, which all men seek. Men have good reason therefore to pursue pleasure, since it perfects for each his life, which is a desirable thing. The question whether we desire life for the sake of pleasure or pleasure for the sake of life need not be raised for the present. In any case they appear to be inseparably united; for there is no pleasure without activity, and also no perfect activity without its pleasure'. In the version used by Giles of Rome we can read: 'Quedam autem delectant nova encia, posterius autem non similiter, propter hoc; primum quidem enim per desideria inclinata est mens et intense circa eadem operatur, quemadmodum secundum visum aspicientes; postea non fit talis operacio, set neclecta; propter quod et delectacio obscuratur. Appetere autem delectaciones existimabit quis utique omnes, quoniam et vivere omnes appetunt, vita autem operacio quedam est, et unusquisque circa hoc et in his operatur que et maxime diligit; puta musicus quidem auditu circa melodias, amator autem discipline mente circa theoremata, sic autem et reliquorum unusquisque. Delectacio autem perficit operaciones, et vivere autem, quod appetunt. Racionabiliter igitur et delectacionem appetunt; perficit enim unicuique vivere, eligibile ens. Utrum autem propter delectacionem vivere eligimus vel propter vivere delectacionem; dimittatur in presenti; coniugi quidem enim hec videntur et separacionem non recipere. Sine operacione enim non fit delectacio'. Aristotle, *Ethica Nicomachea translatio Roberti Grosseteste Lincolniensis*, X, 5, ed. by Gauthier, p. 571.

Like Aristotle, he considers the intimate link between a 'perfect' activity and the best form of pleasure and gives music and the learning of *litteras* as examples of suitable activities which lead to permitted pleasures and prevent illicit acts.[34] Thus, it is essentially through example that children are led to turn away from immediate and unsuitable pleasures. The role of a good educator is therefore essential. He needs to know how to develop in the child the psychic, moral, and intellectual faculties that will guide him towards an ethical ideal and controlled pleasure.

Given the important role of pleasure in a child's nature, a necessary focus of attention should be on the particular child. Through the learning of good habits and the following of correct examples taught by the educator, 'the child, as soon as he learns to speak, has to be guided towards a virtuous life governed not by passions, but rather by his reason'.[35] Giles underlines how much the human being is tempted to commit inappropriate acts. Indeed, it takes time to get used to goodness and to avoid surrendering to forbidden pleasures. The child's soul is perceived as soft wax on which it is very easy to leave the impression of a seal, and so the child must, at as early an age as possible, get used to adopting good morals. Education consists of instilling in the child the habits that will come to be like a second nature to him. Indeed, with the development of reason, the acquisition of good habits constitutes one of the principal elements of education that make it possible to lead the child to act according to what is right and just. By nurturing good habits in the child, it becomes possible, over time, for the child to assimilate moral virtues and appreciate their true value.

Parents and pedagogues must take it upon themselves to make up for the deficiencies in the infant nature that are caused by the sensory instincts that gradually worsen as the child approaches adulthood. The will of young adults should therefore be directed according to the principles of modesty and obedience, on the one hand, and of sexual abstinence on the other. Young people are animated by an immodest desire for pleasure and often have particularly excessive natures. William, Giles's translator, seems to be particularly interested in this question as he adds comments, through interlinear glosses, in this particular passage of the second book of *De regimine principum*. William underlines that this final period of childhood is indeed marked by the entry into puberty

[34] 'Ut per eas prudentiores effecti, magis possent illicita praecavere': Aegidius Romanus, *De regimine principum*, II, II, 7, p. 303.

[35] 'Statim cum pueri sunt sermonum capaces, sunt instruendi ad bonos mores, et debent eis fieri monitiones debitae': Aegidius Romanus, *De regimine principum*, II, II, 6, p. 301 (my translation).

and the first inclinations towards the pleasures of love, and he provides his own insight: 'when [children] love, they love too much and when they start to play, they play in an excessive way too'.[36]

Giles, once again directly inspired by Aristotle, recommends that young people be guided towards a virtuous life by helping them to find a middle position in which they gradually manage to control their impulses.[37] This difficult balance towards which the young adult is led allows him to find, should he reach it, a certain harmony between contrary emotions composed of pleasure and pain.[38] Giles again considers reason to be the most effective instrument for regulating different passions and natural impulses. Controlled by reason, the vices that push young people to do evil can then become virtuous attitudes.

The Role of Pleasure in Intellectual Education

Given their future burdens and in order to avoid their becoming tyrants, according to Giles of Rome, the sons of princes and kings must apply themselves more than others to the study of the sciences. An education in the liter-

[36] 'Quant ils aiment, ils aiment trop et quant ils commencent à jouer, ils jouent trop'. French translation by William (1330), Paris, Bibl. de l'Arsenal, MS 2690, fol. 119v.

[37] It refers specifically to Aristotle, *Nicomachean Ethics*, 1109a, in which Aristotle declares: 'Enough has now been said to show that moral virtue is a mean, and in what sense this is so, namely that it is a mean between two vices, one of excess and the other of defect; and that it is such a mean because it aims at hitting the middle point in feelings and in actions. [...] so that to do these things properly is rare, praiseworthy, and noble' (trans. by Rackam). In the version used by Giles of Rome we can read: 'Quoniam quidem igitur est virtus moralis medietas et qualiter et quoniam est medietas duarum maliciarum, huius quidem secundum superhabundanciam, huius autem secundum defectum, et quoniam talis est quia coniectatrix medii est quod est in passionibus et operacionibus, sufficienter dictum est. [...] quod est bene et arum et laudabile et bonum'. Aristotle, *Ethica Nicomachea translatio Roberti Grosseteste Lincolniensis*, II, 9, ed. by Gauthier, p. 408.

[38] Giles of Rome's view of youth is largely inspired by the portrait that Aristotle outlines in the second book of his *Rhetoric*. The Greek philosopher describes, in particular, the violence and instability of young people's passions. He perceives in them a generous naiveté. He considers the ardour and selflessness of their friendships, but also the excess they put into everything they do. He highlights their capacity to enjoy themselves and their love of laughter. He also shows the deep optimism of young people that results from their inexperience; they know nothing of the risk of failure. Giles of Rome, following Aristotle, understands this optimism as the result of the body's natural heat, which the young possess in great quantity, and which leads them to see the future in a positive way, according to the same principle that governs wine turning drunkards into optimists.

ary disciplines from a very young age is supposed to allow them to demonstrate a certain pleasure in study and to show themselves capable of becoming adults. Moreover, he specifies, nobody will reach a high level of knowledge without 'being initiated from the cradle'.[39] To deal with this question, our author refers again to the role played by habit, recalling that it is the things that we become used to from childhood that please us the most and for which we display the most enthusiasm. In this domain, too, human beings need a lot of time to reach a certain level of perfection. Our writer bases his reasoning on the theory of knowledge developed by Aristotle in the first book of *De Anima* and that of Thomas Aquinas in his *Summa Theologiae* (Ia, Q. 84 to 89), when he observes that the poor natural dispositions of human beings prevent them from having a direct understanding of the different sciences and oblige them to show perseverance in order to be able to feel pleasure, through practice.[40]

Young men also, according to Giles, need to be educated in the disciplines of the liberal arts (grammar, logic, rhetoric, music, arithmetic, geometry, and astronomy). These sciences, especially rhetoric, are particularly useful for those who will one day be called on to rule. In general, music represents an activity appropriate to the nature of children and youth which provides them with harmless pleasure — 'delectationes innocuas'.[41]

Even if Giles's reflections on pleasure in education concern above all boys and young men, he did recognize the right of girls and women to take pleasure in some activities. His pages on the education of girls, at the end of Book II, can be situated within a broader movement which develops, from the thirteenth century, a specific discourse dedicated to this question.[42] Like Aristotle, Giles considers that nature ordained not only physical differences between males and females, but mental differences as well.[43] From this perspective, the educa-

[39] 'Nisi quasi ab ipsis cunabulis vacare incipiat ad ipsam': Aegidius Romanus, *De regimine principum*, II, II, 7, p. 305 (my translation).

[40] Indeed, as Giles underlines, '[Homines] male nati sunt ad sciendum: quia nostra cognitio incipit a sensu et a posterioribus': Aegidius Romanus, *De regimine principum*, II, II, 6, p. 305.

[41] 'Quarum una est, quia pueri nihil tristabile sustinere possunt: quare si debent eis aliqua delectabilia concedi, dignum est quod ordinentur ad delectationes innocuas: quare (secundum eundem Philosphum) musica est consentanea naturae iuvenum, quia habent innocuas delectationes': Aegidius Romanus, *De regimine principum*, II, II, 8, p. 307.

[42] See, for example, *Le Livre du chevalier de la Tour Landry pour l'enseignement de ses filles*, ed. by de Montaiglon. See also '*Aucuns petis enseignemens*', ed. by Drijvers and MacDonald.

[43] For women in the Middle Ages, see particularly, within an extensive bibliography, Duby and Perrot, *Histoire des femmes*, vol. II, *Le Moyen Âge*, dir. by Klapisch-Zuber.

tion of girls requires great care, since they are all particularly prone to lust and unsuitable pleasures, as they are mainly governed by impulses.[44]

Giles advises therefore that fathers keep their daughters at home and keep them from going out walking, in order to keep them away from any chance of giving way to their bad habits. If girls are accustomed to having social relations, they lose their natural modesty which must nevertheless protect their chastity; devoid of any shyness towards men, they are then like wild beasts. Incapable of making use of their reason, it is modesty that must prevent them from seeking out forbidden pleasures. Giles therefore recommends that they be kept permanently occupied. At most, we can give them some suitable activity such as sewing or spinning. Depending on her social status, the woman can devote herself to and take pleasure in reading.[45]

Giles does not specify which texts might divert women; however, they are probably religious. William, Giles's translator, agrees and adds that young girls of noble standing might embroider the altar cloths of the Lord, a suitable pleasure and a sign of 'perfect devotion'.[46]

It is particularly important that girls learn to make moderate use of speech; discretion will be appreciated by their future husbands and keep them happy. Needless to say, Giles condemns the beauty treatments that women indulge in and which he associates with the sins of lust and pride. It is principally important that young girls, like young boys, learn to show modesty in their actions and their nutrition. Food should not, in any case, be a source of inappropriate pleasures.

Food and Reasonable Pleasures

Giles also tackles the notion of pleasure in the passages of his work that he dedicates to how men and women should feed themselves. There, too, it is just a question of moderation. Eating is related to touch and to taste, and these repre-

[44] Aristotle's misogyny had a profound influence on medieval Western thinkers. On this question, see Lett, *Le Genre au Moyen Âge* and Schaus, *Women and Gender in Medieval Europe*.

[45] 'Ut ad amorem literarum affecta, non vacaret ociose, sed saepe saepius librum arripiens, se lectionibus occuparet': Aegidius Romanus, *De regimine principum*, II, II, 20, p. 345.

[46] 'Laquele chose ie ne croi pas car selonc ne doive pas ouvrer des mains une royne ou une princesse pour hoinine par aventure non pour tant eles ne sont pas a reprendre se eles oevres de lour propres mains les aournemenz de l'autel sur lequel l'en sacreste le salveour dou monde aussi sont forment a priser car ce est signe de parfaite devotion mais se si grant dame ne soit pas ouvrer en tele maniere': William (1330), Paris, Bibl. de l'Arsenal, MS 2690, fol. 123^{v}.

sent the sensual forms of pleasure that man shares with animals and which are, for that very reason, highly reprehensible. For Giles, eating should not spring from unreasonable desire, because eating with excessive pleasure and in excessive quantity, as gluttons do, causes damage not only to the body, but also to the soul.

For William the translator, however, eating is not entirely problematic, as it is also perceived as a useful educational instrument. In one of his glosses on Giles's text, for instance, William recalls the Jewish tradition that uses various treats in order to instil in the child the first notions of the alphabet:

> Et li Juys, si tost comme li enfant soivent parler, leur enseignent petit et petit, aussi comme en juant, espeler. Et pour ce qu'il pouissent delectablement aprendre [...] les peres leur donnent pometes et pain chaut, figues et autre fruit [...] et par raison des dons il aient bon cuer de apprendre.[47]

> [The Jews, as soon as they teach their children how to speak, they teach them, little by little, in play, how to spell. To make it possible to take pleasure in learning, [...] the fathers fill their children with little apples and warm bread, with figs and with fruit. [...] With these presents, their hearts are disposed to learning.]

Like William, many preachers and men of the Church advise teachers to play on the greed of children and to use the sweetness of food to transform learning into fun.[48] However, all educators agree on one point: a child should not eat food that is too rich; eating food that is overtly delicate is perceived as a sin if the food does not correspond to that person's social standing. William inserts into his translation of Giles's work a commentary, inspired by observations borrowed from everyday life, in which he gives astonishing details about those meals that William considered to be too deliciously prepared and too subject to pleasure. Such meals threaten the natural equilibrium of the constitution, and children must be taught to abstain from them. The list is long: he tells us of mutton thighs and small stuffed birds; of buttered tarts and almond milk

[47] Paris, Bibl. de l'Arsenal, MS 2690, fol. 119r.

[48] Christiane Klapisch-Zuber underlines how Matteo Palmieri, a wealthy merchant of Florence, in his text *La vita civile* (1430), suggests forming letters using cookies and all kinds of food appeciated by children in order to familiarize them with the learning of the alphabet in an enjoyable way: 'Formate delle lettere in frutte, berlingozi, zucherini et altri cibi puerili, incitate il fanciullo con essi prometterli daglieli, s'egli li conosce, dicendoli: questo torto è un S'. M. Palmieri, *Vita civile* (Venezia, 1534), cited here by Klapisch-Zuber, 'Le chiavi florentine di Barbablu', p. 786, n. 32. See also Alexandre-Bidon, 'Abécédaires et alphabets éducatifs du XIII à la fin du XIVe siècle'; Alexandre-Bidon, 'La Lettre volée'.

sprinkled with delicate powder and decorated with gold leaves, all moistened in daisy oil. It is also better to avoid meat pasties and concoctions that are fried or in jelly.[49] These considerations on children's dietary habits echo the science of dietetics developed in medical literature, such as *regimen sanitatis* (regimen of health), recently studied by Marilyn Nicoud.[50]

In another gloss, William also adds some surprising remarks to Giles's text regarding the form that play can take and the moments of pleasure in the education of children. He also inserts comments which do not exist in the original text. In these additions to Giles's text, William gives a significant place to pleasure. Indeed, he describes in a gloss a nanny playing and laughing with children, taking fun in tying a pan to the tail of a cat — the same nanny who also takes fun in scaring children by pretending to want to devour them and who assures them that she doesn't want to punish them in any way.[51]

This last addition of William takes place in a chapter dedicated by Giles to teachers. Contrary to Vincent of Beauvais, Giles severely criticizes brutal teachers and warns parents to keep their children away. His translator, William, supports this idea in one of his comments. He challenges, as does Giles, the brutality of some teachers. He himself remembers how one of his pupils — whom he calls 'Alexius' — revealed himself to be very good at study, without ever being the subject, he says, of any reprimand. He further emphasizes that if the pupil goes on to prove himself gifted in a diverse range of sciences, it is due to the early education he received. Indeed, like Giles, he underlines as a leitmotif the idea that as adults we show the best understanding and feel pleasure and satisfaction for specific knowledge, even the most complex, if we are used to it from childhood.[52]

[49] 'Ainsi comme quand l'on farcit poulardes, cuisses de mouton et petits oiseaux; et quand l'on fait des pâtisseries avec du beurre, du lait d'amandes, recouvertes de sirop, ornées de feuilles et généreusement arrosées d'huile de marguerite. Ou encore lorsque l'on prépare des gâteaux recherchés d'oiseaux et de fleurs faits de pâte colorée et frite dans le sucre. Cela concerne également la préparation d'un large morceau de viande. Comme sont également les navets sucrés. Premièrement cuits puis frits, ils sont préparés en gelée ou autrement. Ainsi en va-t-il de tant d'autres choses': Paris, Bibl. de l'Arsenal, MS 2690, fol. 115^{r}.

[50] See Nicoud, *Medieval Dietetics*.

[51] 'Translateur. Aussi comme nous veons que les bonnes norrissens se rient aus enffans et les font rire, menant une paëlle environ la queue de un chaton. Et puis, quant li enffes entendent un poi mieux, lor ostent les coutianz des mains ou autre chose inusable et menacent de une paëlle ou baton un autre enffant qui entent qui est de ioste eulz et font un semblant et getent une voiz rude comme se eles voulissent devorer l'enfant qui entent pour ce que li enffens que eles nourrissent le chastie par aucun': Paris, Bibl. de l'Arsenal, MS 2690, fol. 119^{r}.

[52] 'Dont je ai veu en mon tamps un enffant qui out non Alexins, de ix ans, qui estoit de

Conclusion

According to Giles of Rome, princes especially, but also children in general, have to be educated first and foremost through pleasure and not through pain. Pleasure is to be found in various forms of activity and — with moderation — appropriate pleasure may rightly be a part of any activity. The acquisition of virtue nevertheless implies a certain perseverance: to be able to feel pleasure in an activity, such as music or rhetoric, a child should be initiated as young as possible.

As Giles underlines, children's games need special attention since the spontaneous nature of the child is instinctively inclined to follow immoderate pleasures. Giles does not forbid play and fun. On the contrary, he advises making use of them as instruments for helping the child to develop physically and psychically. Play that provides a certain pleasure, exercised within set limits, appears to be like an exercise in self-control that gives the child the means with which to contain his passions and acquire virtues. Playful activities appear to be a way of preparing the child — notably the aristocratic child — to integrate into adult society.

While recognized as having a certain degree of educational effectiveness, pleasure continues, however, to be subject to suspicion in Giles's eyes and for the majority of the thinkers of his time. Aristotle's ambiguous attitude towards pleasure in education has a definite influence on Giles, who follows the Greek philosopher almost to the letter. Pleasure appears as an effective instrument in children's physical and intellectual development as long as it paves the way for the conveyance of virtues, whereas any immoderate pleasure, above all sensual pleasure — related for example to the sin of gluttony — represents a significant impediment to the acquisition of any virtues.

It is to Giles's credit that he not only transfers Aristotle's notions of pleasure from a classical to a medieval context through a 'mirror of princes', but also to

Lombardie de la cité de Pergame, de qui non est entitulé la logique alexine, a Salins en Bourgoigne qui onquez ne fut batuz, ne onques ne out la teste couverte, qui entendit sa gramatique competemment, et ses sillogismes excellentement, et l'argorisme parfaitement tant que a la derreenne espece. Car il avoit este enformé dehnement et benignement, et sanz coaction la quele ne fust ja avenue se il ne eust bien tost commencé de aprendre. Dont il ne convient pas a ceulz qui pevent avoir pedagogue souffisant en mours et en science especialement en benignité et en discrettion, atendre le viij an ains ou quart ou el v an selonc que li enffes sera plus ou moins viguerous, gardant toutes dehues circonstances il pevent abandonner l'enffant au mestre qui soit tel comme dit est. Car se ne sera se l'en procede connue dit est se non un solatiouz excercis et aussi comme un esbatement a l'enffant': William (1330), Paris, Bibl. de l'Arsenal, MS 2690, fol. 120.

have transferred these Aristotelian notions into another social context. Giles's translators — such as William — play a major role in this process. Giles's contribution to the reflection on education in late medieval thought must therefore be considered important, since his adapted Aristotelian ethics and moral philosophy imply a conception of education not only reserved for high nobility — as stated by Aristotle — but for children of different social classes. Indeed, although the monarch is the first intended reader, Giles ideally addresses his reflections to the entire social body. In his mind, those virtues related to pleasure, which should be developed through education, are valid for everyone.

Works Cited

Manuscripts

Berlin, Staatsbibliothek Preußischer Kulturbesitz, MS Ham. 672
Paris, Bibliothèque de l'Arsenal, MS 2690

Primary Sources

Aegidius Romanus, *De regimine principum, Libri III* (Roma: F. Hieronymum Samaritanium, 1607; repr. Frankfurt: Scientia Verlag Aalen, 1967)

Aristotle, *Ethica Nicomachea translatio Roberti Grosseteste Lincolniensis sive 'Liber Ethicorum'. B. Recensio recognita*, ed. by Renatus Antonius Gauthier, Fasc. 4 (Leiden: Brill; Bruxelles: Desclée de Brouwer, 1973)

——, *Éthique à Nicomaque*, ed. by Jules Tricot (Paris: Vrin, 1997)

——, *Nicomachean Ethics*, ed. by Harris Rackham (Cambridge, MA: Harvard University Press, 1982); <http://data.perseus.org/texts/urn:cts:greekLit:tlg0086.tlg010.perseus-eng1>

'*Aucuns petis enseignemens*: "Home-made" Courtesy Books in Medieval France', in *Centres of Learning: Learning and Location in the Pre-modern Europe and the Near East*, ed. by J. W. Drijvers and A. A. MacDonald (Leiden: Brill, 1995), pp. 279–88

Bartholomaeus Anglicus, *De genuinis rerum coelestium, terrestrium et infrarum proprietatibus* ..., (Francofurti: apud Wolfgangum Richterum, sumptibus Nicolaii Steinii, 1601; repr. Frankfurt: Scientia Verlag Aalen, 1964)

Christine de Pizan, *Livre du corps de policie*, ed. by Robert-H. Lucas (Geneva: Droz, 1967)

Giles of Rome, *Giles of Rome on Ecclesiastical Power: The 'De ecclesiastica potestate' of Aegidius Romanus*, trans. by R. W. Dyson (Woodbridge: Boydell, 1986)

'Giles of Rome, On the Rule of Princes (selections)', in *The Cambridge Translations of Medieval Philosophical Textes*, vol. II, *Ethics and Political Philosophy*, ed. and trans. by Arthur Stephen McGrade, John Kilcullen, and Matthew Kempshall (Cambridge: Cambridge University Press, 2001), pp. 200–15

Konrad von Megenberg, *Ökonomik (Yconomica)*, ed. by Sabine Krüger (Stuttgart: Monumenta Germaniae Historica, 1973)

Le Livre du chevalier de la Tour Landry pour l'enseignement de ses filles, ed. by Anatole de Montaiglon (Paris: P. Jannet, 1854)

Secondary Works

Alexandre-Bidon, Danièle, 'Abécédaires et alphabets éducatifs du XIII à la fin du XIVe siècle', *Nouvelles de l'Estampe*, 90 (1986), 6–10

——, 'La Lettre volée: Apprendre à lire à l'enfant au Moyen Âge', *Annales: Économies, Sociétés, Civilisations*, 44 (1989), 953–92

Alexandre-Bidon, Danièle, and Didier Lett, 'Grandeur et renaissance du sentiment de l'enfance au Moyen Âge', in *Éducations médiévales: L'Enfance, l'école, l'Église en Occident (V^e–XVe siècles)*, ed. by Jacques Verger (Paris: Institut National de Recherche pédagogique, 1991), pp. 39–64

Becchi, Egle, and Dominique Julia, *Histoire de l'enfance en Occident*, vol. I, *De l'Antiquité au XVIIe siècle* (Paris: Seuil, 1998)

Bérier, François, 'Traduire en France à la fin du Moyen Âge', in *Grundriss der Romanischen Literaturen des Mittelalters*, vol. VIII.1, *La Littérature française aux XIVe et XVe siècles*, ed. by Daniel Poirion (Heidelberg: Universitätsverlag, 1988), pp. 219–65

Brams, Jozef, 'The Revised Version of Grosseteste's Translation of the *Nicomachean Ethics*', *Bulletin de Philosophie Médiévale*, 36 (1994), 45–55

Classen, Albrecht, ed., *Childhood in the Middle Ages and the Renaissance: The Results of a Paradigm Shift in the History of Mentality* (Berlin: Walter de Gruyter, 2005)

Del Punta, Francesco, Silvia Donati, and Luna Concetta, 'Egidio Romano', in *Dizionario Biografico degli Italiani* (Roma: Istituto dell'Enciclopedia Italiana, 1993), XLII, 319–41

Duby, Georges, and Michelle Perrot, eds, *Histoire des femmes*, vol. II, *Le Moyen Âge*, dir. by Christiane Klapisch-Zuber (Paris: Plon, 1991)

Hanawalt, Barbara A., 'Medievalists and the Study of Childhood', *Speculum*, 77 (2002), 440–60

Kaufmann, Michael, 'Von der Sorge der Eltern für die Erziehung ihrer Kinder von Aegidius Romanus de Colonna', in *Aegidius Romanus de Colonna, Johannes Gersons, Dionys des Kartäufers und Jacob Cadolet, Pädagogische Schriften*, ed. by M. Kaufmann, F. Reifer, and H. Kopp (Freiburg im Breisgau: Herdersche Verlagshandlung, 1904), pp. 3–62

Klapisch-Zuber, Christiane, 'Le chiavi florentine di Barbablu', *Quaderni storici*, 57 (1984), 765–92

Lambertini, Roberto, 'A proposito della "costruzione" dell'*Oeconomica* in Egidio Romano', *Medioevo*, 14 (1988), pp. 315–70

——, 'Il filosofo, il principe et la virtù: Note sulla recezione e l'uso dell'*Etica Nicomachea* nel *De regimine principum* di Egidio Romano', *Documenti e studi sulla tradizione filosofica medievale*, 2.1 (1991), 239–79

——, '*Philosophus videtur tangere tres rationes*: Egidio Romano lettore ed interprete della *Politica* nel terzo libro del *De regimine principum*', *Documenti e studi sulla tradizione filosofica medievale*, 1.1 (1990), 277–325

——, 'The Prince in the Mirror of Philosophy: Uses of Aristotle in Giles of Rome's *De regimine principum*', in *Les Philosophies morales et politiques au Moyen Âge — Moral and Political Philosophies in the Middle Ages*, ed. by Carlos B. Bazàn and others (New York: Legas, 1992), pp. 1523–34

Lanza, Lidia, 'La *Politica* di Aristotele e il *De regimine principum* di Egidio Romano', *Medioevo e Rinascimento*, 15, n.s. 12 (2001), 19–75

Lett, Didier, *Le Genre au Moyen Âge: Hommes et femmes, masculins, féminins (XII–XVe s.)* (Paris: Armand Colin, 2013)

Lusignan, Serge, *Parler vulgairement: Les Intellectuels et la langue française aux XIIIe et XIVe siècles* (Paris: Vrin, 1986)

Marmo, Constantino, '*Hoc autem et si potest tollerari* ...: Egidio Romano e Tommaso d'Aquino sulle passioni dell'anima', *Documenti e studi sulla tradizione filosofica medievale*, 2.1 (1991), 281–315

Mehl, Jean-Michel, *Des jeux et des hommes dans la société médiévale* (Paris: Champion, 2010)

Merisalo, Outi, 'Le *Fidus interpres* et Gilles de Rome', in *Pratiques de Traduction au Moyen Âge: Actes du colloque de l'Université de Copenhague 25 et 26 octobre 2002*, ed. by Peter Andersen (Copenhagen: Copenhagen Museum Tusculanum Press, 2004), pp. 225–32

——, 'Guillaume, ou comment traduire Gilles de Rome en 1330', in *Les Traducteurs au travail — leurs manuscrits et leurs méthodes: Actes du Colloque international organisé par le 'Ettore Majorana Centre for Scientific Culture', 30 septembre — 6 octobre 1999*, ed. by Jacqueline Hamesse (Turnhout: Brepols, 2001), pp. 275–83

Nicoud, Marilyn, *Medieval Dietetics: Food and Drink in 'Regimen Sanitatis' Literature from 800 to 1400*, German Studies in Canada, 5, ed. by Melitta Weiss Adamson (Frankfurt: Peter Lang, 1995)

——, *Les Régimes de santé au Moyen Âge: Naissance et diffusion d'une écriture médicale (XIIIe–XVe siècle)*, Bibliothèque des écoles françaises d'Athènes et de Rome, 333, 2 vols (Roma: École française de Rome, 2007)

Orme, Nicholas, 'The Culture of Children in Medieval England', *Past and Present*, 148 (1995), 48–88

Ortalli, Gerardo, 'Tempo libero e Medioevo: tra pulsioni ludiche e schemi culturali', in *Il tempo libero: Economica e società (loisirs, leisure, tiempo libre, Freizeit), secc. XIII–XVIII*, ed. by Simonetta Cavaciocchi, Serie II: Atti delle settimane di studi e altri convegni, 26 (Firenze: Le Monnier, Istituto internazionale di storia economica 'F. Datini', 1995), pp. 31–54

Perret, Noëlle-Laetitia, *Les Traductions françaises du 'De regimine principum' de Gilles de Rome: Parcours matériel, culturel et intellectuel d'un discours sur l'éducation*, Education and Society in the Middle Ages and Renaissance, 39 (Leiden: Brill, 2011)

Riché, Pierre, and Danièle Alexandre-Bidon, *L'Enfance au Moyen Âge*, ed. by Pierre Riché and Danièle Alexandre-Bidon (Paris: Seuil, 1994)

Schaus, Margaret, ed., *Women and Gender in Medieval Europe: An Encyclopedia* (New York: Routledge, 2006)

Schrübbers, Christiane, 'Regimen und Homo Primitivus: Die Pädagogik des Aegidius Romanus', *Augustiniana*, 32–33 (1982–83), pp. 348–91

Shahar, Shulamith, *Childhood in the Middle Ages* (London: Routledge, 1990)

Sigal, Pierre-André, 'L'Histoire de l'enfant au Moyen Âge: Une recherche en plein essor', *Histoire de l'éducation*, 81 (1999), 3–21

Pleasure as an Affective Tool in Pastoral Care: The Cases of Simone Fidati and Richard Rolle in Fourteenth-Century Italy and England

Xavier Biron-Ouellet

Spiritual writings have some unexpected uses when it comes to understanding medieval culture. Their richness resides in the fact that they not only expose what the spiritual relationship between men and divinity should be, they also teach us a great deal about human relations within a Christian society. The study of emotions allows us to grasp this tripartite relation between God, man, and neighbour. The moral value of an emotion is predominant in the medieval understanding of affectivity: according to the situation, it can be evaluated either as a vice or as a virtue. The affective phenomena of pleasure reflect this situation very well as they can be salvific if they bring one closer to God as much as they can cause damnation if they take one away from God. The moral rightness of an emotional movement, the *motus animi*, is thus critical in the spiritual relation the Christian has with God and with other members of the *ecclesia*.

In this paper I will seek to demonstrate how pleasure is used in pastoral discourse and how it is related to the medieval theories of emotions. For this purpose I will compare the texts of two spiritual writers from opposite parts of fourteenth-century Europe: the *Emendatio vitae* of Richard Rolle of Hampole (†1349), from England, and the *Ordine della vita christiana* of Simone Fidati da Cascia (†1348), from central Italy. These authors are interesting because

---

Xavier Biron-Ouellet (Xbiron@gmail.com) is a PhD student working on emotions and affectivity in medieval culture at Université du Québec à Montréal and École des Hautes Études en Sciences Sociales.

Pleasure in the Middle Ages, ed. by Naama Cohen-Hanegbi and Piroska Nagy, IMR 24 (Turnhout: Brepols, 2018), pp. 225–247 BREPOLS PUBLISHERS 10.1484/M.IMR-EB.5.113469

they have quite a similar pedigree: they attended university before starting a career of spiritual caregiving as hermits. But they are also very different since they come from very contrasting environments: the busy cities of central Italy against the rural areas of Yorkshire. Through their example, I would like to investigate whether the changes that occurred in the Christian anthropological conception of man and emotions throughout the thirteenth century influenced the discourse of pastoral caregivers thereafter. Since Rolle and Fidati were acquainted with philosophical scholarship, we can safely say that they were most probably aware of what natural philosophy brought to the anthropological understanding of man. Before we move on to the analysis of the role of pleasure in the *Emendatio vitae* and the *Ordine della vita christiana*, we need to define the affective implications of these anthropological changes in the thirteenth century with a short theoretical reflection on the notion of pleasure in the Middle Ages.

Defining Medieval Pleasure

Although studies on love are quite common in medieval scholarship, only a few historians have directly worked on medieval pleasure.[1] The one that first comes to mind is the great French historian Jacques Le Goff who wrote an article entitled 'Le Refus du plaisir', first published in 1984 in a thematic issue of the magazine *L'Histoire* dedicated to love and sexuality.[2] As proposed by the theme of the publication, Le Goff discusses pleasure in its affiliation with sexuality. His choice is indicative of how historians generally viewed and analysed pleasure in twentieth-century historiography: from its carnal perspective.[3] Accordingly, Le Goff argues that since Augustine condemns *voluptates* and *delectationes*, pleasure as carnal concupiscence is repudiated throughout the Middles Ages and until our own time. Even though for us moderns bodily pleasure may seem to be the only noteworthy pleasure, we can assume that, especially in the context of a religious anthropology such as that of medieval Christendom, spiritual pleasure is an important source of joy and well-being, one that would certainly not be condemned. So when Jacques Le Goff says that medieval people repudiated pleasure, his idea of pleasure is very restrictive and

[1] More often than not, pleasure is tackled within a study of love; for instance, Kitanov, 'Displeasure in Heaven, Pleasure in Hell' and Wack, 'The Measure of Pleasure'.

[2] Le Goff, 'Le Refus du plaisir'.

[3] See for instance Verdon, *Le Plaisir au Moyen Âge* or Baladier, *Éros au Moyen Âge*.

thus non-representative of the complexity of that affective phenomenon in the Middle Ages.[4] The broadening of the reflection on emotions in different disciplines over the last decades has provided a vision of emotions that includes its cognitive aspects as well as its bodily ones.[5] The two flanks of an emotion, the body and the mind, are closely related, and what we feel as pleasure is directly linked with our cognitive conception of it. That was well understood by medieval spiritual writers when commenting on a somewhat difficult biblical book like the Song of Songs. Although I will not venture into this complex issue, it is worth noting the fact that from Origen to the late Middle Ages, the commentary tradition of the Song of Songs has most often sought to 'spiritualize' in an allegorical fashion the sensual language of pleasure that is found in this famous text.[6]

The way medieval emotion is understood here agrees with the definition given by Piroska Nagy and Damien Boquet: 'the territory of transitive affective phenomena of pleasure-displeasure, desire-repulsion in the infinite diversity of its configurations that are associated by the subject to the appraisal of the lived situation'.[7] There are two semantic indications that allow us to identify an emotion: the notion of movement and the location of this movement within the soul. Affects are transitory psychic moments that change not only the person affected, but also the social environment of the affected. They are highly social and cultural facts that have great impact on human relations; thus the need for

[4] Since pleasure has almost always been analysed from a sensual perspective, it seems as though the Middle Ages have been excluded as being a period where there was no pleasure. This situation is well represented in two books on pleasure in which the Middle Ages are passed over without any justification from the authors; see for example Boulègue and Lévy, *Hédonismes* and Galand-Hallyn, Lévy, and Verbaal, *Le Plaisir dans l'Antiquité et à la Renaissance*. This situation is related to a depreciative and polarizing vision of medieval affectivity, seen as being either overly repressed or totally out of control, as proposed in Johan Huizinga's famous book, *The Waning of the Middle Ages* (1919). In both cases, medieval pleasure seems not worthy of being analysed because of its ineluctable irrationality. Even though this view of affectivity is rigorously contested by historians of emotions (see note 5, below), it is still influential because it fits fairly well with our modern conception of pleasure through which we apprehend this notion in the past.

[5] Rosenwein, 'Worrying about Emotions in History'; Boquet and Nagy, 'Pour une histoire des émotions'; and Kasten, 'Einleitung'.

[6] Renevey, *Language Self and Love*; see also Matter, *The Voice of my Beloved* and Turner, *Eros and Allegory*. See also Constant Mews's paper in this volume, pp. 329–52.

[7] Boquet and Nagy, 'Pour une histoire des émotions', p. 47.

religious authorities to supervise the affective life of human beings, especially when it comes to a thorny affect like pleasure.

In this line of thought, the vision of the Italian historians of philosophy Carla Casagrande and Silvana Vecchio is much more appealing to the historian of emotions, as their understanding of pleasure is comprehensive and goes beyond sexuality to include all kinds of pleasures as well as their relation to pain. They argue that the couple pleasure/pain represents an irreplaceable polarity to which we can relate the entire medieval discourse on emotions. As they note in the introduction to their book *Piacere e dolore*, the emotional pair joy/sadness is narrowly related to the pair pleasure/pain.[8] But, at the same time, it is different because it does not refer directly to bodily sensations. Joy and sadness are, in a way, more spiritual and, unlike pain/pleasure, they are absolute opposites. One must then be careful not to define pleasure in its opposition to pain, for example, 'pleasure is the absence of pain'. In Christian culture, the relation between pleasure and pain is very complex since Christ has chosen to suffer in order to save humanity.[9] Consequently, pain can enhance the greatest Christian pleasure: the pleasure of getting closer to God. Bodily pain can bring pleasure to the soul as much as carnal pleasure can bring pain to the soul. The relationship between the two emotions is very complex because the line of distinction between them is very thin.

Following Casagrande and Vecchio, it is possible to grasp how medieval people considered pleasure because it is so often a central affect in their writings. Monks and preachers speak of pleasure and pain as a way to articulate good and evil in the life of men and to fix their destiny in the life to come. To fully comprehend that lofty notion, one has to, on the one hand, understand how pleasure and emotions were conceived in accordance with its philosophical background and, on the other hand, see how these conceptions were handled in pastoral care. Seeking pleasure and avoiding pain are principles of natural philosophy that define human behaviour. Therefore theologians have developed systems in which pleasure represents a device that generates emotions, and which is also the terminus of those emotional movements.[10] In that context, pleasure can be felt in a variety of manners, but the bulk of the theological investigation is concerned with how to feel it properly.

Even though we can distinguish different kinds of pleasure, for instance, carnal pleasure (*voluptas*), pleasure as a part of the sin process (*delectatio*), or

[8] Casagrande and Vecchio, 'Introduzione', pp. 3–12.

[9] See Cohen, *The Modulated Scream*, pp. 198–227.

[10] Cohen, 'Towards a History of European Physical Sensibility'.

spiritual joy (*gaudium*), we have to consider pleasure as a unique affective phenomenon where all distinctions are interrelated in the operating soul and body. Pleasure has to be considered within a religious anthropology that gives a moral meaning to emotions.

In most, if not all, medieval religious texts, moral goodness is something that brings you closer to God and opens the way to salvation. In Christian anthropology, every emotion, or passion, can be good if its movement is directed towards the love of God, or evil if it is directed towards the love of earthly things. For example, beatitude (*beatitudo*) is a peaceful state of mind that implies pleasurable emotions such as happiness (*laetitia*) and solace (*solatium*); but to rejoice in carnal pleasure (*gaudere in voluptate*) causes unpleasant torments to the soul. The same considerations apply to an emotion commonly considered negative, like anger (*ira*): being angry against your neighbour because of your pride (*superbia*) is bad, but if it is in humility (*humilitas*) against your own sins then it is good. This idea of moving the soul in the right direction is constant in medieval moral philosophy.[11] One gets closer to God while being moved by certain virtues that are also emotions and, at the same time, the achievement of that affective process creates the ultimate pleasurable emotion of joy, that of the *fruitio Dei*.

Before the twelfth century, carnal pleasure was almost always viewed as negative because Augustine had designated *voluptas* as the consequence of the Fall. He said that carnal pleasure was not natural because it did not exist in Eden. It was a *passio carnalis* that could not be controlled by the will and rightly oriented like other emotions; it was a rebel to the *ratio* and needed to be fought.[12] *Delectatio* was absolutely negative as well, because delectation is a sin in itself as it implies delight in a bad thought or suggestion. Consequently Augustine's influential legacy has been the unavoidable connection between carnal pleasure and sin, which is ultimately represented in the vice of luxury. This relation between emotions and sin is central to the twelfth century's psychological inquiry, and pleasure, as *delectatio*, is omnipresent.[13]

[11] Knuuttila, *Emotions in Ancient and Medieval Philosophy*; see also *Passiones animae — Die 'Leidenschaft der Seele' in der mitteralterlichen Theologie und Philosophie*, ed. by Schäfer and Thurner.

[12] Augustine, *De civitate Dei*, lib. 14, cap. 15 and cap. 23, ed. by *Dombart and Kalb*, pp. 436–38, 444–46. See as well Peter Brown's interpretation in *The Body and Society*.

[13] Boquet, 'Des racines de l'émotion', and for a larger perspective Lottin, *Psychologie et morale aux XIIe et XIIIe siècles*.

From the early thirteenth century onwards, carnal pleasure is no longer seen as absolutely wicked; it is a sin only if it is not mediated by the will of the rational soul. It seems that a change occurred in the anthropological conception of pleasure during the central Middle Ages. This change is mainly due to the rediscovery of Aristotle's natural philosophy, which allowed the sensible delectations to regain their natural status and thus be submitted to the power of the will and the rational part of the soul.[14] For Thomas Aquinas, whose thinking was strongly influenced by Avicenna and Aristotle, if the sensible delectations are controlled by the will, or by the rational part of the soul, they can bring spiritual delectation. Similarly, in Aquinas as well as in Albert the Great, sensible pleasures are passions of the sensitive part of the soul that can become spiritualized when they are echoed by the rational part of the soul.[15] Consequently, every pleasurable emotion such as *delectatio*, *iocunditas*, and *laetitia* can contribute to moral goodness if it is related to a *gaudium* that leads to enjoyment of God. In his treatise *De Bono*, Albert the Great says:

> Dicendum, quod gaudium, secundum quod est fructus, est habitus, qui consistit in elevatione cordis ex captu dulcedinis dei, quod delectat fruentem. Secundum autem quod est passio, est affectio cordis ex captu desiderati convenientis. Differt autem autem a voluptate, quia voluptas dicit pasturam appetitus in dulci convenienti, sed gaudium dicit elevationem animae ex tali pastura. Iucunditas autem sonat in hilaritatem quandam vultus et serenitatem procedentem ex tali dulcedine interiori. Exsultatio autem dicit exhalationem spirituum et sanguinis ad exteriora ex calore cordis affecti a tali dulcedine. Laetitia vera quasi latitia dicitur, eo quod consistit in cordis dilatation.[16]

> [It is to be said that joy (*gaudium*), as something enjoyed (*fructus*), is a disposition (*habitus*) that delights enjoyment and consists in the elevation of the heart according to the apprehension of the sweetness of God. As a passion (*passio*), however, it is an affection of the heart according to the apprehension of a suitable desire. It differs from sensuality (*voluptas*) because sensuality is said to feed the appetite in similar sweetness, while joy is the elevation of the soul from such feeding. Cheerfulness

[14] Vecchio, 'Il piacere da Abelardo a Tommaso'. The following philosophical background draws heavily from this study.

[15] Thomas Aquinas, *Summa Theologiae*, 1a 2ae, q. 31, a. 5, ed. by Caramello, I, 238; and Albert the Great, *Super ethica*, lib. 2, q. II, art. 2, ed. by Kubel, p. 97: 'Delectationes sensibiles, cum sint passiones sensitivi appetitus, sunt cum aliqua transmutatione corporali. Quod non contingit in delectationibus spiritualibus nisi per quandam renduntiam a superirori appetitu in inferiorem.'

[16] Albert the Great, *De bono*, 2 q. V, a. 2, ed. by Kühle, pp. 204–05.

(*iocunditas*) resounds in hilarity in some facet or in apparent serenity from such interior sweetness. Exultation is the exhalation of spirits and of the blood towards the exterior by the heat of the heart affected by such sweetness. True happiness (*laetitia*) is pronounced as if it were width (*latitia*) because it consists in the dilation of the heart.]

We see that *gaudium* can be a disposition and a passion. As a disposition, it is a pleasure of the rational soul because it elevates the heart towards God. As a passion, it is a spiritual emotion that differs from carnal sensuality. *Gaudium* is reflected in bodily responses such as the manifestation of hilarity through cheerfulness, which, by a movement of the soul, releases the exultation that dilates the heart and leads to happiness (*laetitia*). From there, we understand that pleasure is not a fierce passion to be fought, even though the danger is still present, but is rather to be dominated by reason in order to become an ordered spiritual pleasure.

We can also see this anthropological change in the typology of vices. According to Silvana Vecchio, the *Summa de vitiis* of the Franciscan John of Rupella (†1245) is a turning point in the development of the doctrine of sin.[17] Based on the Aristotelian-Avicennian theory of the soul, John says that there are three powers of the soul (*vires anime*): vegetative, sensitive, and rational. Each power can be good or bad. So when the soul acts according to its vegetative power, that is, eating and reproducing, it performs a nutritive or generative action aimed at the conservation of the person and of the species.[18] But when those powers of the soul are unordered, they become sins of lust and gluttony.[19] This development of the doctrine of sin was very influential, as it was integrated into the *Summa* of Alexander of Hales, which would in turn influence Thomas Aquinas. This is the basis of the discourse of moderation that is so important in the late Middle Ages.

[17] Vecchio, 'The Seven Deadly Sins between Pastoral Care and Scholastic Theology'.

[18] John of Rupella, *Summa de vitiis*, Paris, BnF, MS lat. 16417, fol. 113^{rb-va}, as cited in Vecchio, 'The Seven Deadly Sins between Pastoral Care and Scholastic Theology', p. 118: 'Tres enim sunt vires anime: vegetabilis, sensibilis, rationalis; triplex est bonum: inferius scilicet bonum carnis, ad hoc se habet anima secundum secundum duplicem actum vegetabilis scilicet nutritive et generative; actus nitritive est ad conservationem singularis et actus generative ad conservationem speciei'.

[19] John of Rupella, *Summa de vitiis*, Paris, BnF, MS lat. 16417, fol. 113va: 'Nam inordinacio amoris boni inferioris scilicet carnis secundum actum nutritive est gula. Inordinatio amoris boni inferioris scilicet carnis secundum actum generative est luxuria'.

For most of the subsequent authors following John of Rupella and Albert the Great, carnal pleasure of the soul (*concupiscentia carnis*) is only a sin when it is felt as a disorderly passion, as a vice. God wants men to procreate and eat, but they must act within certain limits in order not to fall into vice. It is the function of virtue, principally the virtues of temperance and moderation, to limit those natural appetites, and it is the role of caregivers to elevate virtue in men by their preaching and counselling. This vision of sin is much more accurate in its balance between the psychological aspects and the social dimension of sin than the monastic tradition which had been conceived for a rather rigid universe of asceticism. It is important to consider this anthropo-theological development because the two authors I am considering here are well aware of it.

What we just saw is important, as both authors considered here have quite a similar conception of pleasure linked to this theoretical background. In the following section of this paper, I will compare two texts that are directly concerned with spiritual care: Richard Rolle's *Emendatio vitae* and Simone Fidati's *Ordine della vita Christiania*. Yet, as we will see, their account of pleasure is not the same. For Rolle, the greatest pleasure is to be found in the *vita contemplativa*, and for Fidati, it lies in the Franciscan notion of *christiformitas*.[20] Both authors have a different vocabulary of pleasure, which it is important to highlight before analysing how pleasure is embedded in the proposed ways of living.

Pleasure in the Emendatio vitae

Richard Rolle of Hampole was an Oxford-educated man who subsequently became a hermit in the region of Yorkshire. He had an impressive career as a Latin and English author as well as a spiritual caregiver. Rolle is related to the movement of contemplative writing that emerged in the monastic milieu of the eleventh century. This movement is characterized by the commitment of the penitent to an inner self-examination propelled by a revival of interest in the structure of the soul, linked, amongst other things, to natural philosophy and the (mostly Cistercian) *De Anima* tradition.[21] This is the purpose of his main work: the *Emendatio vitae* (dating from 1345–49) of which more than

[20] I leave aside Rolle's idea of *canor* because I see it as a part of the *vita contemplativa* and also since the latter is the specific focus of the *Emendatio vitae*.

[21] See the introduction by Watson in Rolle, *Emendatio vitae*, ed. by Watson, pp. 1–27. For a more general account of Richard Rolle, see Watson, *Richard Rolle and the Invention of Authority* and Allen, *Writings Ascribed to Richard Rolle Hermit of Hampole*.

a hundred manuscripts survive of the original Latin version and sixteen of the English translation. This work is a programme of spiritual transformation that was originally meant for monastic use that Rolle has adapted to the needs of general secular clergy. It is a transmission of traditions inherited by Rolle, in order to make them accessible to a larger audience, which would eventually include women and lay people as it gets translated into Middle English following Rolle's death.

Rolle's references to pleasurable emotions must be understood in the pattern of a language of sensuality as he often refers to the taste of being close to God and its sensual enjoyment. This kind of linguistic style is associated with the mystical tradition stemming from Origen but mediated, most predominantly, by Bernard of Clairvaux.[22] As we will see, the strong sensory rhetoric of Richard Rolle gives pleasure an important role.

In the *Emendatio vitae*, the word *delectatio* is mostly used in reference to sinful pleasure linked to the flesh, as the verb *delectare* and the adjective *delectabile* can both refer to the carnal enjoyment as much as the spiritual enjoyment. He does not use the word *voluptas* very often, but when he does, it is always in a negative fashion. Even if he does not say it explicitly, we understand that those are affects of the sensitive part of the soul. On the contrary, he uses *gaudium* as a spiritual affection, linked to the rational part of the soul. We can see its spiritual potency because, on the one hand, it is almost always used in reference to the proximity of God and, on the other hand, when used in the wrong way it leads to damnation. For example, Rolle says: 'Although you may be seen to be of incredible penitence and continence, as long as you rejoice (*gaudes*) in the glory of men rather than angels, there is nothing left for you in the future except torment';[23] and again: 'he who rejoices (*gaudet*) in earthly goods distances himself far away from the eternal goods'.[24] From a medieval psychology standpoint, *gaudium* is the rational affect of enjoyment of a sensual *delectatio*. It is the affect that one has after having given the *consensus* to a sensation. Rejoicing in worldly things is thus dangerous for the Christian soul because the rational part of the soul consents to a sinful sensation.

[22] Rudy, *Mystical Language of Sensations in the Later Middle Ages*.

[23] Rolle, *Emendatio vitae*, cap. 4, ed. by Watson, p. 43: 'Et quamvis mirabilis penitencie vel continencie videaris, dum enim magis gaudes in Gloria hominum quam angelorum, in futuro nichil tibi restat nisi tormentum'.

[24] Rolle, *Emendatio vitae*, cap. 5, ed. by Watson, p. 46: 'et qui gaudet in terrenis bonis longe distat ab eternis'.

Rolle also says that the more interior *gaudium* we gather, the less we are involved in exterior things;[25] but at the same time one must be careful not to feel 'vana gaudium et solatium'.[26] It is all a question of directing rightly the movements of the soul. One must avoid living in aversion to God in order to shun temptations: 'What can aversion to God be but a turning towards some transitory good, towards the delightful sight of a (female) creature, towards the works of the Devil, towards the pleasures of the flesh and of the world?'.[27] The opposite of aversion is conversion, which is a reordering of the whole man, a change in one's affects and behaviour.[28] The enjoyment of pleasurable sensations not directed towards the love of God is thus always negative just as the enjoyment of pleasurable sensations ordered to the love of God is always positive.

The *Emendatio vitae* is a spiritual progression in twelve steps from conversion to contemplation, and every step is supposed to lead to spiritual pleasure expressed by the words we have just seen. The *vita contemplativa* is then the ordered state of mind and affects in which one can feel positive pleasure and live in *caritas*, which is the key to contemplation. *Caritas* is the most important virtue: the true love, not only of God but also of one's neighbour for the sake of God. The link between *caritas* and pleasurable emotions is obvious, as Rolle says that charity is the only celestial joy,[29] it is the most agreeable and singular joy,[30] and it is a pleasing sweetness.[31] Every emotion that is felt with charity is valued positively; even sensations of the sensitive part of the soul, such as *suavitas* and *dulcor* are rendered positive because they are felt according to the love of God. Richard Rolle also says that the love of God is *dulcis et delectabilis* and

[25] Rolle, *Emendatio vitae*, cap. 11, ed. by Watson, p. 59: 'quia tanto magis internis gaudiis rapitur quanto minus in exterioribus rebus implicatur'.

[26] Rolle, *Emendatio vitae*, cap. 2, ed. by Watson, pp. 36–37.

[27] Rolle, *Emendatio vitae*, cap. 1, ed. by Watson, p. 34: 'Quid etiam est aversio a Deo nisi conversio ad bonum commutabile, ad delectabilem speciem creaturae, ad opera diaboli, ad voluptates carnis et mundi?'.

[28] Rolle, *Emendatio vitae*, cap. 1, ed. by Watson, p. 34: 'Non enim incessu pedum ad Deum convertimur, sed mutatione affectuum et morum'. We can see a similar idea in Bernard of Clairvaux, *Sermones in festiuitate omnium sanctorum*, ed. by Leclercq and Rochais, p. 331: 'Accesserunt non tam incessu pedum quam affectu cordis et imitatione virtutum'.

[29] Rolle, *Emendatio vitae*, cap. 4, ed. by Watson, p. 46: 'caritas est sola celestia gaudia'.

[30] Rolle, *Emendatio vitae*, cap. 11, ed. by Watson, p. 60: 'suavissima et singular gaudium'.

[31] Rolle, *Emendatio vitae*, cap. 11, ed. by Watson, p. 62: 'dulcor placens'.

brings *iubilatio*. This last emotion is of great importance as Rolle, following the Psalmist, declares: 'happy is the man who knows jubilation'.[32]

By using words like *dulcis/dulcor* or *suavitas* to express pleasurable sensations, Richard Rolle employs a vocabulary of sensuality found in the Song of Songs and its tradition of commentaries, which tends to favour the senses of touch and taste as the way to experience union with God in the *affectus*. Largely influenced by Bernard of Clairvaux, this spiritual idea was followed in the scholastic tradition, as Albert the Great says that the *affectus* is the faculty by which we can get closer to God and the senses of taste and touch permit an experience of direct contact with the divine.[33] This use of a sensual language of pleasure implies that Rolle has an anthropological comprehension of the human being that relates the structure of men's sensibility (or *affectus*) to that of God. In Rolle this vocabulary is expressed in a theological language that is different from the scholastic one, but, at the same time, they are both pervaded by a common set of anthropological ideas stemming from the frequentation of a similar body of knowledge.

We can see further scholastic influence in Rolle's definition of contemplation. According to him contemplation is the death of carnal affections through the jubilation of the uplifted mind, and it is a jubilation of divine love, received into the mind with the sweetness of angelic praise.[34] In this definition, we see that restraint of carnal pleasure and desires brings even more pleasurable emotions such as jubilation. But the important point is that the mind is elevated from sensory appetite, thus killing the carnal affections. Following Albert's quotation seen earlier, the carnal affections of the sensitive part of the soul are not a fierce obstacle but simply desires that ought to be dominated. I don't suppose that Rolle would have read Albert; I am only pointing out the fact that they share a common anthropological understanding of the *homo christianus* in which carnal pleasures may be considered bad but they can also be turned around to exalt the mind, thus leading to salvation. What we can see in the *Emendatio vitae* is that the anthropological basis was somehow influenced by

[32] Rolle, *Emendatio vitae*, cap. 12, ed. by Watson, p. 63: 'beatus vir qui scit iubilationem'. Cf. Psalm 88. 16.

[33] Albert the Great, *In III Sententiae*, dist. 13, A, art. 4, ed. by Borgnet, pp. 239–41. As cited in Rudy, *Mystical Language of Sensations in the Later Middle Ages*, pp. 42–43.

[34] Rolle, *Emendatio vitae*, cap. 12, ed. by Watson, p. 63: 'alii dicunt, et optime, quod contemplacio est per sublevantis mentis iubilum mors carnalium affectionum. Michi videtur quod contemplacio sit iubilus divini amoris, susceptus in mente suavitate laudis. [...] Hec est iubilatio, exaltatio mentis habita pro eterno dilecto in spirituali canora voce prorumpens'.

the natural philosophy of the thirteenth century, but it is treated in a way and with a vocabulary closer to that of the twelfth century.

By putting a strong emphasis on pleasurable emotions following the contemplative life, Richard Rolle seems to use pleasure in the *Emendatio vitae* as an affective rhetorical tool to strengthen his position as a pastoral caregiver. Every step towards contemplation, be it prayer, lecture, and meditation, leads to pleasurable things, expressed by words such as *suavitas, iocunditas, dulcis, iubilum*. When he discusses wicked pleasures, it is only to show that they can be overruled by proper spiritual exercises bringing even more enjoyable pleasures. His contemplative and affective experience (full of joy and pleasure) which is reported in the *Emendatio vitae* could thus be seen as an affective rhetoric, aiming to demonstrate the normativity of his experience in order to prove his authority as a caregiver.[35] This is common to the mystical rhetoric that recurrently uses themes such as pleasure, desire, bodily sensation, and death to express the transformative union with God.[36] As a mystical writer, Rolle seeks to express this inexpressible experience with simple, highly affective words. Pleasurable sensations and emotions may be seen as the conditions of effectiveness of spiritual contemplation. If the tendency in the scholastic world is to naturalize religious emotion with a philosophical language, Richard Rolle remains faithful to Bernard's language while sharing the anthropological views of the scholastics.

Pleasure in the Ordine della vita christiana

Simone Fidati da Cascia was also a hermit, but he was part of an official order, the Augustinian hermits, which he entered at a very young age.[37] He acquired philosophical education in Bologna before going back to preaching in the regions of Tuscany and Umbria.[38] He wrote his spiritual works in both Latin and Italian. The work that interests us here is named *L'Ordine della vita christiana*, written in vernacular Italian around 1333.[39] About twenty-five manuscript

[35] I am following here Watson's thesis in *Richard Rolle and the Invention of Authority*.

[36] De Courcelles, *Langages mystiques et avènement de la modernité*. For other examples of analyses of affectivity in Rolle's texts, see Gillespie, 'Mystic's Foot' and Nelstrop, 'The Merging of Eremitic and "Affectivist" Spirituality in Richard Rolle's Reshaping of Contemplation'.

[37] Mattioli, *Il beato Simone Fidati da Cascia dell'Ordine romitano di S. Agostino e i suoi scritti editi ed inediti*.

[38] Oser-Grote, '*Es ist nicht meine Absicht, andere oder falsche Lehrmeinungen zu widerlegen, sondern zu vermitteln, was dem Menchsen zum Heil nützt (De gestis, prol. 1)*'.

[39] Simonis Fidati de Cassia, *L'Ordine della vita christiana*, ed. by Eckermann, pp. 5–120; hereafter *ODVC*.

versions survive, plus one subsequent Latin translation. *L'Ordine della vita christiana* was originally written in Italian to serve as a pedagogical treatise directed at ordinary people (*simplici* as Fidati says). The main idea is that Christian society should be built by lay people and clerics together and that all should be willing to give their lives for the good of others just as Christ did. Fidati wants Christians to become conscious of their responsibilities in the process of salvation. His fundamental notion is *christiformitas*, conformity to Christ's life.[40] This idea of a life lived in conformity to the figure of Christ stems from the life of St Francis himself who, as an *alter Christus*, lived in conformity with Christ up to the point of being stigmatized. The life of Christ is a powerful devotional model, and it is therefore not surprising that the Franciscans had such immense popularity in the late Middle Ages. It is also significant that Fidati was related to the spiritual Franciscans, particularly to Angelo Clareno, but without publicly endorsing their cause.[41] The Franciscan influence on Fidati is thus prominent in subjects such as poverty, ascetic life, and devotion to Christ.

Christiformitas is the idea of reciprocal service between Christians, an interdependence among all the members of the *corpus Christi*. Likewise, living *in christiformitate* requires an affective life modelled in accordance with that of Christ. Fidati says that one ought to love what Christ loved, to hate what Christ hated, to hold in contempt what Christ held in contempt, and to desire what Christ endured.[42] This idea, which is closely connected to the notion of *caritas*, is not only an essential characteristic of salvation but also the key to a moral-ethical way of living. To live in christiformity is to live in virtue, and Fidati defines virtues according to whether or not they bring pleasure (*piacere*) to God. On the contrary, if God is displeased by one's action, then it is a sin.[43] We understand here that the good kind of pleasure is the one that we make others experience and not, as in Rolle, a pleasure that we feel ourselves. This idea

[40] Eckermann, 'Simon Fidati von Cascia OESA (†1348)' and Schwaetzer, '"... dann ist uns unser Vater Augustinus als Beispiel gesetzt!"'.

[41] Corsi, 'Simone da Cascia, un "rebellis ecclesiae"?' and Sensi, 'Simone Fidati e gli Spirituali (Angelo Clareno)'.

[42] *ODVC*, lib. 1 cap. 10, p. 67: 'amare quelle cose, che Cristo amoe, le quali manifestano la sua vita privata d'honore et d'ogni dilecto, ornata d'ogni cosa, che al mondo dispiace. Odiare quello, che Cristo ebbe in odio, et disprezzare quello che Cristo dispreczoe, desiderare quello, che Cristo sostenette'.

[43] *ODVC*, lib. cap. 10, p. 64: 'Et dovemo per questa fede credere, che le virtudi sieno virtudi, perche piaciono a dio et ad noi sono utili, et che le peccata sieno peccata, pero che dispiacciono a dio et a noi sono damnosi'.

is representative of the notion of *ecclesia* defined as a network of spiritual relations that unite Christians through the mediation of God and by the exercise of the theological virtues of *caritas* and *fides*.[44] The fulfilment of this societal project requires an effective politic of emotions that ought to make Christians conscious of their actions and sensations. Simone Fidati's use of pleasure as an affective tool aims at just that.

L'Ordine della vita christiana is divided into two parts: one devoted to the matter of the soul and the other to the matter of the body. The two are related by the idea that virtues are located in the soul but that they are put into action through the body.[45] Fidati stresses that although both parts of the human being are distinct, they must act together in order that 'they render one sweet and suave sound'.[46] Here we see a common theme in medieval spirituality: Fidati says that wisdom permits one to know, when possible, divine things and to taste the sweetness of virtues.[47] Even if these kinds of sensation are not as central in Fidati as in Rolle, sweetness is still seen as a condition of the effectiveness of a good spiritual progression. However, what is important to note is that this idea of a unity of heart is central to Fidati's anthropology, which confers a special influence to the action of the body.[48]

In *L'Ordine della vita christiana* the words that are related to pleasure mostly derive from *piacere*. Therefore, *piacimento*, *piacevoli*, *piacevoleze* can all be understood as pleasures. If the terms derived from *piacere* can be both negative and positive, the terms *dilecto*, *dilectevoli* are mostly negative because they relate to the enjoyment of carnal pleasure. As Rolle uses *gaudium* quite often and *laetitia* rather rarely, Fidati does just the opposite by using more often *letitia* than *gaudio* as a spiritual pleasure.

Fidati dedicates a whole chapter to how to feel happiness (*letitia*) in a spiritually good way. He says that good happiness is felt for the good pleasure (*beneplacito*) of God and of virtue. When that emotion is felt rightly, it allows us to rejoice (*rallegare*) in our own good and in that of our neighbour, which is vir-

[44] Guerreau-Jalabert, 'L'*Ecclesia* médiévale, une institution totale'.

[45] *ODVC*, lib. 2, prol., p. 90: 'la virtude della fede cristiana e nell anima et l'acto et l'opere delle virtu sono di fuori exercitate per lo corpo'.

[46] *ODVC*, lib. 2, prol., p. 90: 'Ad quelle di sopra dette nello exercito della anima accordando l'uno et l'altro insieme. Et queste due corde rendono uno suave et dolce suono'.

[47] *ODVC*, lib. 1, cap. 10, p. 62: 'Il dono della sapientia, cioe saprorosa scientia, per lo qual dono l'anima conoscie, quanto sono possibili di cognoscere le cose divine, et gusta et sapora la dolceza delle virtudi'.

[48] Eckermann, 'Cor novum'.

tuous because it pleases (*piace*) God.[49] On the contrary, happiness in worldly things is a voluntary delectation (*dilecto*) of sin. We see the importance of *christiformitas* as Fidati says that good happiness and enjoyment are conditional to the well-being of one's neighbour, not only to that of oneself.

Fidati demonstrates a good anthropological understanding of the operations of the soul by using a nice metaphor to explain the structure of the soul and its emotions: the soul is a tree, the trunk is reason, the branches are memory, will, and intellect, and the leaves are desires, emotions, and pleasures (*piacimenti*). So when the wind blows, it moves the leaves and the branches but all should be kept in order by the trunk. If the trunk is moved by the wind, it is like a corrupted soul and everything else goes wrong.[50]

Consequently, when emotional movements come from God through control of the rational soul, emotions bring peace to the soul; if they come from the world, they bring war. Peace of mind, which is not to be moved to worldly pleasures (*dilecti*), liberates one's soul from the vice of the flesh. But here Fidati shows the influence of natural philosophy by saying that the natural necessities of the flesh contribute to the peace of the mind only if they rely on common necessities.[51] Therefore, the natural necessities, such as procreating and eating, are good as long as they are done for the common good and not for one's individual pleasure, which is *dilecto*. Once again, the notion of good pleasure is related to others, not to oneself.

Moderation is put forward as the condition of ordered pleasure when Fidati discusses marriage: he warns us to not indulge in inordinate touching, without the flattery and pleasantness that might cause the fire of *luxuria* in the flesh.

[49] *ODVC*, lib. 1, cap. 14, p. 78: 'Et in prima nella nostra letitia overo tristitia dovemo avere respecto a dio et poscia a noi et al proximo, cioe che piu ci dovemo rallegare del bene nostro overo del proximo, perche n e glorificato idio et piace a llui, che perche riceviamo premio noi overo il proximo'.

[50] *ODVC*, lib. 1, cap. 13, p. 76: 'Et di cio porro due exempli. L uno si e dell albero, il quale ae buono pedale et rami et foglie, che verra uno vento, che movera alcuna volta la foglia, alcuna volta i rami, alcuna volta sara si forte, che movera il pedale. L anima si e l albero. Il pedale si e la ragione. I rami e le fogle sono memoria, et volere et desiderii et affecti e piacimenti. Quando questa ragione e mossa, allora l anima sta male, che non rimane veruno bene nell anima. Et se la ragione sta ferma in sua signoria, ogni altra cosa racconcia et ordina'.

[51] *ODVC*, lib. 1, cap. 13, p. 76: 'La quiete della anima si e liberta, che a dal vitio della carne, della necessita della natura, che pogniamo, ch ella non abbia la necessita comune, non ne cura'.

But when virtue is neither confounded nor damaged, which means performing an ordered behaviour, the couple can be together lovingly and pleasantly.[52]

We can further see the influence of Fidati's philosophical studies in his conception of *gaudio*. In Italy, in contrast to Paris or Oxford, Aristotle's natural philosophy was pervasive in different intellectual milieux and was disseminated without strict control from theologians.[53] Fidati had been exposed to this knowledge and was aware of it, as is shown by the fact that he uses the term 'passioni dell'anima' in reference to emotions.[54] Before the scholastic interpretation of Aristotle in the thirteenth century, it was not common to refer to passions *of the soul* as they were considered rather as bodily affections. Affections of the soul, or *motus animi*, were called *affectus* or *affectiones*. As Alain Boureau argues, what changed in the thirteenth century is that scholastics made the distinction between a natural (biological) passion, which is constitutive of human nature, and the unnatural (moral) passion, which is a consequence of original sin.[55] This distinction, coupled with Augustine's equivalence between *motus animi*, *affectus*, *perturbatio*, and *passio*, gives *passiones* a potentiality to be virtuous like the other affections of the soul. This is why Thomas Aquinas asks such a question as 'utrum aliqua passio sit in anima'.[56] Moreover, Fidati says that *gaudio*, *timore*, *speranza*, and *dolore* are passions or *offenses* of the soul which means that they offend the soul when they are unordered passions. In the case of joy, it becomes an offence not only for spiritual reasons but also for medical reasons. Medical knowledge teaches that an outburst of joy (or anger) heats the heart and, as it is said in the *Pantegni*, excessive heat can dry out the body and cause death.[57] Fidati warns married couples in this sense: they must abstain from the warm delectations that fatten the body and never sleep too closely because that brings heat of the flesh.[58]

[52] *ODVC*, lib. 2, cap. 2, p. 97: 'Ne ornare, ne lavare suo corpo et volto et capo contro all ordine honesto delli cristiani, ne fare disordinanti toccamenti l'uno al altro, ne lusinghe, ne piacevoleze, le quali mettano fuoco di luxuria nelle loro carni. [...] In ogni altro modo, che virtude non confonde, ne guasta, sieno insieme amorevoli et piacevoli'.

[53] Piron and Coccia, 'Poésie, sciences et politique', p. 553.

[54] *ODVC*, lib. 1, cap. 13, p. 76: 'Qualunque sio quella, cioe le quattro passioni, overo offesioni dell anima, cioe gaudio, timore, speranza, dolore'.

[55] Boureau, 'Un sujet agité'.

[56] Thomas Aquinas, *Summa Theologia*, 1a 2ae, q. 22, art. 2, ed. by Caramello, II, 185.

[57] Knuuttila, *Emotions in Ancient and Medieval Philosophy*, p. 214.

[58] *ODVC*, lib. 2, cap. 3, p. 99: 'Et fare abstinentia delle cose dilectevoli et che facciano ing-

The key then is to have a moderated joy, and pleasure, so that emotions stay balanced and keep the body healthy. *Christiformitas* implies the well-being of the soul *and* the body.

One can, however, object to this interpretation because in his other writings, Fidati rejects natural philosophy as being vain.[59] I do not think that Fidati despises philosophical knowledge as a whole, but he recognizes the potential theological danger of natural philosophy when it comes to understanding human nature. One of the most common philosophical errors listed in the inquisition records of northern Italy was that of the 'rationalist' vision of man.[60] This vision of man stressed that love is merely a bodily phenomenon that impedes the rational activity of the soul, thus negating the bond between will and love.[61] This was an extreme position which drew many reactions, and an Augustinian spiritual writer like Fidati could in no way have agreed with it because the value of an emotion such as love plays a decisive role as a moral choice in the process of salvation. The kind of opinion that implies that affectivity is an obstacle to intellectual contemplation could not be more opposite to Fidati's theological tradition.[62] Therefore, Fidati had a negative opinion of natural philosophy only when it was not ordered by real knowledge, which is the knowledge of the love of God through the complementarity of *intellectus* and *affectus*. Here lies probably the main resemblance between Richard Rolle and Simone Fidati: they both display an up-to-date anthropological understanding of human beings without using the speculative scholastic language to describe it. They express their spiritual counselling in a highly affective language, with its inherent subtleties, that has a strong rhetorical power, in order to move rightly their public's emotions and fulfil their tasks as spiritual caregivers.

rassare et sieno calde [...] Giamai neuno dovrebbe domire tanto presso, che l calore delle carni si sentisse l'uno dal altro'.

59 See Grassi, 'Simone Fidati e la Scolastica'; Stammkötter, 'Simon Fidati und seine Kritik an der Philosophie'; and Zumkeller, 'Die Augustinertheologen Simon Fidati von Cascia und Hugolin von Orvieto und Martin Luthers Kritik an Aristoteles'.

60 Thompson, *Cities of God*, pp. 419–56, and Zanella, 'Malessere ereticale in valle padana (1260–1308)'.

61 Gentili, *L'uomo aristotelico alle origini della letteratura italiana* and Gentili, 'L'amour entrave-t-il la raison?'.

62 Grossi, 'La teologia affetiva di tradizione agostiana'.

Concluding Remarks

The shrewd reader will notice that I have not directly referred to rhetoric, even though pleasure is an essential part of this art. I think the rhetorical importance of pleasure is implicit in my analysis when it is considered as an affective (rhetorical) tool to move the subject towards a better Christian life as well as to illustrate pastoral ideas and practices. Another reason for not referring directly to rhetoric is that I wanted to restrict myself to the anthropological perspective of pleasure in Christian thought.

In this paper, I have tried to demonstrate how a theoretical understanding of man and his emotions can be related to the practice of pastoral care. Teaching how to use emotions rightly is an essential part of Christian spirituality, and emotions related to pleasure are probably the most important, as they are stimuli as well as results. It is important to understand that the thirteenth century witnessed a substantial overhaul in the anthropological understanding of the human being due in large part to the scientific input coming from the translation of Aristotle's *libri naturales*. The way pleasure is comprehended has thus changed to take into account basic human needs even if they are a source of carnal pleasure. We have seen that although Richard Rolle and Simone Fidati are spiritual authors who have a negative opinion of scholastic knowledge, they seem to be well aware of their ideas concerning pleasure. They both accept that sensible pleasures and delectations can be good if they are controlled by the will towards a morally good end. This was barely conceivable before the thirteenth century. When dealing with a controversial notion such as pleasure, spiritual writers need to take into account all the information available, in order not to mislead Christians into vice.

Nevertheless, the way our authors use pleasure is different in both texts, as they are intended for different publics. The Latin apologetical treatise of Rolle addresses a clerical public; thus it refers to spiritual or mystical experience in a manner exclusively related to the matters of the soul. Fidati's didactical text in vernacular Italian discusses spirituality as well, but since it is aimed at *simplici*, he emphasizes matters, such as interpersonal relationships, judged as relevant to his public. Thus Rolle uses a sensual language with many references to pleasurable sensations while Fidati has more of an ascetic attitude, stressing the further importance of moderation and actions that please God and our neighbours rather than ourselves. For Rolle, pleasure is implied exclusively in relation with inner spirituality, because the *Emendatio vitae* is meant as an individual spiritual progression. On the contrary, Fidati considers pleasure as an important feature of the relation between Christians because the *Ordine della vita christiana* is meant as an ordering of society. This can be explained sociologically by the contexts of each author. Rolle was a solitary hermit living in a rural area: he was concerned with inner experience. Fidati was part of an order, the Hermits of Saint Augustine, and spent his life living in different urban areas of central Italy where social divisions, such as those between rich and poor, lay and religious, men and women, were clearly visible. He was thus much more preoccupied by social care than by personal spiritual progression. For Fidati, salvation cannot be possible without the unity of all Christians, whereas for Rolle, salvation is brought about by one's own unity with the divine through contemplation. Both of them use pleasure as an affective tool in order to bring about unity, the ultimate pleasure, although the type of union is different.

With that in mind, I think these kinds of spiritual texts are witnesses of a form of theological thinking that goes beyond the division between a traditional monastic theology and a speculative scholastic theology. Whether it is named 'vernacular theology' or 'theology of piety', this kind of theology seeks to actualize a primary monastic discourse, while also including some aspects of scholastic intellectual developments, to fit the needs of a larger spectrum of subjects that look to build a relation with the divine.[63] This is therefore more than just a simplification of a more complex thought; it is a rationalization of religious ideas that are structural in a Christian society, which is neither a monastically enclosed world nor a world of highly theoretical speculation. The goal is to gain more effectiveness in the spiritual practices that seek to find God and lead to salvation. In Rolle's *Emendatio vitae* the relation with the divine is built within the self, and in Fidati's *Ordine della vita christiana* it is built through the relation with others. And pleasure is an emotion that definitely helps reach this objective.

[63] For vernacular theology, see McGinn 'Introduction' and Watson 'Censorship and Cultural Change in Late Medieval England'. For the theology of piety, see Hamm, 'Frömmigkeit als Gegenstand theologiegeschichtlicher Forschung'.

Works Cited

Manuscript

John of Rupella, *Summa de vitiis*, Paris, Bibliothèque nationale de France [BnF], MS lat. 16417, fols 69ʳ–172ʳ

Primary Sources

Albert the Great, *De bono*, vol. xxviii of *Opera Omnia*, ed. by Heinrich Kühle (Münster: Aschendorff, 1951)

——, *In III Sententiae*, vol. xxviii of *Opera Omnia*, ed. by Auguste Borgnet (Paris: Vivés, 1890–95)

——, *Super ethica*, vol. xiv of *Opera Omnia*, ed. by Wilhelm Kubel (Münster: Aschendorff, 1987)

Augustine, *De civitate Dei*, ed. and Bernhard Dombard and Alfons Kalb, CCSL, 47–48 (Turnhout: Brepols, 1955)

Bernard of Clairvaux, *Sermones in festiuitate omnium sanctorum*, in *Sancti Bernardi opera*, vol. v, ed. by Jean Leclercq and Henri Rochais (Roma: Editiones Cistercienses, 1972)

Passiones animae — Die 'leidenschaft der Seele' in der mitteralterlichen Theologie und Philosophie, ed. by Christian Schäfer and Martin Thurner (Berlin: Akademie Verlag, 2009)

Rolle, Richard, *Emendatio vitae Orationes ad honorem nominis Ihesu*, ed. by Nicholas Watson (Toronto: Pontifical Institute for Medieval Studies, 1995)

Simone Fidati da Cascia, OESA, *L'Ordine della vita christiana, Tractatus de vita christiana, Epistulae Laude, Opuscula et Johannis de Salerno OESA: Tractatus de vita et moribus Fratris Simonis de Cassia*, ed. by Willigis Eckermann (Roma: Augustinianum, 2006), pp. 5–120

Thomas Aquinas, *Summa Theologiae*, ed. by Pietro Caramello, 3 vols (Torino: Marietti, 1948–50)

Secondary Works

Allen, Hope E., *Writings Ascribed to Richard Rolle Hermit of Hampole and Materials for his Biography* (New York: D. C. Heath, 1927)

Baladier, Charles, *Éros au Moyen Âge: Amour, désir et 'delectatio morosa'* (Paris: Cerf, 1999)

Boquet, Damien, 'Des racines de l'émotion: Les Préaffects et le tournant anthropologique du xiiᵉ siècle', in *Le Sujet des émotions au Moyen Âge*, ed. by Piroska Nagy and Damien Boquet (Paris: Beauchesne, 2008), pp. 163–86

Boquet, Damien, and Piroska Nagy, 'Pour une histoire des émotions: L'Historien face aux questions contemporaines', in *Le Sujet des émotions au Moyen Âge*, ed. by Piroska Nagy and Damien Boquet (Paris: Beauchesne, 2008), pp. 15–52

Boulègue, Laurence, and Carlos Lévy, eds, *Hédonismes: Penser et dire le plaisir dans l'Antiquité et à la Renaissance* (Lille: Presses Universitaires du Septentrion, 2007)

Boureau, Alain, 'Un sujet agité: L'Émergence des passions de l'âme au XIIIe siècle', *Le Sujet des émotions au Moyen Âge*, ed. by Piroska Nagy and Damien Boquet (Paris: Beauchesne, 2008), pp. 187–200

Brown, Peter, *The Body and Society: Men, Women, and Sexual Renunciation in Early Christianity* (New York: Columbia University Press, 1988)

Casagrande, Carla, and Silvana Vecchio, 'Introduzione', in *Piacere e dolore: Materiali per une storia delle passioni nel Medioevo*, ed. by Carla Casagrande and Silvana Vecchio, Micrologus' Library, 29 (Firenze: SISMEL/Edizioni del Galluzzo, 2009), pp. 3–11

Cohen, Esther, *The Modulated Scream: Pain in Late Medieval Culture* (Chicago: University of Chicago Press, 2010)

——, 'Towards a History of European Physical Sensibility: Pain in the Later Middle Ages', *Science in Context*, 8.1 (1995), 47–74

Corsi, Dinora, 'Simone da Cascia, un "rebellis ecclesiae"?', *Archivio storico italiano*, 149 (1991), 739–81

De Courcelles, Dominic, *Langages mystiques et avènement de la modernité* (Paris: Honoré Champion, 2003)

Eckermann, Willigis, 'Cor novum: zur theologischen Anthropologie bei Simon Fidati von Cascia', *Augustiniana*, 56 (2006), 129–47

——, 'Simon Fidati von Cascia OESA (†1348): Europäische Theologie im lateinischen Mittelalter', *Augustiana*, 47 (1997), 339–56

Galand-Hallyn, Perrine, Carlos Lévy, and Wim Verbaal, eds, *Le Plaisir dans l'Antiquité et à la Renaissance: Études réunies* (Turnhout: Brepols, 2008)

Gentili, Sonia, 'L'Amour entrave-t-il la raison?', *Critique*, nos 716–17 (2007), 91–101

——, *L'uomo aristotelico alle origini della letteratura italiana* (Roma: Carocci, 2005)

Gillespie, Vincent A., 'Mystic's Foot: Rolle and Affectivity', in *The Medieval Mystical Tradition in England: Papers Read at Dartington Hall, July 1982*, vol. II, ed. by Marion Glasscoe (Exeter: University of Exeter, 1982), pp. 199–230

Grassi, Onorato, 'Simone Fidati e la Scolastica', in *Simone Fidati da Cascia OESA: un agostiniano spirituale tra Medioevo e umanesimo. Atti del Congresso internazionale in occasione dell'VIII Centenario della nascita, 1295–1347, Cascia, Perugia, 27–30 settembre 2006*, ed. by Caroline M. Oser-Grote and Willigis Eckermann (Roma: Institutum historicum Augustinianum, 2008), pp. 163–76

Grossi, Vittorino, 'La teologia affetiva di tradizione agostiana', *Lateranum*, 61 (1995), 177–87

Guerreau-Jalabert, Anita, 'L'*Ecclesia* médiévale, une institution totale', in *Les Tendances actuelles de l'histoire du Moyen Âge en France et en Allemagne*, ed. by Jean-Claude Schmitt and Otto Gerhard Oexle (Paris: Publications de la Sorbonne, 2002), pp. 219–26

Hamm, Berndt, 'Frömmigkeit als Gegenstand theologiegeschichtlicher Forschung: Methodisch-historiche Überlegungen am Beispiel von Spätmittelalter und Reformation', *Zeitschrift für Theologie und Kirche*, 74 (1977), 464–97

Kasten, Ingrid, 'Einleitung', in *Machtvolle Gefühle*, ed. by Ingrid Kasten (Berlin: De Gruyter, 2010), pp. 1–26

Kitanov, Severine V., 'Displeasure in Heaven, Pleasure in Hell: Four Franciscan Masters on the Relationship between Love and Pleasure, and Hatred and Displeasure', *Traditio*, 58 (2003), 285–340

Knuuttila, Simo, *Emotions in Ancient and Medieval Philosophy* (Oxford: Clarendon Press, 2004)

Le Goff, Jacques, 'Le Refus du plaisir', *L'Histoire*, 63 (1984), 52–59

Lottin, Odon, *Psychologie et morale aux XIIe et XIIIe siècles* (Gembloux, 1942–59)

Matter, E. Ann, *The Voice of my Beloved: The Song of Songs in Western Medieval Christianity* (Philadelphia: University of Pennsylvania Press, 1990)

Mattioli, Nicola, ed., *Il beato Simone Fidati da Cascia dell'Ordine romitano di S. Agostino e i suoi scritti editi ed inediti* (Roma: Tipografia del Campidoglio, 1898)

McGinn, Bernard, 'Introduction: Meister Eckhart and the Beguines in the Context of Vernacular Theology', in *Meister Eckhart and the Beguine Mystics: Hadewijch of Brabant, Mechthild of Magdeburg, and Marguerite Porete*, ed. by Bernard McGinn (New York: Continuum, 1994), pp. 4–14

Nelstrop, Louise, 'The Merging of Eremitic and "Affectivist" Spirituality in Richard Rolle's Reshaping of Contemplation', *Viator*, 34 (2004), 289–310

Oser-Grote, Carolin M., '*Es ist nicht meine Absicht, andere oder falsche Lehrmeinungen zu widerlegen, sondern zu vermitteln, was dem Menchsen zum Heil nützt (De gestis, prol. 1)*: Einführung zum Leben und Werk des Simon Fidati von Cascia', in *Simon Fidati von Cascia OESA: Augustinische Theologie und Philosophie im späten Mittelalter*, ed. by Carolin M. Oser-Grote and Andreas E. J. Grote (Würzburg: Augustinus-Verlag bei Echter, 2006), pp. 13–25

Piron, Sylvain, and Emanuele Coccia, 'Poésie, sciences et politique: Une génération d'intellectuels italiens (1290–1330)', *Revue de Synthèse*, 129.4 (2008), 549–86

Renevey, Denis, *Language Self and Love: Hermeneutics in the Writings of Richard Rolle and the Commentaries on the Song of Songs* (Cardiff: University of Wales Press, 2001)

Rosenwein, Barbara H., 'Worrying about Emotions in History', *American Historical Review*, 107 (2002), 821–45

Rudy, Gordon, *Mystical Language of Sensations in the Later Middle Ages* (New York: Routledge, 2002)

Schwaetzer, Harald, '"... dann ist uns unser Vater Augustinus als Beispiel gesetzt!": Christiformitas bei Nikolaus von Kues und Simon Fidati', in *Simon Fidati von Cascia OESA: Augustinische Theologie und Philosophie im späten Mittelalter*, ed. by Carolin M. Oser-Grote and Andreas E. J. Grote (Würzburg: Augustinus-Verlag bei Echter, 2006), pp. 371–90

Sensi, Mario, 'Simone Fidati e gli Spirituali (Angelo Clareno)', in *Simone Fidati da Cascia OESA: un agostiniano spirituale tra Medioevo e umanesimo. Atti del Congresso internazionale in occasione dell'VIII Centenario della nascita, 1295–1347, Cascia, Perugia, 27–30 settembre 2006*, ed. by Caroline M. Oser-Grote and Willigis Eckermann (Roma: Institutum historicum Augustinianum, 2008), pp. 51–98

Stammkötter, Franz-Bernhard, 'Simon Fidati und seine Kritik an der Philosophie', in *Simon Fidati von Cascia OESA: Augustinische Theologie und Philosophie im späten Mittelalter*, ed. by Carolin M. Oser-Grote and Andreas E. J. Grote (Würzburg: Augustinus-Verlag bei Echter, 2006), pp. 391–95

Thompson, Augustine, *Cities of God: The Religion of the Italian Communes 1125–1325* (University Park: Pennsylvania State University Press, 2005)

Turner, Denys, *Eros and Allegory: Medieval Exegesis of the Song of Songs*, Cistercian Studies Series, 156 (Kalamazoo: Cistercian Publications, 1995)

Vecchio, Silvana 'Il piacere da Abelardo a Tommaso', in *Piacere e dolore: Materiali per une storia delle passioni nel Medioevo*, ed. by Carla Casagrande and Silvana Vecchio, Micrologus' Library, 29 (Firenze: SISMEL/Edizioni del Galluzzo, 2009), pp. 67–86

——, 'The Seven Deadly Sins between Pastoral Care and Scholastic Theology: The *Summa de vitiis* by John of Rupella', in *In the Garden of Evil: The Vices and Culture in the Middle Ages*, ed. by Richard Newhauser, Papers in Mediaeval Studies, 18 (Toronto: Institute for Medieval Studies, 2005), pp. 104–28

Verdon, Jean, *Le Plaisir au Moyen Âge* (Paris: Perrin, 1996)

Wack, Mary Frances, 'The Measure of Pleasure: Peter of Spain on Men, Women, and Lovesickness', *Viator*, 17 (1986), 173–96

Watson, Nicholas, 'Censorship and Cultural Change in Late Medieval England: Vernacular Theology, the Oxford Translation Debate and Arundel's Constitutions of 1409', *Speculum*, 70 (1995), 822–64

——, *Richard Rolle and the Invention of Authority* (Cambridge: Cambridge University Press, 1991)

Zanella, Gabriele, 'Malessere ereticale in valle padana (1260–1308)', in *Hereticalia: Temi e discussioni*, ed. by Gabriele Zanella (Spoleto: Centro Italiano di Studi sull'Alto Medioevo, 1995), pp. 41–47

Zumkeller, Adolar, 'Die Augustinertheologen Simon Fidati von Cascia und Hugolin von Orvieto und Martin Luthers Kritik an Aristoteles', *Archiv für Reformationsgeschichte*, 54 (1963), 15–37

Hell: The Pleasure of the Suffering of Others from Visions of the Afterlife to Religious Theatre

Élyse Dupras
Translated by Sheila Eskenazi

What is an article about Hell doing in a work about pleasure? Is not Hell the place for suffering, the antithesis of pleasure? If a stay in Hell seems to be the time to experience every torment, the evocation of Hell can also be associated with certain dimensions of pleasure, understood here as a feeling of satisfaction, of fascination, of joy that can extend all the way to the jubilation of laughter. Thus, from the evocations of Hell by theologians in the early centuries of Christianity, to representations of this same Hell on the stages of religious theatres in the fifteenth and sixteenth centuries, through the description of infernal torments in some visions of the afterlife, this place of suffering seems to raise, among those who think they will escape it, laughter in the face of violence, the pleasure of watching revenge for their persecutions, and the satisfaction of seeing the triumph of Christendom and its followers over that which threatens them. This pleasure, which has an element

* The translation of this article was made possible by the financial support of the Ministère de l'Éducation, de l'Enseignement supérieur et de la Recherche du Québec. The most recent oral presentation of this work was given in Béatrice Delaurenti's seminar in École des Hautes Études en Sciences Sociales, Paris, 21 March 2014. I would like to thank her for that invitation and for the inspiring discussion that followed the conference. My thanks also go to the seminar participants.

Élyse Dupras (elyse.dupras@mail.mcgill.ca) teaches French literature at Cégep de Saint-Jérôme (Québec). After a PhD thesis exploring the role of devils in medieval hagiographic plays, published under the title *Diables et saints: Rôle des diables dans les mystères hagiographiques français* (Genève: Droz, 2006), her present research focuses on devils, evil, and the representation of otherness in medieval theatre.

Pleasure in the Middle Ages, ed. by Naama Cohen-Hanegbi and Piroska Nagy, IMR 24 (Turnhout: Brepols, 2018), pp. 249–277 BREPOLS PUBLISHERS 10.1484/M.IMR-EB.5.113470

of perversion, seems to me to be close to what is described by the German term *Schadenfreude*; it is interesting to note, too, that, in some languages, a specific term exists to describe this 'nasty' pleasure. We will see how the various sources consulted build a kind of legitimacy for this inversion of compassion.

Early Christianity: Hell and the Pleasure of Vengeance

Justin, a Roman martyr in the second century, is best known for his role in defining the idea of heresy: according to him this is the legacy of both Simon Magus and philosophy.[1] A victim of persecution, Justin defined Hell as 'the vengeance of the persecuted righteous, who contemplate with joy the punishment of their enemies'.[2] Thus, very early in the Christian tradition, the idea asserts itself that the Elect in Paradise will experience watching the torture of the damned as a delight. This idea, far from being marginal, draws its origins from the Jewish tradition: the book of Enoch had already evoked the feelings of joy and triumph that will belong to the Elect watching the punishment of the impious.[3] The New Testament also gives place to this theme through the parable of Lazarus and the rich man (Luke 16. 22–31). Hell therefore becomes the place for a reversal, an inversion whose contemplation causes joy for he who has suffered during his lifetime.[4]

Tertullian, a Carthaginian converted pagan († *c.* 220), was a controversial figure because he was aligned with the Montanist heresy.[5] The author of a large body of work, he wrote a notable treatise against the persecution of the martyrs in the circuses where he asserts that those pagans who had enjoyed the circuses will find themselves in turn the victims of infernal torments, presented as dramatic spectacles for the delight of the Elect:

> How vast a spectacle then bursts upon the eye! What there excites my admiration? what my derision? Which sight gives me joy? which rouses me to exultation? — as I see so many illustrious monarchs, whose reception into the heavens was publicly announced, groaning now in the lowest darkness with great Jove himself, and those,

[1] On this subject, see Poulat and others, *Dictionnaire de l'Histoire du christianisme*, p. 495.

[2] Joly, *Christianisme et philosophie*, quoted by Baschet, *Les Justices de l'au-delà*, p. 21.

[3] Joly, *Christianisme et philosophie*, p. 171.

[4] A Coptic version of the apocryphal Apocalypse of Paul also shows that child victims of infanticide see their parents undergoing punishments that last forever; see Rosentiehl, 'Tartarouchos-Temleouchos', p. 38.

[5] On this subject, see Poulat and others, *Dictionnaire de l'Histoire du christianisme*, pp. 765–71.

> too, who bore witness of their exultation; governors of provinces, too, who persecuted the Christian name, in fires more fierce than those with which in the days of their pride they raged against the followers of Christ. What world's wise men besides, the very philosophers, in fact, who taught their followers that God had no concern in aught that is sublunary, and were wont to assure them that either they had no souls, or that they would never return to the bodies which at death they had left, now covered with shame before the poor deluded ones, as one fire consumes them! Poets also, trembling not before the judgment-seat of Rhadamanthus or Minos, but of the unexpected Christ! I shall have a better opportunity then of hearing the tragedians, louder-voiced in their own calamity; of viewing the play-actors, much more 'dissolute' in the dissolving flame.[6]

The words of Tertullian seem particularly sadistic in their description of the pleasure that the Elect take in watching the suffering of the impious. This pleasure seems even greater given that the drama is not fictional, but rather puts on the stage those damned who enjoyed and sometimes even participated in equivalent pagan 'shows'.

Cyprian († *c.* 258), a Carthaginian fellow-citizen of Tertullian and heir to his thought, became a martyr. Like Justin, he sees the torture of the damned as a just revenge, even retribution, for the pleasure that these same damned took at the spectacle of the persecution of the Christians. He writes:

> And the eternal, infinite torments will torture the souls at the same time as the bodies. Therefore, they will be on show for us, we who had been their show for a day, therefore, the brief cruel pleasure that they got watching us be persecuted will be made up for with an eternal show of fire.[7]

The spectacle of the defeat of enemies, even if it takes place in the afterlife, appears as a consolation to the defeated and persecuted Christians. The idea of spectacle appears in Tertullian as much as in Cyprian. The theatrical shows that these Fathers of the Church think about, those that they know, are obviously not the fictions of the Greek theatre of Sophocles and Euripides. They are more like Roman theatre, even Roman circuses, since theatre had more or less disappeared in Rome, eclipsed by circus games with all the cruelty that they imply.[8]

[6] Tertullian, *The Shows or De Spectaculis*, XXX, trans. by Thelwall.

[7] Quoted by Joly, *Christianisme et philosophie*, p. 174.

[8] The decadence of the theatre in Rome begins in the first century. It will soon be replaced by circus games and dancing. When Tertullian wrote his *De Spectaculis*, the theatre of which he speaks is not Greek tragedy anymore, but either the circus games or the theatrical plays associated with libertinism, pantomime, and discourse on sex and love given by prostitutes on the occasion of celebrations of Flora (28 April). See Mazouer, *Le Théâtre français du Moyen Âge*, p. 15.

The idea of show unavoidably leads back to that of catharsis and the definition of this catharsis (process by which a strong emotion, usually fear or pity, is released, cleaned) given by Aristotle. However, in my opinion, the nature of the Roman circus spectacle was not to cleanse the emotions of terror and pity.[9] The cathartic aspect, if present, consisted more of a purgation of the fear, the anguish, in the face of the threat that the other represents. We can perhaps see the same sort of catharsis among the Christians who attend the spectacles of the tormenting of the damned.

Two Visions of the Afterlife (Eleventh and Twelfth Centuries): Terror and Pleasure

The tradition of the visions of the afterlife is an important one in the Middle Ages. Some theologians of the twelfth and the thirteenth centuries, if they don't see them as a true report of a real journey, acknowledge at least their pedagogical value. It is therefore important to note that all the visions of the afterlife written from the seventh century to the end of the twelfth century describe physical torture.[10] The visions of the afterlife were often, and rightly so, seen as texts aimed at confirming the usefulness of the intercession of the living in favour of the dead. Thus, visions of the afterlife appear as occasions to stimulate the compassion of the living in respect to the souls that are suffering. However, to this undeniable function must be added another that inverts compassion by arousing pleasure/rejoicing at the suffering of the other, or, rather, a certain type of other. It is not about rejoicing at the suffering of the neighbour, this other who springs from sameness and who, because of this, merits the compassion of the person to whom the texts are addressed. These others who merit compassion are certainly Christians; intercessory prayers for the dead cannot save pagans, destined to infernal torment for eternity. Furthermore, the others arising from sameness belong to the same universe both in a religious and in a political sense. To feel compassion for them is also to feel compassion for oneself. To rejoice in their suffering is impossible.

[9] Aristotle's 'catharsis' is not the purification of these emotions, but rather their purgation or expulsion.

[10] According to Baschet, *Les Justices de l'au-delà*, pp. 39 and 41, except for Johannes Scotus Eriugena and his emulators, medieval theologians agree on the aspects, both physical and spiritual, of the punishment of the damned after doomsday.

The real others do not merit compassion: they do not belong to the same universe of meaning. They are radically other. In general, they are not even Christians. Worse still, they are the enemies of Christ. Or else, while being sacramental Christians, they are barred from the Christian community by the radical deviance of their behaviour. These true others, who share neither a religion nor a sense of political belonging, often do not even share a geographical space with the Christians; these others can suffer. Better yet, they must suffer. The description of these tortures holds an important place in the two visions addressed here.

The *Vision of Tnugdal*

In 1149, an Irish monk named Marcus, living in Germany, wrote down a vision that was related to him by Tnugdal, an Irish knight.[11] This knight is surprised by Death while he is feasting with friends. He then visits the afterlife, accompanied by his guardian angel,[12] and he undergoes some punishments that Hell reserves for his sins. The knight's catalepsy lasts three days, after which he is restored and recounts what he has seen and suffered. One of the people listening is the monk Marcus, whose text is presented as a Latin translation of the account given in the vernacular. The Latin text occasioned many translations in Europe and found literary fame. Vincent de Beauvais, notably, took it up in an abridged way in his *Speculum historiale* (1263), where Tnugdal becomes Tondalus.[13] This literary fame is itself evidence of the fascination aroused by its contents. In Marcus's Latin version, approximately half the text relates to the vision of Hell (all areas combined), while two-thirds of the remaining half are devoted to Paradise.[14] The public's fascination is therefore largely attributable to the interest in, if not the pleasure at, the description of Hell that is provided.

The *Vision of Tnugdal* is rather complete: it broaches Upper Hell (which most commentators understand as Purgatory), then Lower Hell (eternal and without appeal), then two places reserved for half-hearted Christians (the

[11] On the context of the writing of this vision, see Yolande de Pontfarcy's introduction to *The Vision of Tnugdal*, ed. by Picard and de Pontfarcy.

[12] In addition to the guardian angel, the *Vision of Tnugdal* also presents an unusual character that I would describe as the 'guardian devil'. The angel blames Tnugdal for having listened to the advice of this particular devil.

[13] On translations and manuscripts, see Palmer, *Visio Tnugdali*, p. 3.

[14] Palmer, *Visio Tnugdali*, p. 48.

'not so bad' and the 'not so good'), and finally several locations in Paradise. However, reading this vision gives the impression that the writer's imagination is demonstrably much more fertile on the subject of infernal penalties (purgatorial or otherwise) than on the delights of Paradise. It is important to distinguish the pleasure and the torments attributed in the story to the elect and to the damned, from the pleasures (and even the torments) that they arouse among the writers/listeners. Among the latter, the torments provoke a morbid fascination that is not devoid of pleasure and, of interest to us here, that tends towards the pleasure in the pain of the other.

If the devils are numerous, cruel, foul-smelling, noisy in the parts of the vision devoted to the various levels of Hell, the emphasis is placed rather on the arsenal of tortures. This is notably made up of a horrifying and teeming phantasmagorical fauna: serpents, dragons, scorpions, snakes, and other vermin. An integral part of the tortures, these beasts are sometimes its only agents. One invariably sees in these devouring monsters the magnified and horribly fantasized memory of the Roman tortures (imperial era) which consisted of delivering criminals and Christians to the beasts, that mode of torture properly called the 'condemnation to the beasts' or even 'damnatio ad bestias'.[15] The tortures associated with this devouring are described more than once: for example, a monster devours members of the clergy who have broken their vows of chastity or who have 'abnormal' relations ('against nature', *contra naturam*, the texts would say).[16] The anguish associated with illicit pleasure expresses itself clearly in the role of this monster. The association between pleasure and eternal torment here takes on the expected dimension of an inversion. But this inversion results precisely from the illicit character of the erotic pleasure in which the clergy have indulged on Earth. And the pleasure, more than a little perverse, engendered by the description of torture, is linked as well to the disgusted rejection by the faithful of a clergy seen as decadent or unworthy.[17]

The description of the monster strikes the imagination: the beast devours sinners, then inseminates them while they are in his stomach, and then gives birth to them (or excretes them). Inside his belly, souls suffer great torments

[15] See Ménard, 'Du prédateur à la proie'.

[16] See Chiffoleau, 'Dire l'indicible'. Chiffoleau indicates that homosexual practices are considered 'abominable' as early as the third century, and against nature from the sixth century.

[17] About the irritation of the faithful towards unworthy priests, and its role in the birth of heresy in the Middle Ages, see Vauchez, *Les Hérétiques au Moyen Âge*, p. 97 and passim. Henriet, *La Parole et la prière au Moyen Âge*, p. 227, highlights that some preachers virulently reprimanded unworthy priests.

and, first destroyed, they take shape again and find themselves pregnant, having been inseminated by the monster. This latter then expels them on a frozen pond, in a violent suffering of the souls. These in their turn give birth to loathsome serpents, which gush, not from the genital organs, but from the whole body: the little monsters coiled up inside shred the body with the sharp blades of their tongues in order to materialize.[18] The dispersal of the pain and the abundance of details are a reminder that lust cannot simply be reduced to copulation, but that it corrupts the total being. The parturition finds itself inextricably tied to the sin of lust, in an infernal world with no end, where torturer and victim, parent and offspring, ingestion and birthing merge and are linked. This punishment, perhaps more than others, appears like the punishment of a pleasure, operating on the anguish of the disorder it generates. Therefore the description, long and detailed, is evidence of the writer's pleasure (and, undoubtedly, of the reader) in contemplating this particular torture. The religious who breaks his vow of chastity, like the believer who devotes himself to abnormal sexual relations, creates disorder in the Christian community. The gravity of the transgression is enough to make them others, and to turn them into radical outcasts. In a universe where the relationship to the body is itself ambiguous, caught between the often carnivalesque pleasure of the body and the morbid anguish related to the rejection of the animality in man, everything that goes beyond the normal codification of physical relationships appears as a threat that weighs on the whole community. In this regard, sinners become enemies of their community. The pleasure taken at the description of such a torment by the recorder and listener can seem legitimate since they are torments that, in his wisdom, God predicted for criminals of sexuality. Hell, yet again, grants to the weak the pleasure of feeling avenged.

[18] See Baschet, *Les Justices de l'au-delà*, p. 111, nn. 94 and 95: 'Le choix des serpents trouve un écho dans la littérature des Bestiaires: au lieu d'attendre la délivrance naturelle, les petits de la vipère rongent les flancs de leur mère pour sortir de force, provoquant ainsi sa mort. [...] Les serpents se comportent donc à l'égard des damnés conformément à la loi de leur espèce. [...] En outre, le non-respect de la chasteté est ainsi puni par un animal auquel on attribue une sexualité particulièrement violente, et même morbide. En effet, selon les Bestiaires, lors de l'accouplement des vipères, le mâle introduit sa tête dans la gorge de la femelle; celle-ci tranche sa tête puis l'avale' (The choice of snakes finds an echo in the Bestiaries: instead of waiting for natural deliverance, the viper's babies gnaw their mother's side in order to force their exit, thus inducing their mother's death. [...] Therefore, the snakes behave towards the damned according to the law of their species. [...] In addition, the disrespect for chastity is punished by an animal which is associated with a particularly violent and even morbid sexuality. According to the Bestiaries, during coupling the male viper puts his head into the female's throat; she then cuts the male's head off and swallows it).

After visiting many torture chambers, Tnugdal finds himself back in Hell, which he leaves in order to be able to give his account. The visit could be seen as interrupted at the moment when Tnugdal leaves Hell: the various zones of Paradise cannot help but follow threat with promise. But since Paradise is a place of infinite delights, its description offers a new form of pleasure to those who are already taken by the writers' and listeners' evocation of Hell. Thus the reader goes from the perverse pleasure associated with *Schadenfreude* to the virtuous pleasure of the contemplation of paradisiacal bliss. However, this bliss does not seem to be completely untinged by perversion. In this regard, a sentence in the *Vision of Tnugdal* catches our attention, in the way that it recalls in the minor mode the idea of vengeance already evoked by Cyprian and Tertullian. It shows that the Elect, from their paradise, can see the entire world:

> Ab illo ergo loco, in quo tunc stabant, non solum omnem, quam ante viderant, gloriam, verum etiam predictarum *supplicia* penarum videbant, miramur, terrarum orbem quasi sub uno solis radio videre valebant.[19] (emphasis added)
>
> [From the place where they had earlier found themselves, they saw not only the complete glory that they could earlier gaze upon, but also the *tortures* related to the punishments described earlier and, a marvel, they were able to see the entire world as under a single ray of sunshine.][20] (emphasis added)

Curiously, some French translators of the *Vision* thought it a good idea to cut out this sentence. Thus the translation by David Aubert (1475) reads:

> Et la ou l'ame estoit ne se veoit point tant seulement toute la gloire que par avant elle avoit veeue, ainshcois se veoit tout le monde ainsi comme se l'enfeust dessoubz ung seul ray de soleil.[21]
>
> [And there where the soul found itself, it saw not only all the glory it had gazed upon earlier, but also saw the entire world, as if revealed beneath a single ray of sunshine.]

No trace of the *supplicia* evoked in Latin. On the other hand, the version produced a century earlier by Jean de Vignay (*c.* 1332–33) in his *Miroir Historial*,

19 De Pontfarcy, *L'Au-delà au Moyen Âge*, p. 144.

20 This is a clear reference to the Vision of Saint Benedict in the *Dialogues* of Gregory the Great, II, 35, trans. by Gardner, p. 97: 'Upon this sight a marvellous strange thing followed, for, as himself did afterward report, the whole world, gathered as it were together under one beam of the sun, was presented before his eyes'.

21 *La Vision de Tondale*, ed. by Cavagna, p. 219, lines 1796–98.

the French translation of the *Speculum historiale* of Vincent de Beauvais, includes a similar allusion:

> Du lieu ou il estoient seurmontoit toute joie, et non pas tant seulement celle que il avoient veue par devant, et si veoient *les devans dis tourmens*; et encore, ce qui estoit plus a merveillier, toute la rondesce du monde et des terres ils veoient aussi comme sous un rai de soleil.[22] (emphasis added)

> [And from the place where they were, he gazed upon all joy and not only that which they had earlier gazed upon, and they also saw the *tortures described above*, and again, what is the most astonishing, they saw the whole sphere of the world and its lands, as though under a single ray of sunshine.] (emphasis added)

Undeniably then, the *Vision of Tnugdal*, in its original version and in some of its translations, states that since their arrival in Paradise, the Elect are capable of seeing the torments of Hell. And yet, in Paradise the Elect not only cannot be afflicted by any suffering (they therefore feel no compassion towards the damned, since that would mean suffering with them) but, furthermore, they cannot experience anything except delights. In consequence, the sensation produced by this encompassing vision, which includes the vision of the torments, is a delicious feeling. For the Elect who find themselves inside the visionary story, seeing the torment of the other constitutes a pleasure, and a not inconsiderable one: it is one of the pleasures of Paradise, one of the rewards provided to the Elect.[23]

The *Vision of Thurkill*

The place of the pleasure aroused by the contemplation of torture is equally important, and in a very special way, in the *Vision of Thurkill* (dated All Soul's Week, October 1206).[24] The recording of this vision is attributed to an English Cistercian, Ralph of Coggestall (abbot of the Cistercian monastery of Coggestall, Essex; he died after 1227). It appears, with some changes, in the *Flores historiarum* by Roger of Wendover (1235) and in his follower Matthieu

[22] *La Vision de Tondale*, ed. by Cavagna, p. 105, lines 962–66.

[23] A very interesting theological and anthropological study could be made of the comparison of the translations produced by Jean de Vignay and David Aubert, in order to discuss what happened between 1333 and 1475, what influenced them, and specifically why Aubert removed this mention, why it may have become incomprehensible or unacceptable for him.

[24] Gardiner, *Medieval Visions of Heaven and Hell*, p. 204.

Paris's *Chronica Majora* (1259).[25] Vincent de Beauvais also takes it up in his *Speculum historiale* (1263). If the *Vision of Tnugdal* fascinates with the details in its descriptions and by its literary impact, that of Thurkill, recorded between 1206 and 1218,[26] is astonishing in its singularity. Thurkill is a pious English peasant. One day, while he is working to dry out his field that had been flooded by a recent rain, Saint Julian the Hospitaler appears to him and warns him that he will be coming to collect him that same evening. When the evening arrives, Thurkill is taken to the afterlife by the saint who, along with Saint Domnin, will act as his guide.

Two notable elements of this vision merit our attention. On the one hand, the demons feel pain and the saints can inflict it on them: thus, when Saint Domnin asks a demon to explain to him who the soul is that the demon enjoys mistreating, and the demon ignores the saint's request, the latter violently flogs the devil, who screams in pain and ends by complying. A new dimension to the saint appears: he is more than just kindly. In this regard, the vision foretells the mystery scenes where angels beat demons, such as the one in the *Miracle de Théophile* where Notre Dame threatens to 'fouler la pance' (trample on the belly) of Satan, or the one in the *Mystère de Saint Barbe* where the young saint beats Satan.[27] The saint is evidently stronger than the demon, frequently in this world, and in the afterlife at the very least. This power of the saint, as we will see, contributes greatly to the pleasure of spectators at mystery plays.

On the other hand, the specific torture that damned souls endure on Sundays appears particularly striking.[28] On Sunday nights, the devils look after their 'theatrical games' and increase the sufferings of the damned by more painful tortures. That night, the damned on stage re-present the sins that caused their damnation. Even the description of the place corresponds to that of a theatre: it is an imposing building equipped with many seats. The seats of the damned, made of blazing metal and pointy nails, act as instruments of torture. As for the devils, they sit on other seats (and they do not appear to be seats of torture) in order to

[25] *Visio Thurkilli*, ed. by Schmidt.

[26] The earlier is the date on which the vision would have taken place; the later is the year in which Ralph of Coggeshall's charge as abbot in the Cistercian monastery ended.

[27] Satan is also badly beaten by the Archangel Michael in *La Pacience de Job* (the stage instructions indicate that the angel hits the devil: vv. 6267–6315, ed. by Meiller).

[28] It seems quite far from the alleviation on Sundays of the punishment described in *Visio Pauli*! See Joly, *Christianisme et philosophie*, p. 177, quoting *Visio sancti Pauli*, chs XXXIII and XL. In *Visio Pauli*, the traveller experiences no pleasure in seeing the suffering of the damned, but rather he feels an intense compassion.

mock the sinners and the tortures that they endure. The first 'actor' is arrogant. Violently pulled from his seat by the demons, he behaves as he did on Earth, which ignites the devils' mirth.[29] Subsequently, the infernal inversion takes over: his clothes catch fire and burn his body. After the performance, the arrogant one is cut into pieces and fried by the devils, then he is put back together, savagely tortured using a variety of instruments, returned to his torture-seat, and a new actor is sent onto the stage, then another, then another again. Each one reproduces the actions associated with the sin for which he was damned and, while he re-presents his sin, the demons mock him and snigger. After that, the sinner metamorphoses during punishment, and the sequence of tortures begins again. The importance of inversion in punishment of the sin is made clear by its great pedagogical power: it shows that sin, which gives pleasure in the world, ends with punishment and is designed to make the sinner understand that when he commits a sin in this world, the devils, invisible, take pleasure in the show he provides, mocking and sniggering. The inversion of the punishment thus shows that even if the reversal seems to take place in a future far from the commission of the sin, in the unified time of the afterlife this reversal is immediate.

Thus, the infernal theatre is both a torture chamber for the actors and a place for pleasure, for laughter, for the devils. Here we find three elements that will return in religious theatre, in the theatre-pain-pleasure relationship. The vision does not indicate feelings of compassion on the part of the visionary; nor does it indicate enjoyment on the part of the guiding saints during the show, no more than it evokes the idea that the Elect can also attend. In a word, in this show everything relates to damnation: the spectators, the actors, and the subject of the theatrical play itself.

It is important to note that in England, when Thurkill has his vision, a particular type of theatre existed. Between 965 and 975 two English bishops, Saint Dunstan, Archbishop of Canterbury, and Saint Ethelwold, Archbishop of Winchester, prescribed a ritual of the disposition of the body of Christ which is comparable to the staging of a show.[30] Thus the theatre at the centre of the

[29] Diller also points out that the York cycle (of medieval religious English drama) mainly uses the words 'laugh' and 'laughter' in association with evil characters such as devils (Diller, 'Laughter in Medieval English Drama', p. 8).

[30] They both wrote a rule for the monasteries of England in which they define the Good Friday ritual in which Christ's body is solemnly laid down in the sepulchre, giving a pedagogical virtue to this performance; cf. Mazouer, *Le Théâtre français du Moyen Âge*, pp. 25–27. Mazouer states that this rule seems to be 'l'acte de naissance du théâtre médiéval' (medieval theatre's birth certificate; p. 27).

liturgy as it is (re)born in the tenth century aims to re-present (present again) an event held as real by Christianity: the disposition of the body of Christ. It is not about building a story to amuse or edify spectators, but to make visible that which had been made invisible by the passage of time, to re-present an event that certainly really happened, in order to impart knowledge of it to the simple who, following Saint Thomas's example, need to see to believe.[31] In the same way, infernal theatrical plays cannot be considered as near to fiction: they also show what the passage of time has rendered invisible — a sin committed in the past — and their description shows the torments to come for the sinners as well as the perverse pleasure that the devils gain from the spectacle of the sin. Thus in liturgical drama as in the infernal theatrical plays equally, the theatre is a tool for the confirmation and reproduction of faith in the multiplicity of its aspects.

Some Mystery Plays from the Fifteenth and Sixteenth Centuries: Torments (of the Martyrs and the Damned) and Pleasures (of the Spectators)

The vision of Thurkill provides theatrical plays with a rich and ample forum for the suffering of the damned and for the pleasure of the devils. Only a few centuries separate this vision from the Mystery plays (both Passion plays and hagiographic plays), which provide an occasion for the spectators' pleasure in watching the representation of the suffering of the devils and of the damned (but also of the martyrs). When edifying theatre develops outside of the Church, in all its scope (plays often run for several days), a new means for the portrayal of Hell emerges. Visions of the afterlife describe the insight that a character could have of Heaven and Hell; the theatre displays it by constructing one set portraying Heaven, and another portraying Hell. In effect, Hell is the most elaborate set in medieval religious theatre, and the most complex, the one that uses the most gadgets and machinery.[32] The theatre not only describes what happens in the other world, it also represents the characters, the places, the

[31] As early as the twelfth century, the Church's position on the performance of these liturgical dramas during religious rituals becomes more reluctant. Gradually, the liturgical drama tends to disappear from a certain number of churches, yet remains in others. Simultaneously, however, religious drama presented in the vernacular rises outside of the Church and develops wonderfully; cf. Mazouer, *Le Théâtre français du Moyen Âge*, pp. 61–62.

[32] For a complete description of the set for the theatrical depiction of Hell, see Runnalls, 'Were They Listening or Watching?' and Runnalls, 'Les Acteurs dans le *Mystère de la Passion* de Châteaudun en 1510', as well as Konigson, *L'Espace théâtral médiéval*, pp. 103–17, and Dupras, *Diables et saints*, pp. 35–41.

atmosphere, the actions: theatre really gives life to what remained only a recitation in the visions. But the redactors were clearly inspired by the stories they read and heard, and among them by the visions of the afterlife.

To my eyes, theatre remains particularly important as evidence of the expectations of an era, through its privileged status as art aimed not at the individual but at a whole crowd, as underlined by Anne Ubersfeld:

> [on] ne peut dire (écrire) au théâtre que ce qui peut être entendu: positivement, le scripteur répond à une voix du public. [...] Tout texte théâtral est la réponse à une demande du public, et c'est sur ce point que se fait le plus aisément l'articulation du discours théâtral avec l'histoire et l'idéologie.[33]
>
> [[Nothing] can be said (written) in the theatre except what can be heard: positively, the writer responds to the public's voice. [...] Every theatrical text is a response to public demand, and it is on this point that it is easiest to link theatrical discourse with history and ideology.]

Therefore, the expectations of the medieval public convey a fascination as much for the torments of the damned as for the tortures inflicted on martyrs. Here again, torments and pleasure intertwine. An exceptional event, the performance of a mystery play, energizes the whole town, as much for the preparations as for the performance. Though costly, it was a very prestigious occasion for a town; the authorities sought the approval and collaboration of the religious establishment. Motivated by the desire to solicit the protection of a saint or to display the economic prosperity of a town, the numerous organizers invested heavily to cover the various costs, from the writing or adaptation of the text (often by an anonymous redactor) to the construction of the sets (temporary, in the town centre). Most of the time, the non-professional actors were citizens of the town and paid for their own costumes. During the performance, the shops were closed, and everyone watched; even the actors, when they were not performing, joined the audience to see the show.[34]

The best-known plays of medieval religious theatre are the great mysteries of the Passion of Christ, such as that of Arnoul Gréban (organist at the Paris Cathedral, author of, among others, a four-day mystery play performed in Abbeville from 23 to 25 May 1455), that tells the story of humanity from the Fall to the Redemption. To the mysteries of the Passion are added numer-

[33] Ubersfeld, *Lire le théâtre* (1977), p. 198.

[34] For the history of French medieval theatre, see Mazouer, *Le Théâtre français du Moyen Âge* and Nagler, *The Medieval Religious Stage*.

ous hagiographic mysteries. Among other things in common, these different mystery plays often feature martyrs. Of the total of twenty-four hagiographic mysteries that I have studied closely, fourteen celebrate the life and death of a martyr. In general, these plays devote considerable importance to tortures, which justifies a large number of special effects, allowing the 'master of secrets' to deploy the range of his art. The ten remaining mystery plays are not lacking scenes of violence: it is the damned who bear the brunt in Hell, and on Earth, the catechumens are tormented by the devils (*Mystère du Roy Advenir*), and the possessed are beaten by the saints who then deliver them from the tormenting devil (*Mystère de l'institution de l'ordre des frères précheurs*).

In an important article devoted to scenes of martyrdom, Élisabeth Lalou speculates on what spectators felt while watching the tortures inflicted on Jesus or the saints and draws a parallel between the well-known public punishments of the era and the tortures in the theatre.[35] It seems to me that this valuable reflection can be completed by a greater examination of torture in the theatre — not only inflicted on (fictional) members of the Christian community or on Jesus himself, but equally on the others. The various types of tortures, like the various types of victims, are intertwined: the martyrdom on the stage is generally followed by the torture of the human torturers by the devils in Hell. It is important, however, to make a clear distinction between the torments that were still used in public punishments, such as boiling in a cauldron, a punishment intended for counterfeiters, and the tortures that were obsolete, such as the *damnatio ad bestias*, used on Christians in Antiquity, for example. The spectator's response to the various types of torment could have been different according to this distinction.[36]

Of course the first martyr in the Christian religion, and the most famous, remains Jesus. In this respect, Gréban's *Mystère de la Passion* accords considerable space to the sufferings inflicted on him, as witnessed in the scenes devoted to his flagellation and then his crucifixion. The dialogue of the torturers is marked by good humour that leaves no doubt about the pleasure that they get from flogging:

Pilate Avant, garçons, vous vous rendez :
reprenez allaine et vertu
et le me rendez tant batu
de tous lez qu'il n'y ait que batre.

[35] Lalou, 'Les Tortures dans les mystères'.

[36] Carlson, *Performing Bodies in Pain*, p. 42, and Lalou, 'Les Tortures dans les mystères', p. 43.

Griffon Empreu.
Orillart Et deux.
Brayart Et trois.
Claquedent Et quatre,
Et le cinquieme de surcroix.
[...]
Griffon, tu comptes sans rabatre :
pour ung cop tu en frappes trois.
Griffon Quand ce sont dix, fais une crois,
je ne le fais que pour esbatre.[37]

[**Pilate** Go, boys, you are weakening;
Catch your breath and your strength
And give him to me so beaten
That on all sides there is nothing more to beat.
Griffon And a-one.
Orillart And a-two.
Brayart And a-three.
Claquedent And a-four,
And a fifth for good measure.
[...]
Griffon, you don't count by half-measures:
For one blow, you give three!
Griffon When you get to ten, make a cross,
I only do it to amuse myself / for a bit of exercise.]

The character of Griffon asserts explicitly that this flogging is, for him, an amusement: the term 'esbatre' is associated with the idea of entertainment, of pleasure. This pleasure does not seem to be uniquely related to the activity (that of whipping), but equally to the suffering inflicted, as suggested by the enthusiasm with which the torturers obey Pilate's order. The dialogue devoted to the crucifixion (vv. 24725–25025) goes the same way. Thus, in this piece as in many others showing martyrdom, the torturers are shown taking pleasure in the suffering that they cause to the other. Pilate underlines, moreover, that once the flogging is finished, Jesus is in a pitiful state, but that his accusers 'sont contens des griefves doleurs | dont [Jésus] es[t] asprement pugny' (are satisfied with the serious pain | with which Jesus is severely punished) (vv. 22874–75). The sergeants-

[37] Christ's flogging scene in Gréban, *Le Mystère de la Passion*, vv. 22850–61, ed. by Jodogne.

at-arms, however, pursue their comedy, decking him out in a crown of thorns and mocking the blood that trickles down his face (vv. 22974–89), to the point that Pilate, moved by pity, puts an end to the scene. Pilate's pity shows that the pleasure taken from the suffering of Jesus finds itself reserved for characters considered to be coarse, whose names — Griffon (Griffin), Claquedent (Beggar), Braillard (Crybaby), Orillart (Big Ears) — call to mind their membership in the paradigmatic group of torturers, a group that, in its behaviour, its gestures, and its language, resembles the infernal hordes. The 'paradigmatic group' designates a group of more or less interchangeable theatrical signs or characters that evoke each other through metonymy.[38] The pleasure taken in the suffering of the other, in this mystery play, seems first to be associated with demonized characters, that is to say, those close to the paradigmatic group of devils. These episodes can seem to have been intended to arouse the most passionate compassion, and doubtless this was the intention of the redactor and the effect often produced in the spectators. Marla Carlson asserts: 'The martyr might be impassible, but the spectator suffered. That was the point of contemplating devotional images or watching dramatic performances'.[39] That may have been the intention of the *fatiste* and the producers of the play; however, the coarse and comical nature of the torturers' retorts, if they do not cause repugnance, can have the effect of defusing, at least in part, this compassion, and of transforming it into a good laugh. The pleasure, which should have come about only through watching the torments inflicted on the enemies of the faith and through the triumph of Christianity, somehow manages to pollute the reception of the tortures imposed on Christ. However, this cannot be separated from the fact that the Parliament of Paris eventually banned these mystery plays, from 1548 onwards. It is important to note here that if the spectators laugh at the torments endured by Christ, this laughter is to be understood as carnival laughter, in Bakhtin's sense; but it is also likely that most of the time the pleasure spectators take at these tortures is not pleasure at comedy but rather the pleasure of a community suffering together, the pleasure of sharing a religious emotion.

While in Gréban's *Mystère de la Passion*, the pleasure taken by contemplating the suffering of the other, or its infliction, is essentially associated with the torturers so that their function contributes to its demonization, this pleasure becomes more ambiguous in many hagiographic mysteries. There are many scenes of martyrdom in these mysteries indicating, if not the spectators' pleas-

[38] See Ubersfeld, *Lire le théâtre* (1996), p. 24.

[39] Carlson, *Performing Bodies in Pain*, p. 43.

ure, then at least the public's taste for these scenes (pleasure from the compassion experienced together, which can become a taste for suffering shared in community). *Le Mystère des trois Doms* performed in 1509, which tells the story of three martyrs, Severinus, Exuperius, and Felician, provides a very good example. The many stage directions in this text (a fairly rare phenomenon at that time) reveal the treatment inflicted on the martyrs. The violence to which they are subjected cannot help but call to mind the Passion of Christ, and this connection is also explicit in the text, since the martyred saints search for the passion that will bring them closer to Jesus. The stoic attitude of the martyrs during the scenes of torture greatly contrasts with the verbal and gestural excess of the torturers and contributes to the comic effect produced by the latter.[40] The tortures inflicted (on dummies, *corps feints*, that stand in for the actors) are terrible: one Christian is sawn in half on the stage (vv. 3295–3311); a second is cut up into three pieces ('*Lors se separera le corps saing en troes pars*' (then the dummy representing the martyr is separated into three parts; p. 182, vv. 3366–67); a third is nailed to a board, one shoulder after the other, then the head (vv. 3420–61). The treatment intended for the three saints celebrated by the mystery play is no more delicate, but it corresponds to a good number of tortures inflicted on Christians under the Tetrarchy: flaying with the help of iron nails, whips, etc.[41] This episode resembles the infernal torments (and vice versa), as much by the iron nails as by the flames used against the poor martyrs. Thus, the coming together between the torturers and the devils, signaled above, finds itself intensified by the coming together of the infernal torments and the martyrdom. Therefore, Hell corresponds to the earthly tortures, as well as being an inversion of them. Are we thus not surprised, a few scenes later, to find the torturers grappling with devils? Soon after the martyrdom of the three saints, the torturers quarrel amongst themselves at the tavern; the dispute turns nasty, one of the torturers is killed, and all finally catch each other by the hair:

> Prant Torchemuseau par les cheveulx. Se tenans tous par les cheveulx, sortira par le tresbuchet tout a l'entour d'eux une fumée qui les enclourra. [...] Le tresbuchet tumbera, et le diable en fouldre descandra sur eux, et puis le tresbuchet se reclourra et le page parlera.[42]

[40] This contrast has been discussed by, amongst others, Lalou, 'Les Tortures dans les mystères', p. 44, and Newbigin, 'Agata, Apollonia and Other Martyred Virgins', pp. 89, 95.

[41] See Baslez, *Les Persécutions dans l'Antiquité*, p. 352 and passim.

[42] Chanoine Pra and Chevalet, *Le Mystère des trois Doms*, vv. 9647–48, 9653–54, ed. by Giraud and Chevalier.

> [He takes Torchemuseau by the hair. While they are all holding each other by the hair, smoke must come out of the trap door located above and engulf them. [...] Then the trap door opens, the devil in the form of lightning descends on them, then the trap door closes again and the page speaks.]

The torturers dedicate themselves to the devils, who hurry to seize them. Divine justice demands immediate punishment for those who cause irreparable wrong to saints; the devils act as zealous instruments of this justice, as the torturers were those of temporal justice. Thus the pleasure which, in the story, the torturers could experience in their torturing activity comes to legitimize, in advance, the pleasure that, in reality, the spectators experience by watching the torments of the torturers who become the damned. Moreover, the martyrdom very often results from a plot hatched in Hell by the devils,[43] which, in contributing to another linking of the paradigmatic group of the infernal hordes with the torturers, also contributes to glorifying the martyred saint. A victim of the machinations of the devils and the pagans, the saint resists, and the physical torments do not make him forget the love of Christ. Apparently vanquished by the pagans since he dies at their hands, the martyr is presented as victorious in reality in the only realm that counts, that of the afterlife. Fictional witnesses and real witnesses of a fictional martyr are present at the same show, and the discourse of the play leaves the message that Christians belonging to one or another category have a shared understanding, which enflames their hearts with an even more ardent faith.

To magnify the victory of Christianity, miracles often attenuate the tortures inflicted on the saints. This is evident, for instance, in *St Crépin et St Crépinien* (composed in the middle of the fifteenth century for the cobblers' brotherhood), where the cobblers' patron saints Crispin and Crispinian are thrown into the water with millstones around their necks, but escape unharmed (the millstones float!, Paris-a, vv. 1669–80). The miracles naturally increase the pleasure that the spectators get from the spectacle of martyrdom, and not only because of the special effects: the public rejoices not at the suffering of the saints but at that of the devils and the torturers, whose ruin is as risible as it is manifest.[44] Thus, by inciting martyrdom, the devils involuntarily cause a mira-

[43] As in *Mystère de St Genis* (Jean Oudin, *L'Ystoyre et la vie de saint Genis*, vv. 2149–51, 2165–70, ed. by Mostert and Stengel), for example.

[44] Diller points out that laughing at the devil's misfortune is a sign of holiness (Diller, 'Laughter in Medieval English Drama', p. 4); I'm convinced that laughing at a pagan torturer's misfortune is also perceived positively.

cle or a divine intervention: once again the Christian public experiences the pleasure of watching its community of faith triumph.

The Torments of the Damned in Hell

This triumph, moreover, is confirmed by the infernal torments that the torturers of the martyrs undergo. Thus, in *St Crépin et St Crépinien*, the punishments of the torturers begin with a turnaround: awls, the long needles of the cobbler (the craft of the two martyrs) are driven into the saints' members by the torturers, then extracted by angels and thrown at the torturers. The torturers die; the devils hurry to seize their souls:

> Lez tyrans se demainent par devant lez martirz comme se il deussent enragier puis chient mors a terre.[45]
>
> [The torturers thrash about in front of the martyrs as if they were at the point of going mad then they fall to the ground dead.]

The description of the agony of the torturers stresses the madness that has a hold on them at the moment of death, which shows that they were unable to repent *in extremis* and cements the link between the devils and the torturers, as madness also characterizes the devils. The torturers constitute the designated prey for the infernal cauldron, even more so because they took pleasure in the pain of the Christians. Thus, by a just turnaround, those who took pleasure in inflicting tortures on Christians will, in their turn, suffer the tortures that the devils will take pleasure in announcing and that the spectators will take pleasure in hearing recounted. These scenes very often start with the comic apparition of devils coming to collect the souls and the bodies of the damned: the devils complain about the weight of the bodies, transport them by handling them roughly, and ask what sauce they will be able to spread on them. By the laughter that they prompt, these episodes contribute to balancing the rhythm of dramatic tension in the mystery plays. This laughter has nothing innocent or pure about it: the spectators laugh at the character of the damned, who is demonized by his religious adherence, and thus express their hatred for what he made the martyr undergo. The spectators, whose faith had been persecuted in the person of the saint, experience the feelings of vengeance.

The carnivalesque character of Hell and the devils, the driving force of laughter, asserts itself notably in *Le Mystère des trois Doms* when Getta, murderous

[45] 'Le Mystère de saint Crépin et saint Crépinien', Chantilly-c, v. 1654, ed. by Lalou.

son of the emperor, is himself murdered. The devils deliver this freshly killed 'wild game' to Prosperine's cauldron, who will serve it to Lucifer. Astaroth first announces it, addressing Lucifer: 'Bon sera pour ton gras potaige' (He will be good to put in your rich soup).[46] Beelzebub remembers the cordon-bleu talents of Prosperine: 'Tout venyn elle scet confire' (She knows how to cook any venom).[47] Moreover, Prosperine has many recipes in mind. She plans to make a chive pâté, or cook him in a lamprey sauce; as for his liver, it will end up in a fricassee.[48] This conversation about the best recipe for the somber Getta doubles its effectiveness because it takes place just before dinner for the spectators and the actors themselves, just before the meal that takes place in the real world! The scene actually precedes a scene entitled '*L'Après disgnée*' (After the Dinner; v. 8581). The allusion to a fictional meal in Hell just before a meal taken in the real world creates a tight bond between the fictional world and the real world, a bond that comes from the superimposition of the temporal and reinforces more strongly the impression that the performance is a 'presentation anew', more than fiction, among the spectators.

Devils therefore act as instruments of divine justice. Themselves beaten by their colleagues when they fail at their ventures, also suffering everlasting damnation, they take a kind of vengeance through the tortures inflicted on humans. But the thing that makes clearest the pleasure taken by the spectators (and the actors!) at the description of the torments is the abundance of a type of diabolical discourse in the hagiographic mysteries. In *Le Mystère de Saint Didier*, three devils strive to outdo each other in their descriptions of the sufferings reserved for various types of sinners (witches, magicians, misers), destined respectively to be cooked in a cauldron, to be roasted, and to suffer the torture of sulphur and melted lead.[49] The boiling inflicted on a witch in *Le Mystère du Roy Advenir* is perhaps most edifying. The first intervention by the devils shows them as kitchen boys, and Lucifer as head chef (thus we see the omnipresence of the food theme in the infernal torments). After asking that she be 'pourbollue' (parboiled to tenderize), Lucifer tastes the witch to check if she is done,

[46] Chanoine Pra and Chevalet, *Le Mystère des trois Doms*, v. 8529, ed. by Giraud and Chevalier.

[47] Chanoine Pra and Chevalet, *Le Mystère des trois Doms*, v. 8540, ed. by Giraud and Chevalier.

[48] Chanoine Pra and Chevalet, *Le Mystère des trois Doms*, vv. 8557–68, 8571–72, ed. by Giraud and Chevalier.

[49] Flamang, *La Vie et passion de monseigneur sainct Didier*, ed. by Carnandet, pp. 25–26.

conveying a comic association of the witch with old meat. Several devils stir the victim and note that she has, since the cooking began, emptied herself of a great quantity of shit.[50] The scalding evoked in *Roy Advenir* — in pitch, oil, or water — appears in many visions from the twelfth and thirteenth centuries and recalls the worldly punishment inflicted on counterfeiters.[51] Psychological cruelty is added to physical tortures, the devils apparently finding much pleasure in overwhelming the soul with their irony and their insults. Hans-Jurgen Diller, as Marla Carlson reports, 'observes that medieval religious depictions of the fate of the damned were intended to induce *Schadenfreude*, a response of which we are now ashamed but they were not'.[52] Associating a positive value with the emotion of *Schadenfreude* felt by the spectators seems to me to be closely linked to otherness. Diller even speaks of a 'pious Schadenfreude', thus insisting on the fact that taking pleasure in the suffering of characters associated with evil is considered as an act of religiosity.[53] The many allusions to infernal torments give the impression that they possess a cathartic function, serving to crystalize, and even to enhance, the status of the hatred of the other.

This hatred of the other is evident in the enjoyment experienced at the reciting of their torments, torments that were perceived as deserved, by contrast to the related torments that were inflicted, by the damned themselves or under their orders, on Christians, with whom the spectators feel a closeness, united by their common belief. Thus the Christian community is able to rejoice in the punishments inflicted on the damned because they do not bear the odium; the responsibility for the violence stays between the claws of the devils. The comic aspect of the infernal torments reveals and increases the spectators' pleasure in the face of Christian vengeance — their vengeance — over the impiety of the pagans. The vengeance is seen as real since the torments are as well: there can be no question of doubt at the reality of the torments inflicted by the demons, on the pretext that they are depicted on the stage of a theatre. To liken the performance to an illusion is outside medieval conception, and, on the contrary, the medieval stage must be considered as a place of Truth where Christianity's foundational myths and the reality of the invisible are embodied.[54] Incidentally,

[50] Jehan du Prier, *Le Mystère du roy Advenir*, vv. 825–26, 839–52, ed. by Meiller.

[51] See Baschet, *Les Justices de l'au-delà*, p. 133.

[52] Carlson, *Performing Bodies in Pain*, p. 41, quoting Diller, 'Laughter in Medieval English Drama'.

[53] Diller, 'Laughter in Medieval English Drama', p. 5.

[54] Baschet, *Les Justices de l'au-delà*, p. 128.

if the spectators perceive the described torments as possessing some reality, so does the threat that weighs on them through sin: the ambivalence of laughter in the face of torture there takes on all its meaning, since the spectator, who knows himself to be a sinner, laughs in order to keep from crying as well, to ward off his or her fear.

Certainly, because of the configuration of the Hell stage set — a giant mouth that opens and shuts to allow the devils and the damned to pass through, although we cannot see into the interior — the infernal torments are found to be evoked more by the script than by the performance. But medieval spectators, who witnessed performances of martyrdom and who were used to public punishments, could easily use their imagination to fill the gap between the instruments of torture displayed on the set of Hell and the descriptions provided by the devils. This is especially because some of the tortures evoked were a horrifying metaphor for what still existed in medieval society.

Punishments Inflicted by the Christians on the Possessed and on Heretics

If the punishments inflicted on martyrs could arouse compassion for the persecuted innocent despite the clownish aspect of the torturers, the same did not apply for the possessed. Both the possessed who were in the real world and those who were part of the theatrical story often endured harsh treatment.[55] Violence appears to be a regular treatment for possession, as shown in many scenes in the hagiographic mysteries. I shall cite two examples here.

In the *Mystère de Saint Rémi* (performed in Reims between 1520 and 1528) the possessed person, a young girl named Fleurie, is beaten by an exorcist. The failure of the first exorcist becomes apparent when this violence is turned back on him and the young girl beats him, undoubtedly to the great amusement of the spectators of Reims, thrilled to see that only Saint Rémi, the city's patron saint, succeeds in saving the unfortunate girl.[56]

Le Mystère de l'institution des frères prêcheurs (a hagiographic play of the early sixteenth century relating the birth of the Dominican Order with especial emphasis on the role of Réginald d'Orléans and addressed to the Dominicans themselves and others close to the monastery)[57] explores the therapeutic vio-

[55] See Closson, *L'Imaginaire démoniaque en France*, p. 225 and passim, and Chave-Mahir, *L'Exorcisme des possédés dans l'Église d'Occident*, p. 303 and passim.

[56] See *Le Mystère de Saint Rémi*, ed. by Koopmans, p. 9 and p. 24.

[57] See *Le Mistère de l'Institucion de l'Ordre des Freres Prescheurs*, ed. by Reyff, Bedouelle, and Gérard-Zai, p. 27.

lence reserved for a rebellious (thus possessed) convert. In the play's speeches, this therapeutic violence serves to punish disobedience and lack of discipline:

S. Regnault Le chef de desobeissance
C'est Sathan, qui a grant puissance,
Et jamais dehors n'ystrera,
Nisi in rigoris disciplina :
Parquoy le fault discipliner !

Le convers Vous me orrés si treshault crier
Que les diables venront en aide !

S. Regnault Tout partout il y a remede:
Frappés fort !

Le convers Haro, à la mort !

S. Regnault C'est le commandement de Dieu ![58]

[**S. Regnault** The cause of disobedience
Is Satan, who is very powerful
And he will never escape this brother
Without harsh discipline
That's why he must be given the good blows of discipline!

The Convert You will hear me screaming so loudly
That the devils will come to save me!

S. Regnault Every problem has a solution
Knock hard!

The Convert Help!

S. Regnault It's God's commandment!]

The convert's principle sin is a scandalous conversation in which he asserts that it was better at the tavern than at the monastery. The treatment reserved for the rebellious brother, although it may seem farcical, remains significant: laughter allows the victim to be kept at a distance, ensuring that the laugher is dissociated from the one who is mocked and beaten. The spectators' pleasure here comes as much from the display of violence as from the disassociation from its victim. As long as he is possessed (and the convert is soon delivered by this energetic treatment), the convert belongs to the domain of otherness: he is no longer a Christian; he is apostate. The violence ceases as soon as he escapes the devils. The public can then move from dissociated laughter to compassionate solidarity.

[58] *Le Mistère de l'Institucion de l'Ordre des Freres Prescheurs*, vv. 3659–76, 3681–87, ed. by Reyff, Bedouelle, and Gérard-Zai.

Conclusion

During the early centuries of Christianity, some theologians assumed that the Elect would see their bliss increased by watching the torments inflicted on the damned. These theologians belonged to a persecuted Church, whose only possible revenge was in the afterlife. Thus emerged the idea that the vision of infernal tortures could arouse more pleasure than compassion. The Middle Ages saw the flourishing of many visionary texts, of which I have shown only two examples: the visions of Tnugdal and of Thurkill. The first clearly evokes this pleasure, at least in its Latin version; as for the second, it is the pleasure of the theatre that it evokes, the visionary becoming not only a spectator at the torturing of the damned souls, but also a spectator at the show provided to the sniggering devils, and therefore a spectator of pleasure. Pleasure in the face of infernal torment is therefore no longer a Christian phenomenon, but is also enjoyed by devils. In other words, taking pleasure in the spectacle of torment consists in sharing pleasure with the devils, and therefore becoming diabolical. What dimension does the pleasure of the narrative take on for the Christians at whom it is aimed? What can their reception be in regard to the pleasure taken by the devils in the face of this infernal theatre except their welcoming of infernal theatre itself? What link can be established between this pleasure and that of the real theatre presented to many spectators? Is there not a real pleasure (morbid, maybe, but no less real) in listening to or reading the cruel details of infernal torments?

On the occasion of the Passion plays and the hagiographic plays, Christian audiences take a further step in their relationship to the pleasure in the pain of the other, since it is no longer about hearing pain recounted, but also participating in it. For the organizers of the mystery plays to have accorded so much importance to the spectacle of martyrdom, it was necessary that these scenes be appreciated by the public. Thus the spectators got their pleasure by watching the re-presentation on stage of the tortures inflicted on the martyred saints and on Jesus himself.[59] It was certainly sometimes an ambiguous pleasure, which could take the form of a sort of compassionate trance allowing the spectators to feel closer to God and to the saints. However, the responses of the torturers,

[59] See in Philippe de Vigneulles's *Les Cent Nouvelles Nouvelles* the relating of a sermon given in Metz by a Franciscan in 1515. The spectators were so deeply moved by compassion that they shed tears. However, the sermon described by de Vigneulles seems quite far from the tormentors' gibes (Philippe de Vigneulles, *Les Cent Nouvelles Nouvelles*, ed. by Livingston, pp. 189–90, quoted by Martin, *Le Métier de prédicateur à la fin du Moyen Âge*, p. 584, n. 75).

often crude, give the impression rather that the pleasure experienced came not only from compassion, but also had a carnivalesque dimension in the face of the violence.[60] The pleasure spectators gain from seeing or hearing the tortures of the damned — particularly the torture of martyrs, or the violence inflicted on the possessed (therefore on devils within the bodies of the possessed) — is less mysterious and less ambiguous. This pleasure hints at paradisiacal bliss, compounded once again, no doubt, with carnivalesque pleasure.[61] Carnivalesque laughter and *Schadenfreude* are therefore not opposed; rather, they complete one another and perhaps even nourish one another.

In his condemnation of theatre, Augustine (who, like Tertullian and Cyprian, was born in Carthage but lived one century after the latter, from 354 to 430) denounced this pleasure felt by the contemplation of the pain of the other:

> Why does man like to be made sad when viewing doleful and tragical scenes, which yet he himself would by no means suffer? And yet he wishes, as a spectator, to experience from them a sense of grief, and in this very grief his pleasure consists.[62]

The perversion expressed in the enjoyment of others' pain did not escape him. In all the texts that we have examined here, this pleasure does not simply arise as the pleasure of the Christian avenging persecution. It is very often, I feel, the inversion of compassion, which seems to correspond perfectly with Hell (the main source of this inversion), since Hell itself is inversion. It is about the pleasure taken from otherness, from differentiation, even at the most elementary level. It is joy at the exclusion of the other, joy at his or her persecution, which contributes to solidifying the Christian community that attends it, not only in a community of shared meaning, but also in shared joy. Medieval theatre, more

[60] In Bakhtin's definition, the 'carnivalesque' is associated with the lower part of the human body (sex and excrement), but also with mockery; the carnivalesque, which typifies both the character of the devils and of the tormentors, is essentially linked to the constant polarization towards the lower body and to the connection often made between lower body and lofty spirit. Carnival ritual, like charivari, includes a form of violence.

[61] Diversion of compassionate emotion to derision is certainly a principal source of the ban on representations of 'sacred mysteries' from 1548.

[62] Augustine, *Confessiones*, bk III, ch. II. 2, trans. by Pilkington. In 'La Tentation de la pitié' (p. 6), Lecler mentions 'Trois siècles après Sénèque, Saint Augustin dénonce le plaisir pris à la souffrance d'autrui, la liaison perverse entre la jouissance (*voluptas*) et la souffrance (*dolor*)' (Three centuries after Seneca, St Augustine denounces the pleasure taken in the suffering of others, the perverse link between enjoyment (*voluptas*) and pain (*dolor*)).

a theatre of complicity between stage practitioners and spectators than a theatre of illusions, allows this complicity that is based on exclusion. This complicity itself is a source of pleasure, pleasure in communion in the same universe of meaning, the same universe of emotions.[63] The spectators at medieval religious theatre, however, seem to be ignorant of the fact that in rejoicing at the tortures inflicted on their enemies, they share an important characteristic with the devils: enjoyment of violence. Their laughter, their joy, demonizes them.

[63] See Boquet and Nagy, 'Émotions communes'.

Works Cited

Primary Sources

Augustine, *Confessiones: The Confessions of St. Augustine*, trans. by J. G. Pilkington <https://en.wikisource.org/wiki/The_Confessions_of_Saint_Augustine_(Pilkington)> [accessed April 22 2015]

Chanoine Pra and Claude Chevalet, *Le Mystère des trois Doms*, ed. by Paul-Émile Giraud and Ulysse Chevalier (Lyon: Auguste Brun, 1887)

Flamang, Guillaume, *La Vie et passion de monseigneur sainct Didier*, ed. by Jean Baptiste Carnandet (Paris: Techener, 1855)

Gréban, Arnoul, *Le Mystère de la Passion*, ed. by Omer Jodogne (Bruxelles: Palais des académies, 1965)

Gregory the Great, *The Dialogues of Saint Gregogry the Great*, trans. by Philip Lee Wagner (1911), ed. by Edmund G. Gardner (Merchantville, NJ: Evolution Publishing, 1991), <http://www.tertullian.org/fathers/index.htm#Gregory_Dialogues> [accessed 22 April 2015]

Jean Oudin, *L'Ystoyre et la vie de saint Genis*, ed. by Wilhelm Mostert and Edmund Stengel (Marburg: Elwert, 1895)

Jehan du Prier, *Le Mystère du roy Advenir*, ed. by Albert Meiller (Geneva: Droz; Paris: Minard, 1970)

Le Mistère de l'Institucion de l'Ordre des Freres Prescheurs, ed. by Simone de Reyff, Guy Bedouelle, and Marie-Claire Gérard-Zai (Geneva: Droz, 1997)

'Le Mystère de saint Crépin et saint Crépinien', ed. by Élisabeth Lalou (unpublished doctoral thesis, École des Chartes, 1980)

Le Mystère de Saint Rémi, ed. by Jelle Koopmans (Genava: Droz, 1997)

La Pacience de Job, ed. by Albert Meiller (Paris: Klincksieck, 1971)

Tertullian, *The Shows or De Spectaculis*, trans. by Sydney Thelwall, <http://www.tertullian.org/anf/anf03/anf03–09.htm#P1011_411386> [accessed 22 April 2015]

Visio Thurkilli, ed. by Paul Gerhard Schmidt (Leipzig: Teubner, 1978)

La Vision de Tondale: Les Versions françaises de Jean de Vignay, David Aubert, Regnaud le Queux, ed. by Mattia Cavagna (Paris: Champion, 2008)

The Vision of Tnugdal, ed. by Jean Michel Picard and Yolande de Pontfarcy (Dublin: Dublin University Press, 1989)

Secondary Works

Baschet, Jérôme, *Les Justices de l'au-delà* (Roma: École Française de Rome, 1993)

Baslez, Marie-Françoise, *Les Persécutions dans l'Antiquité: Victimes, héros, martyrs* (Paris: Fayard, 2007)

Boquet, Damien, and Piroska Nagy, 'Émotions communes', chapter 9 of *Sensible Moyen Âge: Une histoire des émotions dans l'Occident médiéval* (Paris: Seuil, 2015)

Carlson, Marla, *Performing Bodies in Pain: Medieval and Post-modern Martyrs, Mystics and Artists* (New York: Palgrave Macmillan, 2010)

Chave-Mahir, Florence, *L'Exorcisme des possédés dans l'Église d'Occident (xe–xive siècle)* (Turnhout: Brepols, 2000)

Chiffoleau, Jacques, 'Dire l'indicible: Remarques sur la catégorie du nefandum du xiie au xve siècle', *Annales: Économies, Sociétés, Civilisations*, 45 (1990), 289–324

Closson, Marianne, *L'Imaginaire démoniaque en France (1550–1650): Genèse de la littérature fantastique* (Geneva: Droz, 2000)

Diller, Hans-Jürgen, 'Laughter in Medieval English Drama: A Critique of Modernizing and Historical Analyses', *Comparative Drama*, 36.1–2 (2002), 1–19

Dupras, Élyse, *Diables et saints: Rôle des diables dans les mystères hagiographiques français* (Geneva: Droz, 2006)

Gardiner, Eileen, *Medieval Visions of Heaven and Hell: A Sourcebook* (New York: Garland, 1992)

Henriet, Patrick, *La Parole et la prière au Moyen Âge* (Bruxelles: De Boeck et Larcier, 2000)

Joly, Robert, *Christianisme et philosophie: Études sur Justin et les Apologistes grecs du iie siècle* (Bruxelles: Éditions de l'Université de Bruxelles, 1973)

Konigson, Élie, *L'Espace théâtral médiéval* (Paris: CNRS, 1975)

Lalou, Élisabeth, 'Les Tortures dans les mystères: Théâtre et réalité xive–xve siècle', *Medieval English Theatre*, 16 (1994), 37–50

Lecler, Éric, 'La Tentation de la pitié (à propos de la catharsis, Aristote et Saint Augustin)', in *Le Mal et le malheur au théâtre*, Théâtre du monde, 21 (Avignon: ARIAS Éditions, Avignon University Press, 2013), pp. 1–8

Martin, Hervé, *Le Métier de prédicateur à la fin du Moyen Âge, 1350–1520* (Paris: Cerf, 1988)

Mazouer, Charles, *Le Théâtre français du Moyen Âge* (Paris: Sedes, 1998)

Ménard, Hélène, 'Du prédateur à la proie', in *Prédateurs dans tous leurs états, évolution, biodiversité, interactions, mythes, symboles: XXXIe rencontres internationales d'archéologie et d'histoire d'Antibes*, ed. by Jean-Philip Brugal and others (Antibes: Éditions APDCA, 2011), pp. 503–15

Nagler, Alois M., *The Medieval Religious Stage: Shapes and Phantoms* (New Haven: Yale University Press, 1976)

Newbigin, Nerida, 'Agata, Apollonoia and Other Martyred Virgins: Did Florentines Really See These Plays Performed?', *European Medieval Drama*, 1 (1997), 77–100

Palmer, Nigel F., *Visio Tnugdali: The German and Dutch Translations and their Circulation in the Later Middle Ages* (München: Artemis Verlag, 1982)

Pontfarcy, Yolande de, *L'Au-delà au Moyen Âge: 'Les Visions du chevalier Tondal' de David Aubert (Los Angeles, Getty Museum, ms. 30) et sa source la 'Visio Tnugdali' de Marcus (Gand, Universiteitsbibliotheek, ms. 316* (Bern: Peter Lang, 2010)

Poulat, Émile, and others, *Dictionnaire de l'Histoire du christianisme* (Paris: Encyclopaedia Universalis et Albin Michel, 2000)

Rosentiehl, Jean Marc, 'Tartarouchos-Temelouchos: Contribution à l'étude de l'Apocalypse apocryphe de Paul', in *Deuxième journée d'études coptes, Strasbourg 25 mai 1984* (Louvain: Peeters, 1986), pp. 29–56

Runnalls, Graham A., 'Les Acteurs dans le *Mystère de la Passion* de Châteaudun en 1510', in *Et c'est la fin pour quoy sommes ensemble: Hommage à Jean Dufournet. Littérature, Histoire et Langue du Moyen Âge*, ed. by Jean Aubailly (Paris: Champion, 1993), III, 1245–53

——, 'Were They Listening or Watching? Text and Spectacle at the 1510 Châteaudun Passion Play', *Medieval English Theatre*, 16 (1994), 25–36

Ubersfeld, Anne, *Lire le théâtre* (Paris: Éditions sociales, 1977)

——, *Lire le théâtre*, new modified edn (Paris: Belin, 1996)

Vauchez, André, *Les Hérétiques au Moyen Âge: Suppôts de Satan ou chrétiens dissidents?* (Paris: CNRS éditions, 2014)

Pleasures in God

Holy Gluttons: Bede and the Carolingians on the Pleasures of Reading

Zachary Giuliano

Eating and drinking are among the most basic pleasures in all human societies. In cultures influenced by the Jewish and Christian scriptures, this pleasure could even have a biblical warrant, for the joy accompanying consumption was considered part of the goodness of God's creation. For God 'brings forth bread and wine from the earth, that they might gladden people's hearts' (Psalm 104. 15). Indeed, other essays in this collection will no doubt address the frequently articulated pleasures of feasting in the Middle Ages. But eating and drinking was sometimes seen as a precarious thing, all too easily abused. Among the many sins enumerated by authors, one often stood out prominently or even headed the list. 'Gluttony' (*gula* or *gastrimargia*) was thought to be at the heart of all that was wrong in the world. And not only was gluttony bad, it also led to more and more evil.

The Carolingians were not immune to this general discourse on gluttony; indeed, they repeated many aspects of it. But they also began to read and write more and more about a kind of eating and drinking that was not subject to the same dangers as usual refreshment, primarily through their reception of the Venerable Bede's exegesis. At the feast he described, one could stuff oneself to the brim and drink oneself into a stupor, yet only become morally better, not worse. Bede articulated, and the Carolingians learned from him, a 'holy gluttony'.[1]

[1] I borrow the phrase from Jerome's famous letter to Eustochia: 'Disce in hac parte superbiam sanctam, scito te illis esse meliorem' (Learn from me a holy arrogance, know you are better than them). Jerome, *Epistulae*, 22.16.17, ed. by Hilberg, I, 163.

The Rev. Dr. **Zachary Guiliano** (zack@livingchurch.org) is curate at St Bene't's Church, Cambridge, and associate editor of *The Living Church* magazine.

Pleasure in the Middle Ages, ed. by Naama Cohen-Hanegbi and Piroska Nagy, IMR 24 (Turnhout: Brepols, 2018), pp. 281–308 BREPOLS PUBLISHERS 10.1484/M.IMR-EB.5.113471

Food and Drink: Pleasure and Problem

Medieval theories concerning the moral relationship between individuals and their consumption of food depended partially on ancient Graeco-Roman medical traditions concerning how one maintained the proper health of the body, usually through the management of the four humours. Ancient manuals, such as Hippocrates' *A Regimen for Health*, provided comments on what sort of foods should be eaten at what seasons of the year, by what sort of individuals, and during specific times of life, in conjunction with particular activities (like physical exercise, reading, sleeping, or having sex), in order to maintain an internal balance of the body and soul.[2] A basic idea runs through nearly all such literature: food brings about an increase to the body, whether in terms of general matter or of specific humours, an increase that could affect bodily capacities, the mind, and behaviour. Other activities brought about decrease. This understanding is common to authors from the ancient world to the early modern.[3]

Christian ascetic authors transformed and augmented ancient Graeco-Roman medical thought in various ways. They strengthened (or perhaps overemphasized) the connection in the literature between the intake of food and an increase in various desires, including sexual desire, thought to be due to a superfluity of bodily fluid or energy, such that the necessary task of controlling desire was routed primarily through the control of food through fasting.[4] In this way, the earlier concern about balancing specific activities and, at times, managing pleasures (depending on season and age) for the maintenance and proper

[2] For a general discussion of ancient and medieval literature on regimen and dietetics, see Gil-Sotres, 'The Regimens of Health', esp. pp. 308–09, 312. Marilyn Nicoud offers a relatively exhaustive analysis of the literature in *Les Régimes de santé au Moyen Âge*. For a useful and succinct review, see Nicoud, 'Food Consumption, a Health Risk?'. The early medieval period is not well covered in any of these publications, however. Among later authors (like Galen), the emphasis perhaps shifted towards a more intense watch kept over the body and mind/soul. See Foucault, *The Care of the Self*, pp. 99–104, 124–32; Brown, *The Body and Society*, pp. 9–10, 17–20. Teresa Shaw emphasizes the connection that Graeco-Roman medical and philosophical authors and early Christian writers on *askesis* saw between care of the body and care of the soul. See Shaw, *The Burden of the Flesh*, esp. pp. 29–52.

[3] Although the way in which they deploy it can be quite different. On this and other matters, Foucault's chapter 'Forms of Problematization' is useful. See Foucault, *The Use of Pleasure*, pp. 13–24.

[4] They had a specific concern with ending the body's production of semen. See Brown, *Body and Society*, pp. 218–20; Shaw, *The Burden of the Flesh*, pp. 53–64, 92, 99, 124–28 (the latter pages treat modern experiments regarding partial starvation, health, and sexual desire).

health of the body was replaced. Much early Christian literature focuses on a more austere and ideally monotonous regimen of physical deprivations that encompassed all of life. With a few notable exceptions,[5] the activities treated by Christian authors were usually limited to labour, eating, prayer, and sleep in order to manage the energies and matter of the body and return them to their proper state.[6] Another change involved joining theories regarding bodily equilibrium and the humours to an emerging tradition regarding the seven or eight principal vices, sins, or demons, which saw its culmination in classical form in the work of Evagrius of Pontus in the East (AD 345–399) and John Cassian in the West (AD 360–435).[7] Bodily integrity became a battle against hostile forces, both internal and external. I shall briefly examine Cassian's writing on diet and gluttony in the *Institutes* and *Conferences*, as these books were practically 'required reading' in the medieval West, especially among Benedictine monks, and they helped shape Western moral literature in many periods, including the Carolingian.

Cassian outlines three forms of gluttony: a desire to eat 'deliciae' (delicacies) (i.e. expensive, high-quality, or complex foods), a desire to feel full, and a desire to eat outside of set meal times. He retains some of the classical tradition's concern about giving advice that is too specific on issues of diet, saying that diet depends on the character of the person.[8] Regarding dietary moderation (specifically, fasting), he says:

[5] Notably, Clement of Alexandria in his *Paedagogus*. See Shaw, *The Burden of the Flesh*, pp. 48–52 and the literature quoted there.

[6] Brown, *Body and Society*, p. 223 on the *autarchic* state and the postponement of pleasures to the *eschaton*.

[7] For Evagrius and Cassian's works, I refer primarily here to the English translations by John Eudes Bamberger and Boniface Ramsey, noted in the bibliography. At moments of deviation from Ramsey's translation, I have used Dom E. Pichery's and Jean-Claude Guy's Sources chrétiennes editions. Evagrius was the teacher of Cassian, and the language of sins, thoughts, demons, and 'spirits' is often interchangeable in their works, although Evagrius has a rather more precisely delineated theory of their interaction in his *Praktikos* and *Chapters on Prayer* than Cassian has in his *Institutes* and *Conferences*. E.g. Evagrius, *Praktikos*, 35 (trans. by Bamberger, p. 25), 36 (pp. 25–26), and 54 (p. 31), as well as the *Chapters on Prayer*, 68 (trans. by Bamberger, p. 66) and 72 (p. 67). For Evagrius, one way that demons affect the soul is by causing 'violence to the bodily equilibrium' or a specific 'agitation' of 'the cerebral circulation'. See also Shaw, *The Burden of the Flesh*, pp. 129–60, and the literature cited by Ramsey in Cassian, *The Conferences*, pp. 177–78.

[8] As does Evagrius, *Praktikos*, 15, trans. by Bamberger, p. 20: 'All these practices are to be engaged in according to due measure and at the appropriate times'.

> Itaque super ieiuniorum modo haud facile potest uniformis regula custodiri, quia nec robur unum cunctis corporibus inest nec sicut ceterae uirtutes animi solius rigore patrantur. [...] diuersum quidem esse refectionis tempus et modum et qualitatem pro inpari scilicet corporum statu uel aetate uel sexu.
>
> [A uniform rule concerning the manner of fasting cannot easily be kept because not all bodies have the same strength, nor is it, like the other virtues, achieved by firmness of mind alone. [...] There are different times, manners, and qualities with respect to eating that are in accordance with the varied conditions, ages, and sexes of bodies.][9]

By the time Cassian came to write the *Conferences*, however, he readily gave a more specific piece of advice that he and his companion Germanus had supposedly heard from one of the Desert Fathers. Cassian and Germanus expressed a desire never to eat 'carelessly to satiety (*saturitas*)', and they were advised to eat no more than two small loaves of bread a day, weighing perhaps one pound, and never to add to this meal any cooked food.[10] 'This is the general norm for abstinence [...] that each person concede himself as much as [... is required] for sustaining the body and not for satisfying the desire to fill himself up'.[11] This norm is relaxed when showing hospitality to guests or on Saturdays and Sundays, in order not to weary the body unduly.[12] But Cassian exhibits considerable concern over the idea of *saturitas*: satiety or fullness.

> Caro luxuriis ac libidine delectatur, spiritus ne ipsis quidem naturalibus desideriis adquiescit. illa cupit satiari somno, repleri cibo, hic ita uigiliis et ieiuniis saginatur, ut ne ad ipsum quidem necessarium uitae usum somnum cibum que uelit admittere.
>
> [The flesh delights in luxuries and pleasure, but the spirit does not give in even to natural desires. The former wants to be sated with sleep and to be filled with food, but the latter is so replete with vigils and fasts that it does not want to take even the sleep and food that are necessary to life.][13]

Cassian thus has little positive appreciation of the pleasures of eating and drinking.

[9] Cassian, *The Institutes*, 5.5.1, trans. by Ramsey, p. 119; ed. by Guy, pp. 196, 198.

[10] Cassian, *The Conferences*, 2, trans. by Ramsey, pp. 100–101.

[11] Cassian, *The Conferences*, 2, trans. by Ramsey, p. 101. Similarly, Evagrius, *Praktikos*, 16, trans. by Bamberger, p. 21: 'Satiety desires a variety of dishes but hunger thinks itself happy to get its fill of nothing more than bread'.

[12] Shaw, *The Burden of the Flesh*, p. 118.

[13] Cassian, *The Conferences*, 4.11.2–3, trans. by Ramsey, p. 161; ed. by Pichery, p. 175. This is not to say that Cassian fails to recognize the dangers of overzealousness with respect to the needs of the body. Cf. Cassian, *The Conferences*, 2, trans. by Ramsey, p. 100.

He notes, perhaps ironically, many foods eaten and enjoyed by the Egyptian monks, but he judges these foods to be too harsh for most others to endure.[14] He also describes in *Institutes* 4.22 the great pleasure taken by Egyptian cenobites in the occasional consumption of maenomenia: salted fish or sardines. It is their 'summa voluptas' ('highest pleasure').[15] But, generally, the fullness that comes from eating is replaced with a fullness of deprivation, and bodily pleasures are replaced with spiritual ones. The body is only to be given enough food to sustain life and is not to experience pleasure, save perhaps (occasionally) in a sardine for one's weakness. For 'with any change in eating, the quality of our purity is necessarily changed as well'.[16] One should be concerned with what is necessary, not with how much 'the yearning appetite demands'.[17]

Cassian makes it clear that there is only one way that someone may be rid of natural desires: through the attainment of new ones. One extinguishes a desire for food by 'desiderio perfectionis' ('a desire for perfection').

> Nequaquam enim poterimus escarum praesentium spernere uoluptates, nisi mens contemplationi diuinae defixa amore uirtutum potius et pulchritudine caelestium delectetur.
>
> [We cannot possibly scorn the pleasures brought on by the present food unless the mind is fixed on the contemplation of divine things, and is more powerfully delighted by the love of virtue and the beauty of celestial things.][18]

Cassian speaks rather less often of these spiritual desires, but this suggestion regarding the replacement of desires is important, and I shall return to it when I discuss Bede's contribution.

Finally, Cassian joins these ideas regarding bodily pleasure to a schema that places gluttony at the head of seven other sins. It is not seen as the root of these other sins, but it prevents the mind from successfully dealing with them:[19]

14 Shaw notes that much of this ascetic diet consists of 'drying' or 'cooling' foods in the classical tradition. *The Burden of the Flesh*, pp. 120–22.

15 Cf. Jerome's recommendation to Paulinus of Nola: *Epistulae*, 58.8, ed. by Hilberg, I, 535: 'Sit uilis et uespertinus cibus holera et legumina interdum que pisciculos pro summis ducas deliciis' (Let your food be cheap and eaten in the evening: vegetables and legumes and, occasionally, you might bring out some little fish as your greatest delicacies) (my translation).

16 Cassian, *The Institutes*, 6.23, trans. by Ramsey, p. 162.

17 Cassian, *The Conferences*, 5.7, trans. by Ramsey, p. 121.

18 Cassian, *The Institutes*, 5.14.4, trans. by Ramsey, p. 125; ed. by Guy, p. 214.

19 Cf. Cassian, *The Institutes*, 5.11.1, trans. by Ramsey, pp. 122–23, as well.

Quibuslibet escis refectus uenter seminaria luxuriae parit nec praeualet mens discretionum gubernacula moderari ciborum pondere praefocata. Non sola crapula uini mentem inebriare consueuit: cunctarum escarum nimietas uacillantem eam ac nutabundam reddit omni que integritatis ac puritatis contemplatione despoliat. Sodomitis causa subuersionis atque luxuriae non uini crapula, sed saturitas extitit panis [...]. Quodsi illos sola nimietas panis ad tam praeruptum flagitiorum praecipitium uitio satietatis inpegit, quid censendum de his qui uegeto corpore perceptionem carnium ac uini inmoderata libertate praesumunt.

[The mind that is suffocated and weighed down by food cannot be guided by the governance of discretion. It is not an excess of wine alone that ordinarily inebriates the mind. Too much food of any kind makes it stagger and sway and robs it of every possibility of integrity and purity. The reason for the overthrow of the Sodomites and for their lasciviousness was not an excess of wine but a surfeit of bread [...]. But if a mere excess of bread and the vice of surfeit (*saturitas*) drove them so abruptly to such dizzying wickedness, what is to be thought of those who with healthy bodies dare to take meat and wine with unbridled freedom?][20]

This quotation suffices to demonstrate the thoroughgoing issues Cassian thought gluttony could bring on. He was not the only author to write on the nature of food and fasting during the period, but his formulations would prove resilient. Even a more moderate or forgiving author like St Benedict helped solidify the influence of Cassian by making his work part of the regular, public reading of Benedictine communities at the daily *Collation*.[21] But we shall turn now to the specific period with which we are concerned.

For the Carolingians, intemperance with regard to food and drink remained a topic of concern. Rachel Stone has dealt with the moral literature of the period in the most depth in her *Morality and Masculinity in the Carolingian Period*. She has argued that, while a condemnation of gluttony exists in much of the moral literature, it is a more moderate and specific concern about the luxurious eating of 'delicacies', rather than overeating in itself. She also thinks it is assumed in this period that the wealthy will (and are entitled to) eat considerably more and better food than others by virtue of their station, although drunkenness remains an issue of keen concern, especially with regard to its effect on public life.[22] But I should say that I am not convinced the overconsumption of food and drink ceased to be an issue of concern quite in the manner she suggests, save among some authors writing to some lay aristocrats, the main focus

[20] Cassian, *The Institutes*, 5.6, trans. by Ramsey, p. 120; ed. by Guy, pp. 198, 200.

[21] *Rule of Benedict*, 42 and 73.

[22] Stone, *Morality and Masculinity in the Carolingian Period*, pp. 238–39.

of Stone's work. It would be more significant if such an emphasis disappeared from literature aimed at monks. A lengthy examination of this issue would involve a considerable and perhaps unnecessary digression, so I shall only make a few broad points.

First, Cassian (and other similar authors) continued to be read widely, and we have to take into consideration their continuing influence. Second, gluttony was still seen as one of the primordial, 'gateway' sins in much of the moral literature,[23] and the 'gluttony-surfeit-sin' paradigm remained in place.[24] For example, Hincmar of Reims could write to Charles the Bald:

> Qui aliquando multa etiam quae magnae sunt fortitudinis faciunt, sed, dominante gulae vitio, per carnis illecebram omne quod fortiter egerint perdunt: et dum venter non restringitur, per carnis concupiscentiam simul cunctae virtutes obruuntur.
>
> [Whoever, at one time, did many things that were also great deeds of fortitude, but is dominated by the vice of gluttony, loses through the allurement of the flesh everything that he might have done with strength. And when the belly is not restrained, it buries every virtue through the desire of the flesh.][25]

There remained an explicit discourse against gluttony, with a specific vocabulary, indebted to the model of Cassian, himself indebted to other classical and ascetic traditions. As Stone has argued, drunkenness may have remained an especially reviled state in the Carolingian period, and some authors may have softened their particular criticism of excessive consumption of food, taking up instead a more moderate criticism of luxuriant eating. However, many authors did not do so, and the discourse against gluttony did not shift wholly in the period. As I turn now to consider the exegetical literature more, this preceding discourse should be kept in mind, for a great many of its themes will come up again. We will discover, however, that a new discourse was opened up in the exegetical literature on the nature of spiritual desire and satisfaction, one that may have picked up on Cassian's brief mention of the need to replace carnal desires with spiritual ones, yet took it in a surprising direction.

[23] E.g. Alcuin, *Epistola*, 81.14, ed. by Dümmler, p. 124; Alcuin, *De virtutibus et vitiis*, 28, ed. by Szarmach, pp. 29–30; Hincmar, *De divortio Lotharii Regis et Theutbergae Reginae*, Resp. 15.15, ed. by Böhringer, p. 208.

[24] E.g. Alcuin, *De virtutibus et vitiis*, 28, trans. by Szarmach; Hincmar, *De cavendiis vitiis*, 2, ed. by Migne; Sedulius Scottus, *Collectaneum miscellaneum*, 13.5.51, 13.5.98, and 74.25, ed. by Simpson.

[25] Hincmar, *De cavendiis vitiis*, c. 2, ed. by Migne, col. 875C. Notably, Hincmar's text is a quotation from Gregory the Great, *Moralia in Iob*, 30.18.59.35–36, ed. by Adriaen, vol. 143B, p. 1530.

Bede and the Carolingians: Scriptural and Exegetical Texts

A note on our sources is appropriate here. The Carolingian period is notable for its promotion of theological and exegetical texts, whether they were older texts from the patristic period or newly composed works.[26] It is also notable for being a time in which various kings and ecclesiastical figures commissioned special works of exegesis for their own consumption, and many key cultural discussions were conducted through the genre of the commentary and the sermon, including the responsibilities of the king and the elite.[27] We cannot understand the discursive range with regard to gluttony in the Carolingian periods without considering the exegetical literature more thoroughly. This literature remains under-studied, often existing in poor editions or in manuscripts alone.[28] Thus, my comments in the coming pages hope to break some new ground, albeit in a small way. I contend that a new approach or concept to the idea of gluttony and the pleasures of food and drink was articulated in the exegetical literature.

The source for this new concept came from the works of the Venerable Bede, an author whose reception by the Carolingians ensured his reputation in the Middle Ages; his authority was seen as comparable to that of the Church Fathers. More specifically, Bede articulates a concept of *scriptural interpretation* as a form of indulgent eating and inebriation. This concept occurs primarily in the comments he offers on the food miracles of Jesus, namely, the Wedding at Cana, the Feeding of the Five Thousand, and the Feeding of the Four Thousand,[29] though it must be said that he makes similar connections between food, drink, and exegesis in other works as well.[30] It is through the

[26] Contreni, 'Carolingian Biblical Studies'.

[27] See e.g., de Jong, 'Exegesis for an Empress'; de Jong, 'The Empire as *ecclesia*', pp. 191–226; Staubach, *Rex christianus*, pp. 21–104.

[28] For a still incomplete list, last updated in May 2005, see Edwards, 'The Manuscript Transmission of Carolingian Biblical Commentaries'.

[29] For Bede's *Homeliae*, I quote primarily from David Hurst's Latin edition, and the English translation of Martin and Hurst, occasionally modified by my own translations. References to his commentaries on Luke and Mark are to the Hurst edition. The main passages in question are 'Wedding at Cana': Bede, *Homelia* II.2. 'Feeding of 5000', ed. by Hurst, pp. 193–199: Bede, *In Lucae euangelium expositio*, III.1216–1353, ed. by Hurst, pp. 197–201; Bede, *In Marci euangelium expositio*, II.855–1011, ed. by Hurst, pp. 510–14; *Homelia* I.14. 'Feeding of 4000', ed. by Hurst, pp. 95–104: Bede, *In Marci euangelium expositio*, II.1572–1680, ed. by Hurst, pp. 527–31.

[30] E.g. Bede, *On the Tabernacle*, I.7 and I.8, trans. by Holder, pp. 28 and 32. Bede interprets the twelve loaves in the Jewish tabernacle as the apostolic teaching which refreshes the Church until the end of time, and the 'cup' and 'bowl' shapes on the branches of the golden

Carolingian reception of these texts that a new approach to the pleasures of eating and drinking was articulated.

Admittedly, Bede was not the first to make the basic connection between the word of God and food or drink.[31] The connection appears in Christian scripture in the context of Jesus's fasting,[32] and Bede is also indebted to Jerome, Ambrose, Augustine, and Gregory the Great at key moments in his exegesis. But he transforms and augments previous patristic concepts quite heavily, charting an especially different course in his comments on the Wedding at Cana. More importantly, he is a direct source for nearly every Carolingian exegete. When they comment on these passages, they are frequently responding to Bede, even when they add in a detail or quote from another author. And it is his innovations regarding spiritual pleasure that most of them follow, in ways that vary from word-for-word repetition to abbreviation to excerption to subtle adaptation and amplification.[33] But we should turn now to the specifics of Bede's exegesis.

lampstand as 'the minds of hearers [...] filled with the wine of knowledge' by preachers and 'inebriated' with the 'wine of love' for God and neighbour.

[31] See, e.g., in exegetical sources only, Clement, *Stromata*, v, ed. and trans. by Roberts and Donaldson, p. 302; Origen, *Commentarium in euangelium Matthaei*, 11.2, ed. by Girod, pp. 268–75; Ambrose, *Expositio Evangelii secundum Lucam*, 6.84, ed. by Schenkl, pp. 269–71; Jerome, *Commentariorum in Matheum libri IV*, 2.1239–1279, ed. by Hurst and Adriaen, pp. 121–22; Augustine, *In Iohannis Evangelium tractatus CXXIV*, 9 and 24, ed. by Willems, pp. 90–100 and 244–48.

[32] In Matthew 4. 4 and Luke 4. 4, Jesus quotes Deuteronomy 8. 3 while fasting in the desert and tempted by the devil to turn stones into bread: 'Man does not live by bread alone but by every word that comes from the mouth of God'. Bede's own treatment of the passage from Luke only partly highlights the link, though, in quoting Jerome: 'The one who does not feed on the word of God does not live'. Bede, *In Lucae euangelium expositio*, I.4.3010–12, ed. by Hurst, p. 95.

[33] A more thorough investigation would be in order. But the general variation is as follows:

Word-for-word repetition: Alcuin, *Expositio in Ioannem* on John 2. 1–14 and 6. 1–12, ed. by Migne, cols 766B–772B, 819B–824A; Pseudo-Bede, *In S. Joannis evangelium expositio* on John 2. 1–14 and 6. 1–12, ed. by Migne, cols 657A–662B, 704C–708B; Paul the Deacon, *Homiliarium*, I:60, I:92, and II:60, for which there is no critical edition. See Grégoire, *Homéliaires liturgiques médiévaux*, pp. 423–86, which must be used with caution. My own forthcoming study will offer a more accurate reconstruction of this homiliary.

Abbreviation: Christian of Stavelot, *Commentarius in Euangelium Matthaei*, ed. by Migne, cols 1381D–1383D; Christian of Stavelot, *Expositio brevis in Lucam*, ed. by Migne, cols 1503C–1514D; Christian of Stavelot, *Expositiuncula in Ioannem Evangelistam*, ed. by Migne, col. 1516A; Pseudo-Bede, *In Matthaei evangelium expositio*, ed. by Migne, cols 71C–72D, 76–77D; Otfrid, *Glossae in Matthaeum*, 14.13–21 (ed. by Grifoni, pp. 199–202)

For the sake of brevity, I will refer primarily to his comments in *Homilia* II.2 on John 6. 1–14 (the Feeding of the Five Thousand) and *Homilia* I.14 on John 2. 1–12 (the Wedding at Cana), though I will make some reference to his other works as well. My comments on Carolingian material will be limited, again for the sake of brevity, as I have discovered that they follow him to such a great degree that a discussion of his own work will largely suffice.

Reading as Gluttony 1: Filled with the Word

From the beginning of *Homilia* II.2, Bede is concerned to address the connection between the moral life and the hearing or reading of scripture. It is by hearing the word of God that one may be cured from vice; it is by hungering for heaven that one may be healed.[34] But in this homily, Bede first notes the connection between pleasures (earthly and temporal) and the reading of the Word of God in his comments on the circumstances surrounding Christ's feeding of the crowds.[35] He mentions that John 6. 4 places the timing of the Feeding of the Five Thousand as being that of the Passover season, interpreting this timing as a sign that those who would receive salvation must 'pass over' or 'carnis uidelicet concupiscentias mentis sublimitate transcendant' ('transcend the lustful desires

and 15.32–39 (pp. 214–16). Excerption: Smaragdus of Saint Mihiel, *Collectiones in epistolas et evangelia*, ed. by Migne, cols 151B–155B; Rabanus Maurus, *Commentariorum in Matthaeum*, V, ed. by Löfstedt, pp. 416–24, 447, 455; Paschasius Radbertus, *Expositio in Mattheo*, 7.1564 (ed. by Paulus, II, 739–48) and 7.2898–3184 (II, 780–89); Sedulius Scottus, *Kommentar zum Evangelium nach Matthäus*, 14:13–14:21 (ed. by Löfstedt, pp. 369–75) and 15:31–38 (pp. 391–96); and Claudius of Turin's *Commentary on Matthew*, which has yet to be edited anywhere. I have thus consulted CCCC, MS 88 (England, s. x), fols 101v–103v, 109r–112r, to identify its use of texts.

Adaptation/augmentation: Haimo of Auxerre, *Homelia* 28 on John 2. 1–12, ed. by Migne, cols 126C–137B; *Homelia* 49 on John 6. 1–14, ed. by Migne, cols 284B–294B; and *Homelia* 99 on Mark 8. 1–10, ed. by Migne, cols 634D–640D; Heiric of Auxerre, *Homeliae*, I.20 on John 2. 1–11 (ed. by Quadri, I, 160–68); I.49 on John 6. 1–14 (II, 442–56); II.26 on Mark 8. 1–19 (III, 236–46). Unsurprisingly, Eriugena also follows in this pattern, though offering up more of his own, idiosyncratic comments that reveal the influence of pseudo-Dionysius. See Eriugena, *Homelia et Commentarius in Euangelium Iohannis*, on John 6. 1–12, ed. by Jeauneau, pp. 121–37.

[34] Bede, *Homilies*, II.2, trans. by Martin and Hurst, II, 14.

[35] On the interpretation of *circumstantiae* in classical rhetorical handbooks and medieval exegesis, see the recent contribution of Sloan, *The Harmonious Organ of Sedulius Scottus*, pp. 13–33. An excellent example (and slightly alternative schema to that presented by Sloan) is Gregory the Great, *Moralia in Iob*, 2.2, ed. by Adriaen, p. 59, where he lists circumstances like 'position of the place [...] position of body [...] quality of environment [... and] quality of time'.

of the flesh by the loftiness of the mind').[36] These desires include both favourable and unfavourable actions, that is, those that are good for the body and soul and bad for them.[37] This opening gambit places Bede's stance on physical pleasures close to that represented in Cassian's works, discussed above.[38] But he leaves more room for those who may not yet be capable of such transcendence of physical pleasure, but can only desire it. What is necessary is that earthly pleasures be 'scorn[ed]', not that the faithful be wholly successful in trampling them.[39] There is some tension in Bede's account, as he will also state that the reason the crowd is later asked to sit on the grass (John 6. 10) is because grass signifies the flesh and evil desires, which 'everyone who wishes to be satisfied with spiritual nourishment ought to tread under foot and repress'.[40] Indeed, he repeats this idea in other writings,[41] and his language can be quite strong:

> Discumbat ergo super faenum ut florem faeni conterat, id est castiget corpus suum et seruituti subiciat uoluptates carnis edomet luxuriae fluxa restringat quisque panis uiui cupit suauitate refici quisquis supernae gratiae dapibus renouari amat ne infima uetustate deficiat caueat.
>
> [Let he who longs to be refreshed by the sweetness of the living bread, who loves to be renewed by the banquet of heavenly grace, sit upon the grass, that he may crush the flower of the field, that is, let him chastise his body and subject it to slavery, repress the pleasures of the flesh, restrain the changeableness of self-indulgence. Let him beware lest he faints away by a degradation to his former self.][42]

[36] Bede, *Homelia*, II.2.84–85, ed. by Hurst, p. 195.

[37] Bede, *Homilies*, II.2, trans. by Martin and Hurst, II, 16.

[38] Indeed, he also sees gluttony as being among the primordial sins, by which Christ was also tempted. See, e.g. Bede, *In Lucae euangelium expositio*, I.4.3068–70 (ed. by Hurst, p. 97); I.4.3121–32 (p. 98). But he does not make the seven/eight deadly sins or demons central to his moral teaching, though he is aware of the scheme. See Carroll, *The Venerable Bede*, pp. 146–57.

[39] Bede, *Homilies*, II.2, trans. by Martin and Hurst, II, 16.

[40] Bede, *Homilies*, II.2, trans. by Martin and Hurst, II, 17–18. A very common patristic gloss used by Bede is from Isaiah 40. 6 and I Peter 1. 24: 'All flesh is grass, and all its glory as the flower of the field', which most authors tend to apply in scriptural interpretation as 'all grass mentioned in Scriptural stories signifies flesh'. Cf. Jerome, *Commentary on Matthew*, 14.19, trans. by Scheck, p. 172, or the rather different use in *Gregory the Great: Forty Gospel Homilies*, 15, trans. by Hurst, p. 107.

[41] Bede, *In Ezram et Neemiam*, I.956–65, ed. by Hurst, p. 265; Bede, *In Marci euangelium expositio*, 2.8.1961–98, ed. by Hurst, pp. 538–39, quoting Gregory the Great; Bede, *Expositio in Actuum Apostolorum*, 27.63, ed. by Laistner, p. 95.

[42] Bede, *Homiliae*, II.2.145, ed. by Hurst, p. 197 (my translation).

But the fact that success in ascetic denial is not the key to Bede's teaching is important. One need not be wholly given to deprivations.

> In quibus singulis quicumque uiriliter agere et confortari satagunt sobrie et iuste et pie uiuendo ut caelestis sapientiae mereantur dulcedine recreari hi nimirum quinque milibus uirorum quos dominus mysticis dapibus satiauit figurantur.

It is those who 'satagunt' ('attempt' or 'struggle') to live this way for the sake of 'the sweetness of heavenly wisdom' who 'are satisfied by this mystical banquet'.[43] The language Bede uses is also quite significant. What the crowd longs for is a 'banquet', 'living bread', 'refreshment', 'sweetness', and other similar words taken from the context of pleasurable eating. But what is this mystical banquet?

It is the reading of the scriptures or, more specifically, the allegorical interpretation of them that brings heavenly sweetness to those who desire to feast on the living bread and, especially, be morally transformed by it.

> Quinque autem panes quibus multitudinem populi saturauit quinque sunt libri moysi quibus spiritali intellectu patefactis et abundantiore iam sensu multiplicatis auditorum fidelium cotidie corda reficit. [...]
>
> Duo autem pisces [...] psalmistarum non inconuenienter et prophetarum scripta significant [...] futura christi et ecclesiae sacramenta narrabant.

> [The five loaves of bread with which he satisfied (*saturauit*) the multitude of the people are the five books of Moses, by which the hearts of faithful hearers are refreshed daily, when the books are opened up by spiritual understanding and more abundantly multiplied in meaning. [...]
>
> The two fish [...] signify the writings of the psalmists and prophets [...] by which the future sacraments of Christ and the Church were narrated.][44]

Throughout this section of his homily, Bede remains within the discourse of eating. The bread that Christ breaks and the fish that are shared are the scriptures that are opened and distributed in teaching or reading. Through these, Christ 'saturauit' ('fills' or 'satisfies') the crowd; Bede focuses here on a word I noted earlier in Cassian.

There are further significant details. In Bede's *Commentary on Mark*, the fish of the Psalms and Prophets are like a topping added to the bread, a sort of *tartine*, giving 'the new savour of grace' to the rough loaves of the Law.[45] What

[43] Bede, *Homeliae*, II.2. 84–85, ed. by Hurst, II, p. 195.

[44] Bede, *Homiliae*, II.2.112–14, 118–22, ed. by Hurst, p. 196 (my translation).

[45] Bede, *In Marci euangelium expositio*, II.935–52, ed. by Hurst, p. 513. This point is not unlike that of Origen, though inflected quite differently. Origen, *Commentary on Matthew*,

is even more important is that, with regards to the food of the word of God, there is no prohibition here on eating to one's fill, to tasting the savour of one's meal, to being refreshed daily and abundantly. This pleasure is one without limit, unlike other kinds of eating. Indeed, one must eat and be filled to receive the benefit:

> Manducant namque et non saturantur qui panem uerbi dei audiendo degustant sed non faciendo quae audiunt nihil ex his internae dulcedinis quo cor ipsorum confirmetur in uentre memoriae recipiunt.
>
> [For they eat and are *not* filled who only tasted the bread of God's Word by hearing it. And, by not doing what they hear, they receive into the belly of the memory nothing of those things of internal sweetness by which their heart is strengthened.][46]

Indeed, the more advanced are encouraged to eat more, not less, for the apostles 'gathered the fragments and filled twelve baskets full', in order that nothing would be lost (John 6. 12–13).[47] 'Omnis doctorum spiritalium chorus [...] quae per se turbae nequeunt et meditando colligere' ('The whole chorus of spiritual teachers, by meditating, collects what the crowds could not gather'),[48] and such teachers, 'caelestis tamen gratiae sunt pane fecundi' ('fruitful by the bread of heavenly grace'), perpetuate the feast and preserve it by continuing to explain the scriptures in writing and preaching.[49] The key to Bede's exegesis here is the idea of fullness, abundance, and sweetness, and this banquet creates a surfeit in the mind that brings spiritual nourishment for all, rather than a full-

c.11, trans. by Patrick, ed. by Menzies, pp. 431–32. 'Perhaps by the five loaves they meant to make a veiled reference to the sensible words of the Scriptures, corresponding in number on this account to the five senses, but by the two fishes either to the word expressed and the word conceived, which are a relish, so to speak, to the sensible things contained in the Scriptures; or, perhaps, to the word which had come to them about the Father and the Son [...]. Such is the contribution we have been able to give to the exposition of the word about the five loaves and the two fishes; and probably those, who are better able than we to gather together the five loaves and the two fishes among themselves, would be able to give a fuller and better interpretation of their meaning'.

[46] Bede, *In Marci euangelium expositio*, I.1649–1652, ed. by Hurst, p. 530. Or, as Pseudo-Bede, *In Matthaei evangelium expositio* puts it more pithily: 'Saturantur qui internae dulcedinis pastum invenire memoriae commendant' (Those who find the food of internal sweetness and commit it to memory are the ones who are filled) (ed. by Migne, col. 77B).

[47] Bede, *Homilies*, II.2, trans. by Martin and Hurst, II, 20.

[48] Bede, *Homiliae*, II.2.189–91, ed. by Hurst, p. 198 (my translation).

[49] Bede, *Homiliae*, II.2.198–99, ed. by Hurst, p. 198 (my translation).

ness of the body leading to immorality. The incredible fullness of the teachers leads to fecundity, overflowing abundance, so that the 'food of the word may not perish'.[50] By the continual reading of those able to understand and teach more fully, the pleasures of the feast remain eternal.

Reading as Gluttony 2: Drunk on the Word

Bede does not immediately discuss spiritual drunkenness in his homily on the Wedding at Cana. He is concerned at first with commenting on the significance of Christ's appearance at a wedding, before moving to a discussion of scriptural interpretation as drinking wine. He engaged with the Gospel text in this way because his homily was modelled on Augustine's comments in *Tractatus* 9, whose outline and conclusions he followed quite closely.[51] However, he develops his train of thought on scriptural interpretation in a way quite different from Augustine, especially by emphasizing the idea of scriptural interpretation as drunkenness and by focusing on the personal meaning of the text, points not present in Augustine's comments.[52] In other words, Bede is far more focused on discerning and describing the pleasure of the reader described in this passage.

As in the previous homily, Bede notes here the circumstances of the event and signals the importance of seeking virtue. 'Hoc quod in cana galilaeae, id est in zelo transmigrationis' ('This marriage was performed in Cana of Galilee: in the "zeal of emigration"').[53] The location designates a particular group: 'qui zelo feruere piae deuotionis et […] de uitiis ad uirtutes bona operando de terrenis ad aeterna norunt sperando et amando transmigrare' ('those who, aflame with the zeal of pious devotion wish to emigrate from vices to virtues by doing good works, and from earthly to eternal things, by hoping and loving').[54] And, once again, Christ's miracle is seen as an allegory for scriptural interpretation.

Bede's explanation of how this meaning is conveyed textually — that is, how the transformation of water into wine can be seen as signifying allegorical

[50] Bede, *Homiliae*, II.2.184–85, ed. by Hurst, pp. 96–97 (my translation).

[51] Including various heresiological thrusts. See the English translation of Augustine, *Tractatus in Iohannem*, 6. 1–12, trans. by Gibb and Innes, ed. by Schaff.

[52] As well as in his interpretations of the six stone water containers (*hydriae*).

[53] Bede, *Homiliae*, I.14.53–54, ed. by Hurst, p. 96; trans. by Martin and Hurst, I, 136. The etymology undoubtedly comes from Jerome's *Interpretation of Hebrew Names*, as Martin and Hurst note.

[54] Bede, *Homiliae*, I.14.56-9, ed. by Hurst p. 96–97.

exegesis — is quite complex. To sum up his argument briefly, the six stone containers which hold water in the Gospel passage are interpreted as 'the devout hearts of the saints' who lived in the six ages of the world, hearts which hold 'the knowledge of sacred scripture, which both cleanses [...] and gives drink' by proffering examples to readers.[55] In other words, the containers already hold a material that effects virtue and provides refreshment. This, for Bede, is 'the undiluted sweetness of the legal meaning' that was known before the incarnation of Christ. We already have hints of the pleasures to come, in the untransformed water of scriptural meaning. But it is not the final product.

> Sed quantum inter aquam et uinum tantum distare inter sensum illum quo scripturae ante aduentum saluatoris intellegebantur et eum quem ueniens ipse reuelauit apostolis eorum que discipulis perpetuo sequendum reliquit.
>
> [As different as water is from wine is the sense in which the Scriptures were understood before the Savior's coming from that sense which he himself revealed to the apostles [...] and which he left to be perpetually followed.][56]

We could stop here in noting how Bede understands scriptural interpretation as a pleasurable activity. It is all explicit already: a meaning that was cleansing, sweet, and refreshing is made even more so by Christ's incarnation and teaching. The difference between water and wine is quite understandable. But Bede goes further; he does not stop with a theory of exegesis.

He not only mentions the pleasure of scriptural interpretation, but he initiates his readers into it by providing examples of the allegorical exegesis of scriptural episodes that occurred in each of the six ages. In doing so, he performs the pleasure he is describing, and he creates 'a text of pleasure', inducing and exciting pleasure in the reader and giving a taste of the bliss he promises.[57] 'Let us see', he says, 'this water turned into the most delightful aroma and taste of wine'.[58] As Bede provides short exegetical passages on each of the six ages, his rhetoric becomes more and more elevated, such that he describes the reader finding water turned into wine in the first age, marveling at it in the second, becoming intoxicated by its fragrance in the third, looking at it in the fourth,

[55] Bede, *Homilies*, I.14, trans. by Martin and Hurst, I, 138. Bede also differs from Augustine here, regarding how the six ages of the world are related to the water containers.

[56] Bede, *Homeliae*, I.14.24–27, ed. by Hurst, pp. 98–99; trans. by Martin and Hurst, I, 139.

[57] The phrase and concept of a 'text of pleasure' is that of Roland Barthes, first brought to my attention in Burrus, Jordan, and MacKendrick, *Seducing Augustine*, p. 3.

[58] Bede, *Homilies*, I.14, trans. by Martin and Hurst, I, 139.

growing warm from it in the fifth, and, in the sixth, the age of Christ, being granted undiluted and wondrous wine that makes the reader cry out in exultation.[59] And yet, what is quite interesting is that Bede never actually describes the drinking of the cup. It seems that his pleasure is left conditional, open. He invites, he cajoles, he performs, but he leaves the drinking of the cup to the reader. The action can only be completed when the reader succumbs to Bede's invitation, accepts the pleasure, and becomes an allegorical reader.[60]

The Carolingians largely understood this and followed Bede in his exposition.[61] One, Haimo of Auxerre, even extended it hugely. His 'performance' of pleasure is even longer than Bede's, culminating in a catena of biblical quotations and a final exposition:

> Hujus suavissima dulcedine spiritaliter inebriatus, cum propheta dicere possis: 'Et calix tuus inebrians quam praeclarus est!' Et iterum: 'Fluminis impetus laetificat civitatem Dei'. Et rursus: 'Filii autem hominum in tegmine alarum tuarum sperabunt, et inebriabuntur ab ubertate domus tuae, et torrente voluptatis tuae potabis eos'. Hoc vinum desiderabat ille qui dicebat in Canticis canticorum: 'Osculetur me osculo oris sui, quia meliora sunt ubera tua vino, fragrantia unguentis optimis'.
>
> Quicunque ergo per singulas aetates exempla sanctorum considerans, bene vivere et spiritaliter didicerit intelligere eorum doctrinam, in singulis aetatibus inveniet hydrias, de quarum haustum et ablui et satiari possit.
>
> [Spiritually drunk on the most delicious sweetness of the wine, you are able to say with the prophet: 'How excellent is your inebriating cup!' And again: 'The river's flow makes glad the city of God!' And 'The sons of men will hope in the covering of your wings, and they will be inebriated by the plenty of your house, and you will give them drink from the torrent of your desire!' The one who spoke in the Song of Songs desired this wine: 'Let him kiss me with the kisses of his mouth, because your breasts are better than wine, your fragrance better than perfumes'.
>
> Therefore, whoever considers the examples of the saints through each age will learn to live well and to understand their teaching spiritually. He will discover in each age a container, from whose draughts he may be cleansed and satisfied.][62]

[59] Bede, *Homilies*, I.14, trans. by Martin and Hurst, I, 139–43.

[60] This 'seduction' seems intentional. Cf. Barthes, *The Pleasure of the Text*, p. 6: 'The text you write must prove to me *that it desires me*' (author's emphasis).

[61] It was omitted by Eriugena, who went in a very different direction, and slightly abbreviated by Heiric of Auxerre. See Eriugena, *Homelia et Commentarius in Euangelium Iohannis*, 6. 1–6, ed. by Jeauneau, pp. 121–37; Heiric of Auxerre, *Homelia*, I.20, ed. by Quadri, vol. 116B, 160–68.

[62] Haimo of Auxerre, *Homelia* 18, ed. by Migne, col. 135B–C.

It is here we can perceive most clearly the understanding and purpose of the pleasure of spiritual reading. Indeed, Bede is more explicit and direct about the benefit and purpose of allegorical exegesis in *Homilia* I.14 than in many of his other writings. For he distinguishes between basic sorts of meaning one might glean from scripture, which are refreshing and serve as an impetus for moral reformation (the water), and more advanced meanings which must be painstakingly and yet pleasurably drawn out of scripture (the wine). These latter readings, moreover, are readings that permit readers to see themselves reflected in the text. For instance, in the fourth age, Bede discusses David's rule over the kingdom of Israel in place of King Saul. 'He was a humble, innocent, and gentle exile', who suffered under the persecutions of Saul but was given an enduring kingdom.[63] The 'water' of the passage is a simple injunction towards humility, based on David's example. This is 'a draught of the clearest water, by which [the reader] may be refreshed'. But, if the reader sees the sufferings of Christ and the Church prefigured here and realizes that their joint reign remains forever, something new is seen.

> Poculum utique uini de aqua factum sentiet quia se suam que uitam et regnum sed et ipsum regem ibi scriptum legere nouit ubi prius quasi de aliis ueterem legebat historiam.
>
> [He will perceive a cup of wine made from the water, for he will know that he is reading not only about that king but about his own life and reign, where before he read the story as if it were an ancient history about others.][64]

Bede differs here from Augustine quite strongly, who leans more in his *Tractatus* 9 towards finding a Christological meaning. Bede, instead, is concerned about the reader finding their self in the text, joined to Christ through the Church, and thus becoming intoxicated with the pleasure of reading. One who reads scripture in this way 'unquestionably marvels at wine [...] for in the history of the ancient deeds [the reader] contemplates their own cleansing, sanctification, and justification being prophesied'.[65]

The culmination of this pleasure comes when the spiritual reader learns to discern how the life of Christ foreshadowed his or her own life. The example Bede proffers is Christ's circumcision and presentation in the Temple.[66]

[63] Bede, *Homilies*, I.14, trans. by Martin and Hurst, I, 141.

[64] Bede, *Homiliae*, I.14.193–95, ed. by Hurst, pp. 100–01; trans. by Martin and Hurst, I, 141.

[65] Bede, *Homilies*, I.14, trans. by Martin and Hurst, I, 140.

[66] Bede, *Homilies*, I.14, trans. by Martin and Hurst, I, 142–43.

The 'water' of the passage comes from seeing that Christ subjected himself to the Law and 'consecrated first' the activities and sacraments he would enjoin to his faithful, thus spurring the reader to place themselves willingly under the Gospel mysteries. But the wine comes when the reader discerns their participation in Christ's circumcision and presentation, when they consider their own baptism 'into the mystery of the Lord's resurrection' and their 'entering from the baptistery to the holy altar and needing to be consecrated by an exceptional sacrificial victim, the Lord's body and blood'.[67] In other words, to see baptism and Eucharist as a participation in Christ's life gives the reader 'undiluted wine', the pleasure of the sixth age, in which they participate both textually and sacramentally by regular ritual participation. The pleasure of the sixth age extends beyond the page in a particular way. But Bede offers a further cup of wine from the exegesis of the sixth age, one that extends its pleasures not only beyond the page, but beyond the boundaries of this life.

> Porro si circumcisionis diem ad generalem humani generis resurrectionem [...] et circumcisos induci in templum cum hostiis intellexeris quando post resurrectionem uniuersali expleto iudicio sancti iam incorruptibiles facti ad contemplandam perpetuo speciem diuinae maiestatis cum bonorum operum muneribus intrabunt.
>
> [You can interpret the day of circumcision as the general resurrection [...] and the leading of the circumcised into the temple with sacrificial offerings as the time after the resurrection when, the universal judgment completed, the saints, then made incorruptible, will enter with their offerings of good works to contemplate forever the divine majesty.][68]

Then the reader not only reflects on and participates in the joy of understanding past events, but they anticipate the eschatological pleasures of the future. Transfixed by the two, the reader moves beyond the contemplation of their own life in the interpretation of the text, moves even beyond the task charted out in the previous homily of preserving and teaching the obscure meanings of the text to others.[69] The reader is instead, finally made drunk by their wallowing in the depths of scripture, intoxicated by its excellent wine and crying

[67] Bede, *Homilies*, I.14, trans. by Martin and Hurst, I, 143.

[68] Bede, *Homiliae*, I.14.231–38, ed. by Hurst, p. 102; trans. by Martin and Hurst, I, 143.

[69] Thus, in one sense, this is the antithesis of Barthes's characterization of Flaubert's proffered literary pleasure of 'no longer anything but language'. Barthes, *The Pleasure of the Text*, p. 9. A reality beckons on the other side of textual play and interpretation, a stupefying, ecstasy-inducing reality, even if the human response is only to quote more text.

out in their ecstasy: 'How excellent is your inebriating cup!' (Psalm 22. 5).[70] Pleasure has reached its apex in the promise of further 'pleasures evermore' (Psalm 16. 11).

What Sort of Pleasure?

But what are these pleasures? I have thus far only spoken of 'spiritual reading' or 'allegorical interpretation' and said little about the actual process, activity, or method that Bede is commending and that Carolingian authors so enthusiastically took up. A lengthy exploration of the tradition of allegorical interpretation is, of course, not possible here, but there is room for some brief explication of just what Bede meant by this pleasure, before some further analytical consideration of this activity as a 'pleasure'.[71] I will draw examples from *Homiliae* I.14 and II.2, though they could be multiplied by reference to many other places in Bede's works.

The beginning of this satisfying and intoxicating pleasure is rooted by Bede in the teaching activity of Jesus, as he opened the scriptures to the apostles. Christ made wine from water when he appeared to the two disciples on the way to Emmaus, whose hearts he caused to 'burn' with intoxication when he opened scripture to them.[72] Christ's disciples, in turn, gave explanations to their followers, such that there has been 'nullum [...] tempus saeculi a sanctis alienum doctoribus' ('no time among the ages of the world that was without its holy teachers').[73] In other words, the feasting and drinking initiated in the apostolic generation was continued by the apostles in their speaking and writing, when they 'non pauca legis et prophetarum dicta mystica suis interpretatione addita inserendo opusculis' ('included quite a number of mystical sayings of the law and prophets in their works, with the addition of their own interpretations').[74] This process was and, for Bede, is continued by those who

[70] Cf. Barthes, *The Pleasure of the Text*, pp. 12–13.

[71] We are still dependent on Henri de Lubac's 1959 work *Exégèse mediévale*, though it is more of a synthetic exploration than a rigorously historical investigation of any single author, as de Lubac himself notes. For the earlier period, see Young, *Biblical Exegesis and the Formation of Christian Culture*. We still await full investigations of most early medieval exegetes like Bede and the Carolingians, though see S. Shimahara, *Haymon d'Auxerre, exégète carolingien*.

[72] Bede, *Homilies*, I.14, trans. by Martin and Hurst, I, 143–44.

[73] Bede, *Homiliae*, I.14.262–64, ed. by Hurst, p. 102; trans. by Martin and Hurst, I, 144.

[74] Bede, *Homiliae*, II.2.193–95, ed. by Hurst, p. 198; trans. by Martin and Hurst, II, 20.

follow in the footsteps of their teaching, carrying on the clarification of the scriptural text: 'integros [...] libros diligentiore explanatione discutiendo' ('by scrutinizing complete books of both testaments').[75]

These interpreters Bede identifies elsewhere as the Church Fathers, in whose footsteps he and others follow.[76] The pleasure of reading is thus seen as a continual activity of the Church, a tradition that is continued in each generation, as the writings of the New Testament are used to interpret the Old, and the writings of the Church Fathers extend those interpretations, multiplying and breaking up the scriptures to feed and intoxicate more and more readers and hearers. The pleasure Bede envisions, then, is a quite rigorous process of study, of absorbing scriptural texts and patristic commentaries until one is capable of extending their teaching even further to other books of scripture, catching mere glimpses, perhaps, of the meaning of these texts. But this only raises more questions. Given that Bede will elsewhere recount such an activity as including a great deal of 'sweat' (*sudor*) and struggle, just what sort of pleasure is this?[77] Moreover, given our earlier discussion of how the language Bede uses to describe this pleasurable activity is that taken from an already existing moral discourse on the dangers of fleshly pleasures, how do we understand this activity?

A simplistic and textually warranted explanation could be that Bede is exalting spiritual desires at the expense of the fleshly, eternal joys for temporal, 'true' pleasure for 'false'. He does use this sort of language, as do many medieval authors. As I noted earlier, the starting point for both of his homilies is the desire to 'pass over' and 'emigrate' from or 'trample' upon destructive pleasures. But I believe something subtle is taking place in the specific deployment of the paradigm taken from an older Graeco-Roman tradition, as well as the ascetic redeployments and transformations of it, regarding *saturitas* and its attendant effects. Bede redirects an already transformed discourse on the management of life and pleasure. What is most striking is that Bede shares the general goal of the ascetic literature (i.e. reaching the moral life, heaven, eternal joys), but that he goes about reaching that goal quite differently. Cassian had spoken of the necessity of focusing on spiritual pleasure, but he mostly then described fasting,

[75] Bede, *Homiliae*, II.2.196–97, ed. by Hurst, p. 198; trans. by Martin and Hurst, II, 20.

[76] Thus, for Bede, his work is in the same continuum as that of the Church Fathers. See DeGregorio, 'Footsteps of his Own'.

[77] Bede, *Expositio in Actuum Apostolorum*, preface, ed. by Laistner, p. 3: 'In explanationem quoque beati euangelistae Lucae iuxta uestigia patrum quantum ualeam sudoris expendam' (In the explanation of the blessed evangelist Luke, following the footsteps of the Fathers, I have expended as much sweat as I could).

reading, vigils, and varied deprivations as the activities to engage in, without going much further. Bede, on the other hand, provides the description of an integrated programme of spiritual reading and transformation, oriented towards satisfaction and pleasure, by using the terms of an older pleasure. Rather than simply replacing old desires and pleasures with new ones (Cassian's position), Bede will describe the new set of desires as the old ones. Rather than replacing eating with fasting, vigils, and reading, he replaces eating with a new form of eating. He constructs a schematization or ordering of desire and pleasures that differs subtly from Cassian, that differs from many understandings of pleasure.

The articulation of this pleasure not only relies on the vocabulary and logic of the Graeco-Roman medical tradition, and its ascetic transformation, but also on the 'normal' categories of desire and pleasure, even as it subverts and redirects them: hunger and satiation, thirst and drunkenness, with all their consequences. The allegorical categories are glimpsed in the regular. In this sense, Bede's articulation of the pleasure of reading is of a piece with his understanding of the whole purpose of scripture and scriptural figures. One thing is said, and another is meant. One pleasure is described, and another is offered. The pleasure of the allegorical reader depends on having other, more basic and familiar pleasures close at hand, teasing the physical senses with their cloying fragrance, before the vigour of their seductive draw can be redirected into the allegorical. These include the pleasures the reader may be trying to shun, like physical drunkenness. There is a constant play, then, between the temporal and the eternal, the false and the true, the fleshly and the spiritual, which cannot banish the memory and experience of the former pleasures too swiftly. It depends on them. It must evoke them constantly, teasing them into the open, fanning their flame into an open blaze before translating them into a different idiom. This translation — 'the effective switching of the bait' between one pleasure and another — makes difficult the distinction between the two.[78] This difficulty, admittedly, appears to play into what Bede sees as the general purpose of allegorical interpretation, in which the heart is moved and shaped 'more firmly [...] and sometimes more sweetly' by 'figurative examples' that are explained and redirected, rather than 'by simple telling'.[79] But the difficulty remains. For if the experience of the pleasure to be embraced is based upon the pleasure to be shunned, how can one be attracted to the spiritual without knowing first the fleshly? Can the allegorical stand on its own?

[78] Burrus, Jordan, and MacKendrick, *Seducing Augustine*, p. 18.

[79] Bede, *Homilies*, I.16, trans. by Martin and Hurst, I, 165.

Textually, we must answer in the negative. It is the interplay that counts.[80] As Gregory the Great will put it in his commentary on the Song of Songs:

> Allegoria enim animae [...] quasi quandam machinam facit, ut per illam leuetur ad deum. Interpositis quippe enigmatibus, dum quiddam in uerbis cognoscit, quod suum est, in sensu uerborum intellegit, quod non est suum [...] ex sermonibus huius amoris discimus, qua uirtute in diuinitatis amore ferueamus.
>
> [Allegory supplies the soul [...] with a kind of mechanism by which it is raised to God. By means of dark sayings in whose words a person can understand something of his own, he can understand what is not his to understand [...]. We learn from the words of this lower love with what intensity we must burn with love for God.][81]

Similarly, the pleasure and practice of reading scripture, as discussed by Bede, takes its language from a previously existing source. For Bede, this is the lesson of the food miracles. Christ multiplies already existing food to show that his deeds and teaching do not do away with the former things. He transforms water into wine that he may show he acts in consonance with all the Law and the Prophets.[82] He is prefigured by the former things, and even the allegorical reader is 'prophesied' by the contents of the scriptures. There is no immediate undoing of what came before; there is a transformation.

[80] Barthes, *The Pleasure of the Text*, p. 10: 'It is intermittence [...] which is erotic: the intermittence of skin flashing between two articles of clothing [...] it is this flash itself which seduces'. The allegorical pleasure, like the pleasure of reading described by Barthes, 'is not the pleasure of the corporeal striptease', even if it gestures towards a historical *denouement*.

[81] Gregory the Great, *Expositio in Canticum Canticorum*, Preface 14–15, 34, ed. by Verbraken, p. 3; Gregory the Great, *Exposition of the Song of Songs*, Pref. 1, trans. by Turner, p. 217.

[82] Bede, *Homilies*, I.14, trans. by Martin and Hurst, I, 139; II.2, trans. by Martin and Hurst, II, 17; Bede, *In Lucae euangelium expositio*, III.1335–1343, ed. by Hurst, p. 201; Bede, *In Marci euangelium expositio*, II.952–1011, ed. by Hurst, pp. 512–14. The meaning of the multiplied ('opened') loaves in the Feeding of the Four Thousand is slightly different, however, as they are partly meant to signify the bread of gospel teaching and the giving of the sacraments. Bede sees the significance of the multiplied loaves as consisting in the Son's unique transmission of knowledge of the Father. Bede, *In Marci euangelium expositio*, II.1512–1680, ed. by Hurst, pp. 527–31. But these loaves also signify Christ's unlocking of the 'secret things' (*arcana*) of scripture, implicitly including the Old Testament: 'Indocti quaesierunt pabulo uerbi dei quo ad uirtutem bonae operationis conualescerent refici nec erat magistris deficientibus qui eis scripturae archana patefaceret eos que ad uiam ueritatis institueret' ('The unlearned seek the food of God's Word, by which they are greatly strengthened for the virtue of good works, and, with the failing masters [of the Law], there was no one who could open to them the secret things of Scripture and institute for them the way of truth' (II.1616–21, ed. by Hurst, p. 530; my translation).

Can we say, then, that the allegorical pleasure is contained within the 'normal' pleasure? While Bede does not put things this way, it seems that an answer in the affirmative is possible. The 'normal' pleasure dimly casts the shadow of the pleasure of the allegorical reader. Within the quotidian pleasures of breaking too much bread and drinking too much wine, which must be known or experienced pleasures in order for their allegorical counterparts to 'work', Bede sees the figure of the reader who gathers the fragments of meaning and savours the fragrance both of former times and of the age to come. The allegorical pleasure is constrained by the shape of the former pleasure, even in its transformation. This is not the abandonment of pleasure. Bede believes humanity was created to dwell in a 'place of pleasure' (*locum voluptatis*),[83] even that 'humanity was placed [in paradise], that, in the presence of their creator, they might forever enjoy there the most blessed and holy delights of the flesh and the soul'.[84] Moreover, the blessed will partake in 'pleasures evermore' in contemplation of the divine face.[85] But Bede's understanding of pleasure in the current time certainly involves the training of desire, a specific means of reorienting one towards new pleasures.

Conclusion

Perhaps this is the reason that the Carolingians embraced Bede's understanding of the nature of feasting and drinking as a pleasure that improved one's moral character, why nearly all of them repeated or augmented his interpretation of Christ's miracles.[86] Beyond recognizing his authority as a spiritual teacher, they

[83] Bede, *Libri Quatuor in principium Genesis*, I.2.1501, ed. by Jones, p. 408. Cf. I.2.1430–33 (p. 45) and II.4.284–88 (p. 81).

[84] Bede, *Libri Quatuor in principium Genesis*, II.4.586, ed. by Jones, p. 89. See the whole context in II.4.570–609 (pp. 88–89), where Bede offers an interpretation of the Hebrew name 'Naama' as 'pleasure'.

[85] Bede, *Retractatio in Actus Apostolorum*, II.174–84, ed. by Laistner, p. 114.

[86] A way they elaborated his teaching, which I have not had time to discuss, was by furthering the link between the allegorical pleasure and moral improvement. Rabanus Maurus, Sedulius Scottus, Paschasius Radbertus, and Heiric and Haimo of Auxerre, when commenting on the Feeding of the Four Thousand, tacked on a quotation from Augustine's *On Diverse Questions* regarding the four virtues, a quotation in which the author himself states that the four thousand are those who, unlike the five thousand, have conquered their subjection to the five senses through their adherence to the four virtues. In this addition of a specific set of comments on the four virtues, I believe these authors were making the link explicit between shifting the desires from carnal to spiritual feasting, with the result of the inculcation of the virtues.

found an account of a pleasure that was both old and new, close at hand and reaching into the future. It was in an indulgent pleasure of scriptural interpretation, figured as feasting and drinking, in which they found satisfaction. Bede offered a spiritual system that went beyond the previous ascetic paradigm of conquering vices and embracing virtues primarily through bodily deprivation. Without giving up the idea of passing beyond temporal pleasures, he crafted a new arrangement or ordering of the pleasures, such that one could advance by pursuing another kind of feasting and drinking, by pursuing pleasure. He spoke of a surfeit within the mind that led to fecundity and virtue, rather than a fullness of the body that led to every vice. He guided them away from a dissipating drunkenness and towards one that stretched the reader towards all the pleasures of the past and the future.

The Carolingians, then, who were quite aware of the preceding ascetic paradigm and who reproduced it to some extent, took on board Bede's new paradigm of pleasure quite enthusiastically, becoming allegorical readers themselves, breaking the bread and drinking the cup anew in imitation of Bede. They took on his task in a new generation. And, in this way, we may have another explanation for why the Carolingians so exuberantly produced new works of exegesis. They loved to do so, for they had learned from Bede a 'holy gluttony', the pleasures of the allegorical reader.

Rabanus Maurus, *Commentariorum in Matthaeum*, 5.66, ed. by Löfstedt, p. 454; Paschasius Radbertus, *Expositio in Mattheo*, 7.1816–23, ed. by Paulus, 747; Claudius, *In Matthaeum*, 15.38 in CCCC, MS 88, fol. 111v; Heiric of Auxerre, *Homelia*, II.26, ed. by Quadri, 289–99; and Haimo of Auxerre, *Homelia* 99, ed. by Migne, col. 640C. There is also a further discursive link in the Augustinian quotation's connection of the 'boys' with various biblical passages related to gluttony.

Works Cited

Manuscript

Cambridge, Corpus Christi College [CCCC], MS 88 (England, s. x): Claudius of Turin, *Commentary on Matthew*

Primary Sources

Alcuin, *De virtutibus et vitiis*, ed. by Paul E. Szarmach, in 'The Latin Tradition of Alcuin's *Liber de virtutibus et vitiis*, cap. xxvii–xxxv, with special reference to Vercelli Homily XX', *Mediaevalia*, 12 (1989), 13–41

——, *Epistola* 81, ed. by Ernst Dümmler, in *Epistolae Karolini aevi*, II, MGH Epistolae, 4 (Berlin: Monumenta Germaniae Historica, 1895)

——, *Expositio in Ioannem* in *PL*, C, cols 737–1008

Ambrose, *Expositio Evangelii secundum Lucam*, ed. by C. Schenkl, CSEL, 32.4 (Wien: Verlag der Österreichischen Akademie der Wissenschaften, 1902)

Augustine, *In Iohannis Evangelium tractatus CXXIV*, ed. by R. Willems, CCSL, 36 (Turnhout: Brepols, 1954)

——, *Tractatus in Iohannem*, trans. by John Gibb and James Innes, ed. by Philip Schaff, Nicene and Post-Nicene Fathers, ser. 1, 7 (Edinburgh: T&T Clark, 1888), <http://www.ccel.org/ccel/schaff/npnf107.html> [accessed 20 June 2013]

Bede, *Expositio in Actuum Apostolorum*, in *Bedae Venerabilis Opera. Pars II:4*, ed. by M. L. W. Laistner, CCSL, 121 (Turnhout: Brepols, 1983)

——, *Homeliae evangelii*, in *Bedae Venerabilis Opera. Pars III*, ed. by David Hurst, CCSL, 122 (Turnhout: Brepols, 1955)

——, *Homilies on the Gospels*, trans. by Lawrence T. Martin and David Hurst, Cistercian Studies, 110–11, 2 vols (Kalamazoo: Cistercian Publications, 1991)

——, *In Ezram et Neemiam*, in *Bedae Venerabilis Opera. Pars II:2A*, ed. by D. Hurst, CCSL, 119A (Turnhout: Brepols, 1969)

——, *In Lucae euangelium expositio*, in *Bedae Venerabilis Opera. Pars II:3*, ed. by David Hurst, CCSL, 451 (Turnhout: Brepols 1960)

——, *In Marci euangelium expositio*, ed. by David Hurst, CCSL, 451 (Turnhout: Brepols 1960)

——, *Libri Quatuor in principium Genesis usque ad nativitatem Isaac et eiectionem Ismahelis adnotationum*, in *Bedae Venerabilis Opera. Pars II:1*, ed. by Ch. W. Jones (Turnhout: Brepols, 1967)

——, *On the Tabernacle*, trans. by Arthur Holder, Translated Texts for Historians, 18 (Liverpool: Liverpool University Press, 1994)

——, *Retractatio in Actus Apostolorum*, in *Bedae Venerabilis Opera. Pars II:4*, ed. by M. L. W. Laistner, CCSL, 121 (Turnhout: Brepols, 1983)

Cassian, John, *Conférences*, ed. Dom E. Pichery, Sources chrétiennes, 42, 54, 65 (Paris: Éditions du Cerf, 1955–59)

——, *The Conferences*, trans. by Boniface Ramsey, OP, Ancient Christian Writers, 57 (New York: Newman Press, 1997)
——, *The Institutes*, trans. by Boniface Ramsey, OP, Ancient Christian Writers, 58 (New York: Newman Press, 2000)
——, *Institutions cénobitiques*, ed. Jean-Claude Guy, Sources chrétiennes, 109 (Paris: Éditions du Cerf, 1965)
Christian of Stavelot, *Commentarius in Euangelium Matthaei* in *PL*, CVI, cols 1261–1504
——, *Expositio brevis in Lucam*, in *PL*, CVI, cols 1503–14
——, *Expositiuncula in Ioannem Evangelistam*, in *PL*, CVI, cols 1515–20
Clement, *Stromata*, ed. and trans. by A. Roberts and J. Donaldson, Ante-Nicene Fathers, 2 (Edinburgh: T&T Clark, 1885); <http://www.ccel.org/ccel/schaff/anf02.html> [accessed 30 May 2013]
Eriugena, Iohannes Scottus, *Homelia et Commentarius in Euangelium Iohannis*, ed. by Édouard A. Jeauneau, CCCM, 166 (Turnhout: Brepols, 2008)
Evagrius Ponticus, *The Praktikos & Chapters on Prayer*, trans. by John Eudes Bamberger, OCSO, Cistercian Studies Series, 4 (Kalamazoo: Cistercian Publications, 1981)
Gregory the Great, *Expositio in canticum canticorum*, ed. by P. Verbraken, CCSL, 144 (Turnhout: Brepols, 1963)
——, *Exposition of the Song of Songs*, Pref. 1, trans. by Denys Turner in *Eros and Allegory*, Cistercian Studies, 156 (Kalamazoo: Cistercian Publications, 1995), pp. 215–55
——, *Forty Gospel Homilies*, trans. by David Hurst, Cistercian Studies Series, 123 (Kalamazoo, MI: Cistercian Publications, 1990)
——, *Moralia in Iob*, ed. by M. Adriaen, CCSL, 143A and 143B (Turnhout: Brepols, 1979)
Haimo of Auxerre, *Homeliae*, in *PL*, CXVIII, cols 9–816
Heiric of Auxerre: *Heirici Autissiodorensis Homeliae per cicrulum anni*, ed. by Richard Quadri, CCCM, 116–116B, 3 vols (Turnhout: Brepols, 1992–94)
Hincmar, *De cavendiis vitiis et virtutibus exercendiis*, in *PL*, CXXV, cols 857–930
——, *De divortio Lotharii Regis et Theutbergae Reginae*, ed. by Letha Böhringer, MGH Concilia, 4, suppl. 1 (Hannover: Monumenta Germaniae Historica, 1992)
Jerome, *Commentariorum in Matheum libri IV*, ed. by D. Hurst and M. Adriaen, CCSL, 77 (Turnhout: Brepols, 1969)
——, *Commentary on Matthew*, trans. by Thomas P. Scheck, Fathers of the Church, 117 (Washington, DC: Catholic University of America Press, 2008)
——, *Epistulae*, ed. by Isidor Hilberg, CSEL, 54–56.2, 4 vols, 2nd edn (Wien: Verlag der Österreichischen Akademie der Wissenschaften, 1996)
Origen, *Commentarium in euangelium Matthaei*, ed. by R. Girod, Sources chrétiennes, 162 (Paris: Éditions du Cerf, 1970)
——, *Commentary on Matthew*, trans. by J. Patrick, ed. by A. Menzies, Ante-Nicene Fathers, 10 (Edinburgh: T&T Clark, 1895); <http://www.ccel.org/ccel/schaff/anf09.html> [accessed 10 June 2013]
Otfrid, *Glossae in Matthaeum*, ed. by C. Grifoni, CCCM, 200 (Turnhout: Brepols, 2003)
Paschasius Radbertus, *Expositio in Mattheo*, ed. by Bedae Paulus, CCCM, 56–56B, 3 vols (Turnhout: Brepols, 1984)

Pseudo-Bede, *In Matthaei evangelium expositio*, in *PL*, XCII, cols 9–132
——, *In S. Joannis evangelium expositio*, in *PL*, XCII, cols 633–937
Rabanus Maurus, *Commentariorum in Matthaeum*, ed. by B. Löfstedt, CCCM, 174A (Turnhout: Brepols, 2003)
Sedulius Scottus, *Collectaneum miscellaneum*, ed. by Dean Simpson, CCCM, 67 (Turnhout: Brepols, 1988)
——, *Kommentar zum Evangelium nach Matthäus 11,1 bis Schluss*, ed. by Bengt Löfstedt, Aus der Geschichte der lateinischen Bibel, 19 (Freiburg im Breisgau: Herder, 1991)
Smaragdus of Saint Mihiel, *Collectiones in epistolas et evangelia*, in *PL*, CII, cols 14–551

Secondary Works

Barthes, Roland. *The Pleasure of the Text*, trans. by Richard Miller (New York: Noonday Press, 1975)
Brown, Peter, *The Body and Society: Men, Women, and Sexual Renunciation in Early Christianity* (London: Faber and Faber, 1988)
Burrus, Virginia, Mark Jordan, and Karmen MacKendrick, *Seducing Augustine: Bodies, Desires, Confessions* (New York: Fordham University Press, 2010)
Carroll, M. Thomas Aquinas, *The Venerable Bede: His Spiritual Teachings* (Washington, DC: Catholic University of America Press, 1946)
Contreni, J.J., 'Carolingian Biblical Studies', in *Carolingian Essays: Andrew W. Mellon Lectures in Early Christian Studies*, ed. by U.-R. Blumenthal (Washington, DC: Catholic University of America Press, 1983), pp. 71–98; repr. as Contreni, *Carolingian Learning, Masters and Manuscripts* (Aldershot: Variorum, 1992), ch. 5
DeGregorio, Scott, 'Footsteps of his Own: Bede's Commentary on Ezra-Nehemiah', in *Innovation and Tradition in the Works of the Venerable Bede*, ed. by DeGregorio (Morgantown: West Virginia University Press, 2006), pp. 143–68
Edwards, Burton Van Name, 'The Manuscript Transmission of Carolingian Biblical Commentaries', <https://emf.pages.tcnj.edu/early-medieval-forum/carolingian/> [accessed 15 December 2017; previous URL accessed 25 June 2013]
Foucault, Michel, *The Care of the Self*, vol. III of *The History of Sexuality*, trans. by Robert Hurley (New York: Vintage Press, 1986)
——, *The Use of Pleasure*, vol. II of *The History of Sexuality*. trans. by Robert Hurley (New York: Vintage Press, 1985)
Gil-Sotres, Pedro, 'The Regimens of Health', in *Western Medical Thought from Antiquity to the Middle Ages*, ed. by Mirko d. Grmek (Cambridge, MA: Harvard University Press, 1998), pp. 291–318
Grégoire, Reginald, *Homéliaires liturgiques médiévaux: Analyse de manuscrits* (Spoleto: Centro italiano di studi sull'alto medioevo, 1980)
Jong, Mayke de, 'Exegesis for an Empress', in *Medieval Transformations: Texts, Power, and Gifts in Context*, ed. by Esther Cohen and Mayke de Jong (Leiden: Brill, 2001), pp. 69–100

——, 'The Empire as *Ecclesia*: Hrabanus Maurus and Biblical *Historia* for Rulers', in *The Uses of the Past in the Early Middle Ages*, ed. by Matthew Innes and Yitzhak Hen (Cambridge: Cambridge University Press, 2000), pp. 191–226

Lubac, Henri de, *Exégèse mediévale: Les Quatre sens de l'Écriture*, trans. by Mark Sebanc (vol. I) and by E. M. Macierowski (vols II–III) as *Medieval Exegesis: The Four Senses of Scripture*, 3 vols (Grand Rapids, MI: Eerdmans, 1998–2009)

Nicoud, Marilyn, 'Food Consumption, a Health Risk? Norms and Medical Practice in the Middle Ages', *Appetite*, 51 (2008), 7–9

——, *Les Régimes de santé au Moyen Âge: Naissance et diffusion d'une écriture médicale, XIIIe–XVe siècle*, Bibliothèque des écoles françaises d'Athènes et de Rome, 333, 2 vols (Roma: École française de Rome, 2007)

Shaw, Teresa M., *The Burden of the Flesh: Fasting and Sexuality in Early Christianity* (Minneapolis: Fortress Press, 1998)

Shimahara, Sumi, *Haymon d'Auxerre, exégète carolingien*, Collection Haut Moyen Âge, 16 (Turnhout: Brepols, 2013)

Sloan, Michael C., *The Harmonious Organ of Sedulius Scottus: Introduction to his 'Collectaneum in Apostolum' and Translation of its Prologue and Commentaries on Galatians and Ephesians* (Berlin: De Gruyter, 2012), pp. 13–33

Staubach, Nikolaus, *Rex christianus: Hofkultur und Herrschaftspropaganda im Reich Karls des Kahlen*, vol. II, *Die Grundlegung der 'religion royale'*, Pictura et Poesis, 2 (Köln: Böhlau, 1993)

Stone, Rachel, *Morality and Masculinity in the Carolingian Period* (Cambridge: Cambridge University Press, 2011)

Young, Frances, *Biblical Exegesis and the Formation of Christian Culture* (Cambridge: Cambridge University Press, 1997)

On Leeks and Onions: Pope Gregory VII and the Rejection of Pleasure

Ken A. Grant

An examination of Pope Gregory VII does not usually engage the subject of pleasure. This is not only due to the fact that the subject does not receive significant explicit treatment in his only extant work, the Register, which it does not, but more likely that most people would simply not think to entertain the notion. Pope Gregory VII and pleasure may seem a rather incongruous pairing in a sentence; Gregory VII and power, or politics, or papal prerogatives, or authority, these are terms that resonate in far more complementary measures in standard examinations of Gregory and his papacy. Yet, in order to more fully explore Pope Gregory VII, and through him the late eleventh century, perhaps it is time to move beyond the traditional avenues of exploration. For in exploring Pope Gregory VII's understanding of pleasure, we may more clearly understand his ideology and actions.

This move is, in part, motivated by the most fruitful turn in Gregorian studies over the last two decades, which has been the effort to turn our attention towards addressing the questions of how and why Pope Gregory VII, as well as the other eleventh-century reformers, developed, promoted, and attempted to bring to fruition their ideas about Church and society. Maureen Miller, in examining Gregory's papacy specifically, and the Investiture Contest generally, noted that we needed to 'set aside questions of whether a belief or development was right or wrong, good or bad, and concentrate on how and why ideas and

Ken A. Grant (grantka@udmercy.edu) is an adjunct professor in History at the University of Detroit Mercy.

Pleasure in the Middle Ages, ed. by Naama Cohen-Hanegbi and Piroska Nagy, IMR 24 (Turnhout: Brepols, 2018), pp. 309–327 BREPOLS PUBLISHERS 10.1484/M.IMR-EB.5.113472

practices developed'.[1] This methodological step is an important attempt to move away from the many confessionally, or ideologically, based interpretations that have been offered since the polemicists began the debate in the late eleventh century, a debate that continued on through at least the middle of the twentieth century. Operating under similar analytical structures, many scholars have recently produced exemplary work that expands our understanding of the late eleventh-century reformers, and the reformers' impact on subsequent centuries.[2]

I argue that we need to broaden this conceptual engagement even further, pushing Gregory VII, and others, into areas that encourage our exploration in new interpretive pathways so that we might continually search for a broader understanding of Gregory's papacy and ideas. If we read Gregory only in light of discussions of power, politics, canon law, and authority, we might miss a discussion that more completely engages his actions, policies, ideals, and self-identity. Because the traditional pathways into the person and ideas of Gregory VII are so well worn, I argue that it is beneficial to explore alternate routes that might reveal new insight. This new set of interpretive lenses challenges us to look at someone that we think we know so well with a new perspective, perhaps in ways that the traditional interpretive lenses of power and authority might not be able to discern. In light of this new directional effort, this article offers an examination into the way in which Gregory developed and explained his ideas regarding pleasure, and the way in which his worldview affected the way he understood pleasure, which, in turn, shaped the way he dealt with the Church, secular officials, and the world.

Pope Gregory VII's ideas and actions stem from a particular worldview, one that discerns a world and Church teetering on the brink of ruin, and that the only way to save the Church and world is through a relentless focus on what truly matters, the eternal. The way in which he understands and reacts to this problem is directly related to his religious worldview, which repeatedly returns to the claim that only those singularly focused on the eternal, and the needs of others, can possibly right the ship. For Gregory, pleasure, especially this-worldly pleasure, is a fatal distraction that the Church cannot afford. While seemingly articulated in a hyperbolic manner, this is how Pope Gregory VII sees the world, and it is this intensity and vehemence, coupled with the singular reach of his office, that makes Gregory unique in a medieval world filled with those con-

[1] Miller, 'The Crisis in the Investiture Crisis Narrative', pp. 1570, 1577.

[2] Blumenthal, *The Investiture Controversy*; Cowdrey, *Pope Gregory VII*; Cushing, *Reform and the Papacy in the Eleventh Century*; Frassetto, *Medieval Purity and Piety*; *The Papal Reform of the Eleventh Century*, ed. by Robinson; Stroll, *Popes and Antipopes*.

cerned about earthly pleasures. A comment in Gregory VII's 24 January 1074 letter, requesting Archbishop Sigehard of Aquileia's attendance at the Lenten Synod, serves as a representative introductory taste of his rhetoric:

> Non ignorare credimus prudentiam tuam; quantis perturbationum fluctibus ecclesia sit usquequaque concussa et pene desolationis suę calamitatibus naufraga et submersa sit facta. Rectores erum et principes huius mundi, singuli quęrentes quę sua sunt, non quę Iesu Christ, dominam et matrem suam, videlicet sponsam Christi omni reverentia conculcata quasi vilem ancillam opprimunt eamque confundere, dum cupiditates suas explere valeant, nullatenus pertimescunt.
>
> [We believe that you in your prudence are not unaware of by how great waves of confusion the church is everywhere being stricken and is almost made shipwreck and caused to founder by the disasters of her desolation. For the rulers and princes of this world, each one of them seeking things that are their own and not those of Jesus Christ, have abandoned all reverence and oppress their lady and mother, that is, the bride of Christ, like a common slave-girl; and they in no wise fear to destroy her, for just so long as they can satisfy their own desires.][3]

The question that is asked at this point, and rightly so, is this: How does this examination of Gregory VII's understanding of the proper perspective on pleasure involve an exploration of leeks and onions? Trundling down new interpretive pathways is commendable, but only if the exploration makes some modicum of sense. By examining the role these two seemingly random vegetables play in the discussion of pleasure and carnality, we note a fascinating and important connection between 'carnal pleasures' and the proper Christian life as expressed by Gregory VII. This connection is not as random or arbitrary as one might think, as a brief, but telling, anecdote about Hildebrand connects these seemingly disparate areas of inquiry in a manner that illuminates our understanding of Gregory and, in an ancillary digression, offers a fascinating, albeit brief, examination of the transmission of a particular piece of folklore.

A seemingly inconsequential comment offered by Peter Damian in his letters provides the starting point: a comment that prompted this exploration about the way in which Hildebrand dealt with the idea of pleasure, as well as the search for the meaning of leeks and onions in ancient and medieval thought. In the *Register*, examples from which I will offer shortly, it is safe to argue that Gregory determined that the idea of earthly pleasure, or of any focus on this world, was a grave distraction from all that was important. For Gregory,

[3] Gregory VII, *Das Register*, ed. by Caspar, II.1, 64–65; Gregory VII, *The Register*, trans. by Cowdrey, pp. 46–47.

anything that distracted from what he saw as that far more important focus or purpose, the eternal, over and against the temporal, was to be actively shunned or overcome. The brief anecdote we find in letter 160 of Peter Damian's letters sheds some light on the way in which Hildebrand saw the people who live in this world, the way they are supposed to act, and why they are supposed to act in that manner.

In letter 160, Peter writes at some length, after the season of Lent in 1069, to Hildebrand, Cardinal Archdeacon of Rome, and Alberic, the deacon of Monte Cassino, regarding the meaning and observance of Lent. Most salient for our purposes is the brief opening reflection on fasts and fasting. Damian begins by exploring the activities of a particular 'servant of God' who observed many fasts throughout the year, and would, when not fasting, still be exceptionally cautious about what he consumed.[4] Damian noted, 'as soon as his appetite tempted him to eat, he at once applied restraint, lest these foods become an addiction'.[5]

This leads Damian to note that Hildebrand had recently told him that he abstained from eating leeks and onions, because he was 'especially fond of these pungent foods'.[6] Damian develops a fascinating and psychologically astute argument, commenting:

> In his itaque despicabilibus rebus et gravior abstinentia, et minor est gloria. Facilius enim carne quam sale quis abstinet, gravius est abicere fructus arborum quam aspersas patinis fraglantias pigmentorum.
>
> [Indeed, with regard to those items that are of small concern, abstinence is more difficult and brings little renown. As you are aware, it is easier for one to give up meat than salt, more difficult to turn down fruit than dishes sprinkled with fragrant spices.][7]

[4] Damian, *Letters 151–180*, trans. by Blum and Resnick, p. 103. Damian, *Die Briefe*, ed. by Reindel, p. 101.

[5] Damian, *Letters 151–180*, trans. by Blum and Resnick, p. 104. Damian, *Die Briefe*, ed. by Reindel, p. 101: 'Sed mox ut gula provocatur ut comedat, disciplina protinus adhibetur, ne desiderata a contingat'.

[6] Damian, *Letters 151–180*, trans. by Blum and Resnick, p. 104. Damian, *Die Briefe*, ed. by Reindel, p. 101. 'Ipse quoque michi nuper confessus es, quoniam ideo te funditus a porrorum sive ceparum perception compescis'. Blum translates *porrorum* as 'chives', though it can be translated either as chives or leeks. 'You yourself also recently told me that you abstained from using onions or chives because you were especially fond of these pungent foods'.

[7] Damian, *Die Briefe*, ed. by Reindel, p. 101; Damian, *Letters 151–80*, trans. by Blum and Resnick, p. 104.

Thus, for Hildebrand to forego leeks and onions — seemingly insignificant to our eyes, I will illustrate shortly that they did have significance to medieval audiences — is the perfect object for a lifetime fast, as it is these types of foods that, while they may seem inconsequential, represent the very problem that confronted the world, distractions that led one away from a focus on the eternal. Damian argued that precisely because they did seem inconsequential to most, they were particularly treacherous. For Hildebrand, leeks and onions were so desirable and enjoyable that they served as a significant distraction, therefore he fasted from them — not because he would gain any kind of plaudits from others, but because he knew that such a distraction was contrary to everything that he believed about the proper action one undertakes in the service of God and the Church. From his own fasting from leeks and onions to stern denunciations of those who 'pant after their own gains or desires for present glory',[8] Gregory constructs a consistent understanding about the perils of worldly pleasures that serve as distraction. Gregory notes, as I will show, that any distraction from the eternal had deleterious effects; such a distraction would lead, inevitably, to crisis for the Church, and therefore the world.

Before proceeding with Gregory's concern, though, it is beneficial to explore the idea that while the perception of the nature of leeks and onions is one a modern reader may regard as innocuous, trivial, or perhaps even irrelevant, medieval audiences would likely have found this reference far more intriguing, and would perhaps more immediately have understood the reference as implying a graver concern. 'These pungent foods',[9] as Damian describes them, are significant in ways that are worth exploring and detailing, especially in light of Gregory's understanding of pleasure, and his particular attitudes and concerns regarding obedience to the Church, including obedience to the Church's stance on clerical marriage.

By the Middle Ages, leeks and onions were well known and popular. Leeks and onions (with garlic, from the species *allium*) can be traced back in the history of cultivation at least four thousand years to Central Asia and the Middle East and are referenced in Egyptian, Sumerian, Indian, Arabian, Greek, Roman, and European sources.[10] As noted by R. E. Kaske, and later Chauncey

[8] Gregory VII, *The Register*, trans. by Cowdrey, p. 9. Gregory VII, *Das Register*, ed. by Caspar, II.1, 14: 'dum suis aut lucris aut presentis glorię desideriis inhiant'.

[9] Damian, *Letters 151–80*, trans. by Blum and Resnick, p. 104. Damian, *Die Briefe*, ed. by Reindel, p. 101: 'his acruminibus uberius delectaris'.

[10] Kiple, *A Moveable Feast*, pp. 32–33; Kiple and Ornelas, *The Cambridge World History of Food*, pp. 249–65; Zohary and Hopf, *Domestication of Plants in the Old World*, pp. 168–70.

Wood, the medieval perspective of such seemingly innocuous vegetables was anything but trivial,[11] and through their exploration of these items we can comfortably draw a thematic connection to Gregory's perspective on pleasure, as well as to his reforms of Church and society, for such a perspective stems from his broader worldview. While not directly related specifically to eleventh-century attitudes, Kaske and Wood illustrate a more general medieval depiction that serves as a better known entry point for a discussion of these items. Kaske and Wood note that a component of the description of the Summoner in the General Prologue to the *Canterbury Tales* by Geoffrey Chaucer was that 'Wel loved he garleek, oynons, and eek lekes'.[12] Kaske's and Wood's articles are most directly focused on ascertaining the rationale for using this verse in the description of the Summoner in an effort to understand the Summoner's physical and spiritual depravity. In this description, Kaske notes a connection to medieval biblical commentary, specifically in both Pope Gregory I's *Moralia in Job* and the eighth-century collection *Clavis Scripturae*, on Numbers 11. 5, wherein the Israelites are complaining in the wilderness and voicing a desire to go back to Egypt: 'We remember the fish we use to eat in Egypt for nothing, the cucumbers, the melons, the leeks, the onions, and the garlic' (NRSV). Kaske further points to the interpretive connection that Pope Gregory I drew between this fond remembrance of the culinary pleasures of Egypt and what Wood called the 'backsliding Christian's rejection of the life of grace for a life of carnal pleasure'.[13] Pope Gregory I's interpretation, as found in the *Moralia in Job*, paints a provocative image:

> Quod aperte in semetipso nobis israeliticus populus ostendit, qui dum refectionem mannae desuper perciperet, ab Aegypto ollas carnium, pepones, porros cepasque concupiuit. Quid enim signatur in manna, nisi esca gratiae, suaue sapiens, ad refectionem interioris uitae bene uacantibus desuper data? Et quid per ollas carnium, nisi carnalia opera, uix tribulationum laboribus quasi ignibus excoquenda? Quid per pepones, nisi terrenae dulcedines? Quid per porros ac cepas exprimitur, quae plerumque qui comedunt, lacrimas emittunt, nisi difficultas uitae praesentis, quae a dilectoribus suis et non sine luctu agitur, et tamen cum lacrimis amatur? Manna igitur deserentes, cum peponibus ac carnibus porros cepasque quaesierunt, quia uidelicet peruersae mentes dulcia per gratiam quietis dona despiciunt, et pro

[11] Kaske, 'The Summoner's Garleek, Oynons, and Eek Lekes'; Wood, 'The Sources of Chaucer's Summoner's "Garleek, Onyons, and Eke Lekes"'.

[12] Chaucer, *The Canterbury Tales*.

[13] Kaske, 'The Summoner's Garleek, Oynons, and Eek Lekes', p. 481; Wood, 'The Sources of Chaucer's Summoner's "Garleek, Oynons, and Eke Lekes"'.

carnalibus uoluptatibus laboriosa huius uitae itinera, etiam lacrimis plena, concupiscent; contemnunt habere ubi spiritaliter gaudeant, et desideranter appetunt, ubi et carnaliter gemant.

[In which his people Israel openly show, that even while receiving the refreshment of the manna from above ardently desired the flesh-pots, melons, leeks, and onions of Egypt. What is meant by manna but the food of grace, having a sweet taste, given from above for the refreshment of the interior life of the people now free? And what of the flesh-pots, except carnal works, that which tempers through the labours of tribulations, as if by fire? What is meant by melons, but earthly sweets? What is meant by leeks and onions, but that those who eat shed tears because of the difficulty of the present life, who though they love it, do not without a sense of grief and tears. Therefore, they reject manna, seeking together with melons and meats, leeks and onions, because they despised, due to bad minds, the gifts of grace, and in the desire of the carnal pleasures of this toilsome life, even though full of tears, they reject what they should rejoice spiritually, and eagerly desire where they may groan carnally.][14]

Pope Gregory I's influence throughout the medieval period is undisputed, the *Moralia* especially widely and carefully read, and thus it is safe to assume that this explication was known. Complicating matters of transmission for this case, though, it seems that Gregory I's concern is not one always shared by Peter Damian. Letter 160 addresses, at great length (following the mention of leeks and onions), the Israelites wandering after the Exodus, but never directly or indirectly addresses the concerns, allegorical or literal, of the dangers of leeks and onions as a sign of carnal appetites or spiritual backsliding as found in Numbers 11. 5. This seems to be an odd omission, for if this was a concern that Damian shared with Gregory I, this letter would have been an ideal opportunity to explore those concerns. Indeed, Damian does explore the topic in letters 96 and 100, both from 1063, wherein he references Numbers 11. 5 as a component of a scathing critique of lust and gluttony, but he does not make the connection to any form of spiritual backsliding.[15] Christian Lohmer explains that Damian, interestingly, and perhaps surprisingly, permitted his monks to eat onions and leeks, along with other vegetables and fruits, on non-fasting days.[16]

[14] Pope Gregory I, *Moralia in Job*, pt. IV, bk XX, XV, 40, lines 78–95, p. 1032.

[15] Damian, *Letters 91–120*, trans. by Blum and Resnick, pp. 58–59.

[16] Lohmer, 'Ausgewählte Aspekte der mittelalterlichen Ernährung für Mönche, untersucht am Beispiel der monastischen Bestimmungen des Petrus Damiani'.

Pope Gregory I's concern about the potential carnal pitfalls for those who consume leeks and onions was shared, if not in the specific case of Numbers 11. 5, in a more general, but consistent, line of thought with a wide variety of ancient, late antique, and early medieval authors. U. P. Hedrick mentions that all segments of Egyptian society consumed and enjoyed onions, all, that is, but priests, who were prohibited from eating them.[17] Likewise, E. Hyams noted that according to the second-century Hindu physician Charaka, onions were prohibited for those on the spiritual path.[18] The concern about onions and garlic raised in each case stems from the supposed aphrodisiacal nature of the vegetables.[19] Traditional folklore surrounding onions and garlic states that their olfactory and gustatory potency implied sexual potency, which made the vegetables off limits for spiritual leaders of numerous religious traditions. The suspect nature of onions and garlic is even referenced by a legend attributed to Mohammad when he noted that as Satan left the Garden of Eden after the Fall, onions grew from the spot where his right foot touched the ground, and from the place where his left foot touched the ground, garlic grew.[20] Of less legendary nature, and certainly not at all concerned with the potential aphrodisiacal nature of onions and garlic, focusing on a far more immediate concern,

[17] Hedrick, *Sturtevant's Edible Plants of the World*.

[18] Hyams, *Plants in the Service of Man*.

[19] Similarly, Albertus Magnus suggested that onions 'were to have favorable effects on fertility by generating sperm in men and lactation in women'. Mauron, 'Food, Mood, and Health'.

[20] The search for the source of this legend has been an instructive case-study in the difficulty of tracking the transmission of folkloric fragments. Throughout the twentieth-century historiography, including Kiple, Hedrick, and Hyams, the fragment of the legend of Satan's footprints is simply restated, without attribution. Additional numerous print and Internet works focusing on culinary or agricultural history and folklore cite the legend as deriving from 'Eastern', 'Muslim', 'Islamic', or 'Turkish' sources, but none offer a source for the legend, let alone for the origin of the legend. In fact, most do not even provide a footnote directing the reader to a secondary source. The sources simply repeat the legend as an accepted narrative fragment. The modern sourcing for the narrative fragment is traced back, through Wilson, 'The Onion in Folk Belief' to Glasspoole, *The History of Cultivated Vegetables*, p. 123. Continuing to work backward, the next significant citation of the legend is found in Çelebi, *Seyâhatnâme*, trans. by von Hammer, p. 151. Çelebi references the legend in a section describing the various food stalls of the market at Constantinople, noting, 'I have seen it recorded in history, that when Satan stepped out from Paradise on the earth, garlic sprung up from the spot whereon he had put his left foot, and onions from the place he had set his right upon; but both are indeed very pleasant food'. Çelebi does not provide a reference or source for the legend, except the tantalizing comment, 'I have seen it recorded in history'. Efforts to track the transmission of the legend prior to this reference have thus far not yielded positive results.

Muhammad, in the Hadith, states that 'Whoever has eaten garlic or onion should keep away from us (or should keep away from our mosque)'.[21] While this injunction clearly does not imply any nefariousness, or even Mohammad's dislike, to or of onions and garlic, it does recognize, at the very least, the potency of their aroma.

This cursory exploration of the various cross-cultural injunctions regarding leeks, onions, and garlic, while fascinating, is important mainly because it suggests that the use of leeks and onions in the anecdote from Damian about Hildebrand would not likely have been read simply as a tale of basic fasting. Either it would be read as Hildebrand abstaining from vegetables with known allegorically troubling or physically scandalous implications, or as Hildebrand/Gregory VII's zeal to believe that anything that served as a distraction created the potential for disaster, even something as perfectly normal as a craving for harmless vegetables, and must be regarded as something from which to abstain for life.[22]

As with Peter Damian, Pope Gregory VII never directly or indirectly referenced Numbers 11. 5, even as he regularly referenced both scripture and the writings of Pope Gregory I throughout the Register. Gregory never referenced the leeks and onions story, either. This is not surprising in that specific anecdotes are not usual fodder for his correspondence. His writing style tends towards brusque concision, not loquacious storytelling. That said, the way in which he develops his ideas about the rejection of pleasure is consonant with Gregory I's concern with temporal and carnal pleasures. Thus, while a direct link from Gregory I to Damian and Gregory VII cannot be discerned regarding the Numbers passage, or references to leeks and onions, those who read Damian and Gregory VII would likely have known about Gregory I's concern, and thus drawn the conclusions linking certain carnal pleasures with the rejection of the 'life of grace'[23] or perhaps disobedience to the Church. More

[21] *Sahib Bukhari*, bk LXX, hadith 80.

[22] C. H. Kneepkens offers important hermeneutical advice, suggesting that the modern reader 'take into consideration that the quoting author might have meant not only to import the context of the quotation into his own text, but also the contemporary knowledge that was commonly associated with it'. Kneepkens, 'There Is More in a Biblical Quotation than Meets the Eye', pp. 90–91. In this case, while we are not dealing with a particular quotation, there is a specific enough concept — leeks and onions — that we need to at least entertain the possibility that it might have been understood by a medieval reader rather differently than a modern reader, whether it was intended or not.

[23] Wood, 'The Sources of Chaucer's Summoner's "Garleek, Oynons, and Eke Lekes"', p. 240.

importantly though, Gregory moves beyond the scope of Gregory I's concern for backsliding, seeing in any carnal pleasure the potential for catastrophe. Gregory VII is a more linear, less nuanced, thinker than Gregory I, and thus the more sophisticated metaphorical or allegorical readings of scripture are not as prevalent in Gregory VII's work. For Gregory VII, the most obvious reason to forgo leeks and onions is not due to their representation of Israelite spiritual backsliding, but because they were a distraction from what should be the true focus in life. In this light, the story of leeks and onions is about Hildebrand/Gregory's single-mindedness.

For Pope Gregory VII, the focus was not so much on the rejection of pleasure, per se, but the rejection of those things which served as fundamental stumbling blocks or distractions, especially if that distraction served to undermine the authority of the Church or created an environment where disobedience could bloom. If leeks and onions became an impediment to proper action, due to the fact that he was 'especially fond' of them, whether they carried implications of carnality and disobedience or simply represented distractions, then abstention was the only proper course. Gregory's argument reasons that if we focus on what gives pleasure to ourselves, it is problematic not because it is pleasurable, but because it focuses on what we want, on what we desire, which diverts our attention from the true object of our attention and affection.

It is Gregory's perspective on the condition of the world, a world he routinely stated was gripped by catastrophe and calamity, which prompted his strict consistency on insuring that all focus should remain on that which is eternal. In his 6 May 1073 letter to Duke Godfrey of Lower Lorraine, written in response to a letter from Godfrey in which he extends his good wishes on Gregory's election, Gregory provides an important statement about his view of the condition of the world. In fact, this statement may be one of the most important early statements from Gregory because everything that follows throughout his papacy can be said to be traced to the concern voiced here:

> Peccatis enim facientibus ita pene totus mundus in maligno est positus, ut omnes et precipue qui in ecclesia prelati sunt, eam potius conturbare quam fideli devotione defendere vel celebrare contendant et, dum suis aut lucris aut presentis glorię desideriis inhiant, omnibus quę ad religionem et iustitiam Dei pertinent, se velut hostes opponant.

> [For as a result of sins, almost the whole world is so placed in the power of the evil one that all, and especially those who hold high office in the Church, strive rather to confound it than with faithful devotion to defend or honour it; while they pant

> after their gains for present glory, they set themselves as enemies against all things that belong to the religion and righteousness of God.][24]

Gregory highlights all of the central crises he sees confronting the Church — the wretched condition of the world due to rampant sin (most clearly exemplified by the canonical abuses of simony, clerical marriage, and lay investiture), the catastrophic leadership of corrupt Church office holders, and the problem of leaders's self-centredness, that is, those not dedicating themselves to the task of tending to the flock — and intimates that only through strict obedience to the commands of the Holy See, to the vicar of St Peter, can the crises be averted. He argues that the proper focus should, therefore, not be on this world, as it seems to be careening out of control, and cannot provide what the people need most, in any event. While this is a standard trope in the medieval Church, it is the depth of Gregory's zeal and idealism that shapes his worldview, and the extent of his reach as Pope which imparts greater effect on the world around him. Any compromise introduced the possibility of disaster, and only the constant effort of the Church, and all Church officials, prevented this from happening.

Interestingly, Gregory was not convinced that he had the ability to right the ship: his letters are littered with keening statements regarding his lack of worthiness or talent to be pope, and that he sat on the see only because he followed the commands of Peter, the Prophets, and God.[25] The question of whether this was simply a tactical rhetorical device to create a sense of modesty to cover for the innovative nature of his papacy can be raised. Indeed, an argument forwarded in the renunciation of Gregory by a collection of German bishops at

[24] Gregory VII, *Das Register*, ed. by Caspar, II.1, 14; Gregory VII, *The Register*, trans. by Cowdrey, p. 9.

[25] Importantly, Gregory uses this argument, his compulsion to act by Peter and the Prophets, to justify many of his actions throughout his papacy. This is especially true when he is advocating particularly innovative or revolutionary actions in his struggle with temporal or religious leaders who did not obey papal directives. By appealing to Peter and the Prophets, he is articulating the belief that his actions are not innovative or revolutionary, for they derive from an unassailably ancient source, St Peter, and therefore, God. This is best exemplified in the 7 March 1080 record of the Lenten Synod of 1080. Gregory addresses the record to St Peter: 'I say these things thus, because I have not chosen you but you have chosen me, and you have placed upon me the most heavy burden of your church. And because you have ordered me to ascend upon a high mountain and to proclaim and announce to the people of God their offences and to the sons of the church their sins, the members of the devil have begun to rise up against me and have presumed to lay their hands upon me to the point of shedding blood'. Gregory VII, *The Register*, trans. by Cowdrey, p. 342.

the Synod of Worms in 1076 develops the idea that Gregory was actually the opposite and is stated with blunt clarity:

> Our Lord and Redeemer impressed the goodness of peace and love upon his Faithful as their distinctive character [...]. But by way of contrast, you have inflicted wounds with proud cruelty and cruel pride, you are eager for profane innovations, you delight in a great name rather than in a good one, and with unheard-of self-exaltation, like a standard bearer of schism, you distend all the limbs of the Church which before your times led a quiet and tranquil life, according to the admonition of the Gospel.[26]

The problem, of course, in choosing who to believe in the polemical conflict between Pope Gregory VII and King Henry IV is that it shapes the way we read Gregory VII, which, in turn, shapes our understanding of Gregory's worldview. While endlessly fascinating, trying to discern who was right or wrong places us back in the old confessional or polemical fights, which distracts us from the more salient exploration of trying to understand Gregory from his own perspective, which is most likely to shed light on why he actually did what he did. In this case, Gregory's self-identification, whether rhetorical device or not, is consistent throughout the Register, and thus important to track. For example, in a 4 April 1074 letter to King William I of England, Gregory explores his own perceived weaknesses:

> Navem inviti ascendimus, quę per undosum pelagus violentia ventorum et impetu turbinum et fluctibus | ad aera usque insurgentibus in incerta deicitur; saxis occultatis et aliis a longe in altum apparentibus, licet cum periculo, obviat tamen et ex animo h. Sancta quippe Romana ecclesia, cui licet indigni et nolentes presidemus, diversis temptationibus quam i plurimis persecutionibus ypocritarum et hereticorum i insidiis et dolosis obiectionibus continue et cotidie quatitur, mundanis vero potestatibus occulte et evidenter per diversa distrahitur.
>
> [We have ascended unwillingly a ship which, through a billowing sea, is cast into uncertain courses by the battering winds and by the force of tornados and by waves rising up to the very skies; it is avoiding, although with peril, rocks that are hidden and other things that appear in the deep from afar — yet also near exhaustion. For the holy Roman Church, over which we though unworthy and willing preside, is continually and daily shaken by diverse trials, by very many harassments of hypocrites, and by the snares and guileful reproaches of heretics; she is, in truth, for different causes rent asunder secretly and openly by this world's powers.][27]

[26] *Imperial Lives and Letters of the Eleventh Century*, trans. by Mommsen and Morrison, pp. 147–48.

[27] Gregors VII, *Das Register*, ed. by Caspar, II.1, 101; Gregory VII, *The Register*, trans. by Cowdrey, p. 74.

Gregory's sense of inadequacy, in conjunction with the belief that the world is on the brink of disaster, shapes his view of the world (whether we believe him or not), which helps to explain why he reacts so dramatically. His argument is that if the world is running headlong into disaster, the Church should, at the very least, be about the business of making certain that the souls are prepared when the day of judgement dawns. He sees himself as woefully inadequate for the job at hand, but attempts to fulfill what has been required of him at all costs. All efforts of the Church should be bent to the desired end, including endeavouring to direct the people to that which is eternal, and away from temporal distractions.

Not surprisingly, we see that Gregory, in the Register, focuses on a particular temporal distraction, one that he, and the other eleventh-century reformers, sought to extirpate: clerical marriage, or as Gregory often categorizes the problem, uncanonical marriage. As H. E. J. Cowdrey comments, it is important to note that Gregory's letters regarding clerical marriage are sent mostly to German or Italian audiences, and that most are sent before the first excommunication and deposition of Henry IV.[28] The conclusions to be drawn from those details may point to a less than purely pastoral concern for righteousness, but certainly no less a concern for proper control of actions. That said, if Gregory VII's motivations are derived from a pastoral concern for righteousness, it is rooted in a desire for purity, which is directly related to temporal pleasure. Gregory VII, Damian, and the other reformers noted that the carnal or familial pleasures of the married clergy distracted them from their eternal calling.

We see these concerns at the end of an 18 November 1074 letter to Archbishop Anno of Cologne; a letter that deals mostly with the attempt to settle a dispute between Bishop Benno II and Abbot Werner of Corvey. Gregory reminds Anno to continue to admonish his 'priests, deacons, and subdeacons to live chastely' and buttresses this reminder with a comment from the *Moralia* about the importance and value of chastity.[29] A letter to Dukes Rudolf of Swabia and Berthold of Carinthia, urging them to take immediate steps against simony and clerical unchastity, on 11 January 1075, unpacks the concern:

> Qui dum nihil aliud nisi gloriam et voluptates seculi querunt, sine sua et populi confusione vivere nequeunt, quoniam in malefactis prava sectantes desideria et suę auctoritatis iura per culpam ligant et aliis peccandi per exemplum frena relaxant.

[28] Cowdrey, 'Pope Gregory VII and the Chastity of the Clergy', pp. 271–72.

[29] Gregory VII, *The Register*, trans. by Cowdrey, p. 116.

> [When they seek nothing other than the glory and pleasures of the world, they cannot but live to their own and other people's confusion; for those who in evil deeds follow base desires both bind through their guilt the rights of their own authority and relax for others through their example the reins of sinning.][30]

The concern is twofold: the focus on this-worldly pleasure and glory not only erects impediments to a focus on the actual task at hand for those priests and others, but also creates confusion for the laity. They see the priests with wives or concubines, knowing that such behaviour is unacceptable, and rationalize that if the priests can so blatantly engage in sinful behaviour, without any seeming condemnation or judgement, then they too can engage in sinful behaviour. How can the clergy preach about a focus on eternal pleasures, when they are so regularly engaging in temporal pleasures?

For Gregory, the focus of the clergy should be on, at the very least, working for the salvation of the people; that in the midst of the crumbling world the people need to know that their religious leaders are directing them correctly, and without hypocrisy. In fact, this reinforces a belief held by certain segments of the laity, most notably the Patarenes of Milan, who strongly supported a more rigorously righteous clergy, clergy who lived as they ought, and who would demand such proper living from all under their care.[31] Gregory, throughout his papacy, argued that the religious leaders must continually demand such righteousness of the laity because they were responsible for those under their care at the time of judgement. Gregory's regular use of Jeremiah 48. 10 in the Register, 'cursed is the man who withholds his sword from the blood' (NRSV), and Gregory I's interpretation, found in the *Regula Pastoralis*, of that passage, 'meaning one who holds back the word of preaching from the rebuking of carnal men',[32] is a direct command for religious leaders to at least make the attempt to extirpate sin.[33] What differentiates Gregory from many in the Middle Ages is his desire and ability to act in innovative ways to extirpate those sins which focused on temporal pleasure.

[30] Gregors VII, *Das Register*, ed. by Caspar, II.1, 183; Gregory VII, *The Register*, trans. by Cowdrey, p. 135.

[31] For a thorough overview of the important relationship between Gregory and the Patarenes, see Cowdrey, 'The Papacy, the Patarenes and the Church of Milan'.

[32] Pope Gregory I, *Liber Regula pastoralis*, trans. by Barmby, pp. 97–98.

[33] Gregory references Jeremiah 48. 10 on nine occasions in the Register, three of these references are supported by Gregory I's commentary on the passage.

In a 2 January 1079 letter to Abbot Hugh of Cluny, reproving him for admitting Duke Hugh of Burgundy to profession at the abbey without the Duke providing for the welfare of his subjects, Gregory states, rather baldly, that 'the shepherds flee as do the dogs that defend the flocks; wolves and robbers invade Christ's sheep while no one challenges them'.[34] The responsibility to insure that the people know what righteousness is and what is sinful is clear, and Gregory laments that this distinction must be stated with great clarity and has not been.

Gregory attempts to make clear that these demands are not of his own devising, that the seemingly innovative castigation of the canonical abuses, especially clerical marriage and, later, lay investiture, derives from God and the Church Fathers. In a 29 March 1075 letter to Archbishop Anno II of Cologne, Gregory argues 'that we do not fashion these orders by our own whim, but by the compulsion of our office we make public binding laws of the ancient fathers which are established through the preaching of the Holy Spirit'.[35] As an aside, Gregory, and this is not uncommon in the Register, provided himself some cover, in the very same letter, for his own bluntly honest pronouncement of new laws, noting that 'the Roman church has always been permitted, and always will be permitted against newly growing transgressions to provide new decrees and remedies'.[36]

Regarding the differentiation between the world above and this world, between the eternal and the temporal, Gregory comments on a number of different occasions how to proceed. For example, in a 17 April 1075 pastoral letter to the people of Bohemia, Gregory encourages the people to 'flee carnal desires; raise up your minds to the heavenly and everlasting joys of the heavenly country'.[37] In a 15 December 1078 pastoral letter to King Olaf III of Norway, Gregory states:

[34] Gregory VII, *The Register*, trans. by Cowdrey, p. 299. Gregory VII, *Das Register*, ed. by Caspar, II.2, 423: 'Fugiunt pastores fugiunt et canes, gregum defensores, invadunt oves Christi nullo contradicente lupi latrones'.

[35] Gregory VII, *The Register*, trans. by Cowdrey, p. 161. Gregory VII, *Das Register*, ed. by Caspar, II.1, 223: 'quia precepta hęc non de nostro sensu exculpimus, sed antiquorum patrum sanctiones Spiritu sancto predictante prolatas officii nostri necessitate in medium propalamus'.

[36] Gregory VII, *The Register*, trans. by Cowdrey, p. 161. Gregory VII, *Das Register*, ed. by Caspar, II.1, 224: 'quamquam huic sanctę Romanę ecclesię semper licuit semperque licebit contra noviter increscentes excessus nova quoque decreta atque remedia procurare'.

[37] Gregory VII, *The Register*, trans. by Cowdrey, p. 167. Gregory VII, *Das Register*, ed. by Caspar, II.1, 233: 'carnalia desideria fugite, ad cęlestia et semper duratura patriæ cęlestis gaudia mentes erigite'.

> Sit cursus vester fides amor et desiderium sit iter vestrum mundi gloriam assidue meditari esse caducam et ideo cum amaritudine potius quam delectatione tenendam.
>
> [Let your course be faith, love, and desire; let your way be constantly to reflect that the glory of the world is fading and so to be possessed with distaste rather than with delight.][38]

He then encourages him to help the oppressed, to defend and protect widows and orphans, and to love and defend righteousness.

> His nanque vestigiis hoc thesauro his opibus de terreno ad cęleste regnum, de fluxo et fragili ad certum et perenne gaudium, de caduca et transitoria ad æternam et semper mansuram pervenitur gloriam.
>
> [For by these steps, by this treasure, by these resources lies the way from an earthly to a heavenly kingdom, from a fleeting and fragile joy to one that is sure and eternal, from a fading and passing glory to one that is eternal and ever abiding.][39]

A 1079 pastoral letter to King Harold Hein of Denmark reinforces the fleeting joys of earthly life,[40] as does a letter to Queen Matilda of England, wherein he asks, 'for what gold, what gems, what precious things of this world, are more to be looked for by me from you than a chaste life, the distribution of your goods to the poor, and love of God and your neighbors?'.[41]

Finally, in Pope Gregory VII's most famous letter, the second letter to Bishop Hermann of Metz, 15 March 1081, wherein he provides his most detailed argument in support of papal prerogatives, Gregory ties his call for a focus on eternal things to his argument against secular authority:

> Scimus enim, quia mundana gloria et secularis cura eos permaxime, qui presunt, ad elationem trahere solet, qua semper neglecta humilitate propriam querendo gloriam fratribus cupiant preminere.

[38] Gregory VII, *Das Register*, ed. by Caspar, II.2, 417; Gregory VII, *The Register*, trans. by Cowdrey, p. 294.

[39] Gregory VII, *Das Register*, ed. by Caspar, II.2, 417; Gregory VII, *The Register*, trans. by Cowdrey, p. 294.

[40] Gregory VII, *The Register*, trans. by Cowdrey, p. 329. Gregory VII, *Das Register*, ed. by Caspar, II.2, 465.

[41] Gregory VII, *The Register*, trans. by Cowdrey, p. 358. Gregory VII, *Das Register*, ed. by Caspar, II.2, 507: 'Quod enim aurum, quę gemme, quę mundi huius pretiosa mihi a te magis sunt expectanda, quam vita casta, rerum tuarum in pauperes distributio, Dei et proximi dilectio?'.

> [For we know that worldly glory and secular care are prone most particularly to draw those who rule into a swelling up by which, putting away humility, they always by seeking their own glory desire to tower above their brothers.][42]

Pope Gregory VII, throughout his papacy, regularly, and with great fervour, attempted to focus on the eternal as opposed to the temporal. These are, of course, standard tropes, a common refrain from a medieval religious figure, but Gregory was zealously consistent on this issue, and this zeal had decisive implications for his entire pontificate. Additionally, it is Gregory's position as pope that gives his ideological agenda an unrivaled platform to be turned into actual Church policy. Gregory attempted to show all Christians that the focus on the temporary pleasurable gain would lead them astray, and that if they focused on satisfying their temporal desires, either for sensual pleasures or the pleasure of temporal power and authority, the Church and the world would fall into utter ruin.

Gregory's reasoning about his concern regarding temporal and eternal pleasures is revealed in everything from the issue of clerical chastity to condemnations of secular authorities regarding their proper role in the protection of the people.[43] Throughout his papacy, Gregory maintained the clear understanding that anything that distracted from living out God's commands was contrary to righteousness and added to the world's deterioration and ultimately to final condemnation, and should therefore be shunned or cast aside, even something as seemingly inconsequential as leeks and onions.

[42] Gregory VII, *Das Register*, ed. by Caspar, II.2, 558; Gregory VII, *The Register*, trans. by Cowdrey, p. 393.

[43] This concern is most explicitly argued in his second letter to Bishop Hermann of Metz in 1081, wherein Gregory argued, most strenuously and at great length, that secular rulers, because they focused only on the temporal, simply could not do what was most necessary for the people, and thus Gregory, or any pope, was justified in excommunicating and deposing a king or emperor, as Gregory had done for the second time in 1080, should they not obey the dictates of the Church. Only a secular ruler following the orders of the Church, because it was the eternal institution, allowed them the ability to act righteously. See Gregory VII, *The Register*, trans. by Cowdrey, pp. 387–95.

Works Cited

Primary Sources

Çelebi, Evliya, *Seyâhatnâme*, trans. by Joseph von Hammer as *Narrative of Travels in Europe, Asia, and Africa in the Seventeenth Century* (London: W. Nicole, 1848)

Chaucer, Geoffrey, *The Canterbury Tales*, Project Gutenberg Etext of The Canterbury Tales and Other Poems, prepared by Donal O'Danachair, 2000, <http://www.gutenberg.org/cache/epub/2383/pg2383.html>

Damian, Peter, *Die Briefe des Petrus Damiani*, ed. by Karl Reindel, vol. iv, MGH Die Briefe der deutschen Kaiserzeit, 4 (Berlin: Monumenta Germaniae Historica, 1993)

——, *The Letters of Peter Damian, 91–120*, trans. by Owen J. Blum and Irven M. Resnick, The Fathers of the Church, Medieval Continuations, 5 (Washington, DC: Catholic University of America Press, 1998)

——, *The Letters of Peter Damian, 151–180*, trans. by Owen J. Blum and Irven M. Resnick, The Fathers of the Church, Medieval Continuation, 1 (Washington, DC: Catholic University of America Press, 2005)

Pope Gregory I, *Liber Regula pastoralis*, trans. by James Barmby (Charles River Editors), <http://www.newadvent.org/fathers/3601.htm>

Pope Gregory I, *Moralia in Iob*, ed. by M. Adriaen, CCSL, 143 (Turnhout: Brepols, 1979)

Gregory VII, *Das Register Gregors VII*, ed. by Erich Caspar, MGH Epistolae selectae, 2, 2 vols (Berlin: Monumenta Germaniae Historica, 1920–23)

——, *The Register of Pope Gregory VII, 1073–1085*, trans. by H. E. J. Cowdrey, (Oxford: Oxford University Press, 2002)

Imperial Lives and Letters of the Eleventh Century, trans. by Theodore E. Mommsen and Karl F. Morrison (New York: Columbia University Press, 2000)

The Papal Reform of the Eleventh Century: Lives of Pope Leo IX and Pope Gregory VII, ed. by Ian S. Robinson (Manchester: Manchester University Press, 2004)

Sahih Bukhari (Complete: 1–97), <https://archive.org/stream/SahihBukhariComplete/Sahih%20Bukhari%20(Complete)_djvu.txt>

Secondary Works

Blumenthal, Uta-Renate, *The Investiture Controversy: Church and Monarchy from the Ninth to the Twelfth Century* (Philadelphia: University of Pennsylvania Press, 1988)

Cowdrey, H. E. J., 'The Papacy, the Patarenes and the Church of Milan', *Transactions of the Royal Historical Society*, 5th Ser., 18 (1968), 25–48

——, *Pope Gregory VII, 1073–1085* (Oxford: Clarendon Press, 1998)

——, 'Pope Gregory VII and the Chastity of the Clergy', in *Medieval Purity and Piety: Essays on Medieval Clerical Celibacy and Religious Reform*, ed. by Michael Frassetto (New York: Garland, 1998), pp. 269–302

Cushing, Kathleen G., *Reform and the Papacy in the Eleventh Century: Spirituality and Social Change* (Manchester: Manchester University Press, 2005)

Frassetto, Michael, ed., *Medieval Purity and Piety: Essays on Medieval Clerical Celibacy and Religious Reform* (New York: Garland, 1998)
Glasspoole, H. G., *The History of Cultivated Vegetables: The Onion* (London: Hardwicke's Science Gossip, 1874)
Hedrick, U. P., *Sturtevant's Edible Plants of the World* (New York: Dover, 1972)
Hyams, E., *Plants in the Service of Man: 10,000 Years of Domestication* (London: Dent, 1971)
Kaske, R. E., 'The Summoner's Garleek, Oynons, and Eek Lekes', *Modern Language Notes*, 74.6 (June 1959), 481–84
Kiple, Kenneth, *A Moveable Feast: Ten Millennia of Food Globalization* (Cambridge: Cambridge University Press, 2007)
Kiple, Kenneth F., and Kriehild Coneè Ornelas, eds, *The Cambridge World History of Food* (Cambridge: Cambridge University Press, 2000)
Kneepkens, C. H., 'There Is More in a Biblical Quotation than Meets the Eye: On Peter the Venerable's Letter of Consolation to Heloise', in *Media Latinitas: A Collection of Essays to Mark the Occasion of the Retirement of L.J. Engels* (Turnhout: Brepols, 1996), pp. 89–100
Lohmer, Christian, 'Ausgewählte Aspekte der mittelalterlichen Ernährung für Mönche, untersucht am Beispiel der monastischen Bestimmungen des Petrus Damiani', *Aktuelle Ernährungsmedizin*, 13 (1988), pp. 179–82
Mauron, J., 'Food, Mood, and Health: The Medieval Outlook', *International Journal for Vitamin and Nutrition Research*, 29 (Supplement 1986), 9–26
Miller, Maureen C., 'The Crisis in the Investiture Crisis Narrative', *History Compass*, 7.6 (2009), 1570–80
Stroll, Mary, *Popes and Antipopes: The Politics of Eleventh-Century Church Reform* (Leiden: Brill, 2012)
Wilson, Eddie W., 'The Onion in Folk Belief', *Western Folklore*, 12. (1953), 94–104
Wood, Chauncey, 'The Sources of Chaucer's Summoner's "Garleek, Oynons, and Eke Lekes"', *Chaucer Review*, 5.3 (Winter 1971), 240–44
Zohary, Daniel, and Maria Hopf, *Domestication of Plants in the Old World* (Oxford: Clarendon Press, 1988)

Intoxication and the Song of Songs: Bernard of Clairvaux and the Rediscovery of Origen in the Twelfth Century

Constant J. Mews

To modern readers, the opening of the Song of Songs appears to celebrate erotic love in a wonderfully physical and sensous way: 'Let him kiss me with the kisses of his mouth, because your breasts are better than wine', rendered in the Latin Vulgate as 'Osculetur me osculo oris sui, quia meliora sunt ubera tua vino'. In a world of suffering, what greater celebration could there be of a moment of long anticipated pleasure, the fullness of union between lover and beloved? The common perception of medieval Christian reading of the Song of Songs, however, tends to assume that their exegesis was always allegorical, in the way they read its celebration of love as not about pleasure in our sense of the term, but in an allegorical sense as a celebration of the mutual love of Christ and the Church. This blanket generalization of the 'medieval' reading of the Song as fundamentally hostile to physical pleasure is inadequate for several reasons, not least because it fails to acknowledge the complexity of competing interpretations of the Song within the Latin Christian tradition, in particular its evolution in the twelfth century. There have been some significant studies of this exegetical tradition, notably by Ann Matter, in speaking about a shift in the twelfth century away from an allegorical to a tropological or moral reading of its text.[1] Of particular importance in promoting this shift is Bernard of

[1] Matter, *The Voice of my Beloved*. See also Ohly, *Hohelied-Studien* and Astell, *The Song of Songs in the Middle Ages*, helpful on the later medieval period. Denys Turner's important study,

Constant J. Mews (constant.mews@monash.edu) is director of the Centre for Religious Studies, School of Philosophical, Historical & International Studies, Monash University, Australia.

Pleasure in the Middle Ages, ed. by Naama Cohen-Hanegbi and Piroska Nagy, IMR 24 (Turnhout: Brepols, 2018), pp. 329–352 BREPOLS PUBLISHERS 10.1484/M.IMR-EB.5.113473

Clairvaux (1090–1153), who initiated a project of composing sermons on each of its verses. Because Bernard never got beyond the first two chapters of the Song, this project would subsequently be continued by two other Cistercians, Gilbert of Hoyland (d. 1172) and John of Ford (d. 1214).[2] The highly personal reading of the Song, initiated by Bernard, continues to attract attention, not just within studies of Christian mysticism, but within the perspective of comparative theology, as comparable to devotional writing within Hinduism. Poetic writing about desire for future pleasure cans also be about the journey of love in the experience of darkness.[3]

In this paper, I wish to examine the multiplicity of potential readings of the Song in the medieval period, in order to better appreciate why the interpretation offered by Bernard of Clairvaux was so important in shaping subsequent understanding of the Song of Songs as about the mystical journey of the soul. I would argue (*pace* Jean Leclercq) that there was no single monastic theology in the medieval period.[4] I would take further, however, Leclercq's important observations of Bernard as a writer who recovered and developed perspectives initially raised in the third century by Origen, a figure who became so controversial by the late fourth century that most of his writings would survive not in Greek, but through the translations of his great admirer in the fourth century, Rufinus.[5] While neither Jerome nor Augustine wrote commentaries on the

Eros and Allegory, focuses more on the later medieval period, exploring in particular the contribution of Dionysius the Areopagite, whose reflection on apophatic discourse only starts to become influential in the thirteenth century. For a helpful anthology of translations of excerpts of patristic and medieval commentaries on the entire text of the Song, see *The Song of Songs*, ed. by Norris.

[2] Bernard's *Sermones in Cantica* are edited in vols I–II of *Sancti Bernardi Opera* [*SBO*], ed. by Leclercq, Talbot, and Rochais; those of Gilbert of Hoyland in *PL*, CLXXXIV, cols 11–298, and of John of Ford, *Sermones super extremam partem Cantici Canticorum*, ed. by Mikkers and Costello.

[3] Clooney, *His Hiding Place Is Darkness*. Clooney compares the exposition of Bernard, Gilbert and John of Ford and a Hindu devotional text, *Holy Word of Mouth* (*Tiruvaymoli*).

[4] The notion that Bernard embodied monastic theology as a contemplative, more personal mode of reflection, in contrast to the analytic emphasis of scholasticism, was put forward by Leclercq, *L'Amour des lettres et le désir de Dieu* (trans. by Misrahi as *The Love of Learning and the Desire for God*).

[5] On the textual transmission of Origen's writings in the Latin West and the transformation that took place in the twelfth century, see Leclercq, 'Origène au XIIe siècle'. For the translation by Rufinus, see Origen, *Commentarium in Canticum Canticorum*, ed. by Baehrens, pp. 61–241, and Origen, *Homélies sur le Cantique des Cantiques*, ed. by Rousseau, pp. 46–49

Song of Songs, Gregory the Great played an important role in keeping alive the perspectives of Origen in a commentary that survives only in relation to the first eight verses of the Song of Songs. Bernard of Clairvaux would find his voice by continuing what he saw as Gregory's unfinished project. For Bernard, the mystical kiss, better than wine, became a statement of imagined desire, escaping the constraints of suffering in this world by looking forward to a moment of ecstasy and intoxication in the world to come. Origen helped Bernard recover the personal dimension of the Song of Songs as first of all about longing of the soul and its capacity to transcend the world of sin, through the magnitude of love.

The opening lines of chapter 5 of the Song of Songs provide what may seem for us a particularly evocative invitation to pleasure: 'comedi favum cum melle meo, bibi vinum meum cum lacte meo; comedite amici, bibite et inebriamini, carissimi' ('I have eaten the honeycomb with my honey, I have drunk my wine with my milk: eat, O friends, and drink, and be inebriated, my dearly beloved') — the final phrase of which is rendered in the Jerusalem Bible simply as 'drink deep, dearest friends'.[6] The Latin reading of Psalm 22. 5, often rendered in the Hebrew version of Psalm 23. 5 as 'My cup brims over' or 'My cup is overflowing', is penetrated by imagery of intoxication: 'calix meus inebrians' ('which inebriateth me', according to the Douay version).[7] This imagery of an intoxicating cup pervades Latin Christian liturgical understanding of the Last Supper, celebrated every time the priest drank from the cup. The exclamation of the bride in the Song of Songs (Canticles 2. 4), 'introduxit me in cellam vinariam, ordinavit me in caritatem' ('He brought me into the cellar of wine, he set in order charity in me'), similarly foreshadows the close connection between inebriation and love.

The spiritualizing emphasis of medieval exegetes to the celebration of conviviality in scripture is evident, not just from its reading of the Song of Songs, but from the way it avoids those verses that seem to celebrate the enjoyment of food and drink. Thus Psalm 103. 14 ('et vinum laetificat cor hominis'; 'And that wine may cheer the heart of man') was never a verse that provoked significant patristic response, and would not be mentioned once by Bernard of Clairvaux.

(on the manuscript transmission). The brief *Expositio sancti Hieronimi presbiteri in libro Cantici canticorum* is a summary of Aponius, a late fifth-century follower of Origen, ed. by de Vregille and Neyrand, pp. 315–90.

[6] English translations of the Vulgate given here are those of the Douay-Rheims (1899) Bible, unless otherwise indicated.

[7] *Biblia sacra*, ed. by Fischer and others, *Psalmi iuxta LXX* and *Psalmi iuxta Hebreos*, pp. 794–95.

Within the Platonizing framework of scriptural interpretation initiated by Origen of Alexandria, and taken over from the Jewish Alexandrian exegesis of Philo, there was always a tendency to privilege the role of the soul giving life to the mind over life to the body. Scriptural references to intoxication tended to be moralistic when interpreted physically, as when Jeremiah chides Israel (Jeremiah 25. 27): 'et dices ad eos haec dicit Dominus exercituum Deus Israhel bibite et inebriamini et vomite et cadite neque surgatis a facie gladii quem ego mittam inter vos' ('And thou shalt say to them: Thus saith the Lord of hosts the God of Israel: Drink ye, and be drunken, and vomit: and fall, and rise no more, because of the sword, which I shall send among you'). St Paul famously warned against drunkenness (Ephesians 5. 18): 'et nolite inebriari vino in quo est luxuria sed implemini Spiritu' ('And be not drunk with wine, wherein is luxury; but be ye filled with the holy Spirit'), contrasting physical intoxication with spiritual inspiration. These passages combined to influence the way the Song of Songs was understood in a Christian context.

Allegory and Tropology among the Fathers

Bernard explains his preference for moral over allegorical exegesis in a sermon on the opening of the Song: 'I rush for us to go through the shady and dark wood of allegories to the clarity of moral senses in the journey as if of a single day'.[8] He was here expanding upon a comment that Gregory the Great had made in the opening of his incomplete commentary on the Song of Songs about allegory as making shady the mountain of the Lord.[9] Gregory was here using allegory in the way that it had been used by Origen, as a device not so much for teaching doctrine as for lifting the soul to God: 'Hence in this book, written about the Song of Songs, words of physical love are placed so that a soul cooled through words of habit may be aroused through words of the love that is

[8] Bernard of Clairvaux, *Sermo* 16.1, ed. by Leclercq, Talbot, and Rochais, *SBO*, I, 89: 'Putavi, fateor, unum ad hoc sermonem sufficere, silvamque istam umbrosam latebrosamque allegoriarum pertransire nos cito, et ad planitiem moralium sensuum itinere diei quasi unius pervenire; sed secus contigit Biduum quippe iam in eo expendimus, et adhuc restat via'. See also *Sermo* 17.8, ed. by Leclercq, Talbot, and Rochais, *SBO*, I, 102: 'Transivimus allegoriarum umbras; ventum est ad indaganda moralia'.

[9] Gregory the Great, *Expositio in Canticum Canticorum*, 5, ed. by Verbraken, p. 5: 'De quo monte per prophetam dicitur: deus a libano ueniet et sanctus de monte umbroso et condenso iste mons et condensus est per sententias et umbrosus per allegorias'.

below to the love that is above'.[10] Origen never systematized his teaching about different senses of scripture, preferring to speak of both the literal or historical meaning and the allegorical or mystical sense of scripture, but incorporated into the letter emphasis on its moral sense. Gregory the Great would systematize the notion that there were three layers of meaning to scripture, namely historical, allegorical, and moral, in his *Moralia in Job*, the title of which asserts the importance he gives to Job as offering not just an allegory of Christ, but a moral exemplar, from whose encounter with suffering we can all benefit.[11] In the case of the Song of Songs, the bride also offers not just an allegorical meaning, namely the Church, but the moral example of a soul.

The notion that all medieval exegesis was based on a fourfold interpretation of scripture, namely historical (about events), allegorical (about belief), tropological or moral (about behaviour), and anagogical (about heavenly realities), is based on a misunderstanding. This perspective was first formulated in the early fifth century by Eucherius of Lyons and John Cassian, drawing on Jerome and Evagrius as authority for introducing the Greek terms *tropologia* and *anagoge* into Latin.[12] In the early eighth century Bede repeated Cassian's teaching when explaining the distinction between these various meanings by giving the example of Jerusalem as allegorically the Church, tropologically the soul, and anagogically the heavenly city.[13] The fourfold theory, however, as Henri de Lubac

[10] Gregory the Great, *Expositio in Canticum Canticorum*, 3, ed. by Verbraken, p. 4: 'Hinc est enim, quod in hoc libro, qui in canticis canticorum conscriptus est, amoris quasi corporei uerba ponuntur: ut a torpore suo anima per sermones suae consuetudinis refricata recalescat et per uerba amoris, qui infra est, excitetur ad amorem, qui supra est'.

[11] Gregory the Great, *Moralia in Job*, *Epist. ad Leandrum*, ed. by Adriaen, p. 4: 'Sciendum uero est, quod quaedam historica expositione transcurrimus et per allegoriam quaedam typica inuestigatione perscrutamur, quaedam per sola allegoricae moralitatis instrumenta discutimus, nonnulla autem per cuncta simul sollicitius exquirentes tripliciter indagamus'. Cf. Origen, *In Genesim homiliae*, 2.6, trans. by Rufinus, ed. by Baehrens, p. 36; Origen, *In Leviticum homiliae*, 5.5, trans. by Rufinus, ed. by Baehrens, p. 344; cf. Ambrose, *Expositio evangelii secundum Lucam*, 3.20, ed. by Adriaen, p. 86. This passage of Gregory's letter to Leander, prefacing the book of Job, is translated as *Registrum* 5.53a in Gregory the Great, *The Letters*, trans. by Martyn, p. 382.

[12] Cassian, *Conlationes*, 14.8, ed. by Petschenig, p. 405; see also Eucherius of Lyons, *Formulae spiritualis intelligentiae*, ed. by Mandolfo, p. 4.

[13] Bede, *In Cantica canticorum*, 3.4, ed. by Hurst, p. 260: 'Ut enim unum demus exemplum, psalmista dicit: *Lauda Hierusalem dominum*, quod iuxta litteram quidem ciues urbis ipsius in qua templum Dei erat ad laudes ei dicendas hortatur; at uero iuxta allegoriam Hierusalem ecclesia Christi est toto orbe diffusa; item iuxta tropologiam, id est moralem sensum, anima

acknowledges in his classic study of the subject, always competed with a more popular threefold model, initiated by Origen and given classical formulation by Gregory the Great.[14] Augustine followed Ambrose in confining himself to the literal and allegorical meanings of scripture, but focused more on its teaching as about Adam's fall, the redeeming work of Christ, and the *Ecclesia*, present in germ throughout history as the people of God. Jerome gave greater emphasis to 'the Hebrew truth', but also expounded (through the influence of Evagrius) not just its tropological (or moral) meaning, but what he calls its highest, or anagogical meaning.[15] Not the least original aspect of the exegesis of Gregory the Great was to quietly drop the anagogical or doctrinal sense and reassert the superiority of the moral sense of scripture.[16] Before Gregory, the one exegete to comment both on Job and the Song of Songs had been Julian of Eclanum, a married bishop who had accused Augustine of being excessively Manichaean in his denigration of human sexuality.[17] Where Augustine attributed all growth in virtue to divine grace, Gregory the Great reasserted the importance of scriptural models as guides for a moral life, without going as far as Julian of Eclanum, perhaps the most articulate of all the supporters of Pelagius.

quaeque sancta Hierusalem recte uocatur; item iuxta anagogen, id est intellegentiam ad superiora ducentem, Hierusalem habitatio est patriae caelestis quae ex angelis sanctis et hominibus constat'. Cassian invokes the fourfold model in *Conlationes*, 14.8, ed. by Petschenig, pp. 404–05.

[14] De Lubac, *Exégèse médiévale*, translated into English as *Medieval Exegesis*, by Sebanc (vol. I) and by Macierowski (vols II–III). De Lubac comments on this division, *Exégèse médiévale*, I, 139–69, noting on p. 158 that the threefold theory was the more commonly cited. He notes how Origen prefers the threefold model on pp. 201–02.

[15] Jerome reformulates Origen's threefold path of exegesis in *Commentiaria in Ezekielem*, 5.16, ed. by Glorie, p. 195, placing the mystical mode above the tropological: 'legimus in prouerbiis: tu autem describe ea tripliciter, ut respondeas sermones ueritatis qui proponuntur tibi, et iubetur nobis ut eloquia ueritatis, id est scripturas sanctas, intellegamus tripliciter: primum, iuxta litteram; secundo, medie, per tropologiam; tertio, sublimius, ut mystica quaeque cognoscamus'.

[16] The literature on Gregory the Great is vast. A helpful introduction to his thought is still Straw, *Gregory the Great*. See also the essays in Neil and Dal Santo, *A Companion to Gregory the Great*, including on his influence, Mews and Renkin, 'The Legacy of Gregory the Great in the Latin West'.

[17] A single manuscript survives of Julian's *Expositio in Job*, ed. by De Coninck. Most of his other writings are only known from excerpts, such as through Augustine, *Contra duas epistolas Pelagianorum*, 1.15.31, ed. by Urba and Zycha, p. 448: 'Ad hoc respondemus motum genitalium, id est ipsam uirilitatem sine qua non potest esse commixtio, a deo dicimus institutam, ut nihil haberet pudendum' (To this we reply that movement of the genitals, namely virility itself, without which there cannot be intercourse, is instituted by God).

Gregory's interest in a moral reading of the Song of Songs was shaped by Origen's interpretation of the bride as *Ecclesia vel anima*.[18] Fully familiar with philosophical discussion of love, he reads the Song of Songs as providing a rich analysis of the longing and desire of the soul as much as of the Church. Origen sees the Song as articulating contemplative enquiry into wisdom, rivalling the philosophical schools.[19] More specifically, he compares the bride to the disciple of Jesus, whom he identifies as Mary (of Bethany), who used ointment on the feet of Jesus, wiping them with her hair.[20] Gregory's empathy for Origen is all the more remarkable given the condemnation of his teaching at the Council of Jerusalem in 400, reasserted at the Second Council of Constantinople in 553. Origen had been consistently (although inaccurately) accused of holding heretical views about the pre-existence of souls and universal redemption.[21] Jerome, once an admirer of Origen and a friend of Rufinus, similarly became much more cautious in his attitudes. The so-called Gelasian Decree declared that only certain works of Origen, acceptable to Jerome, could be accepted as orthodox, condemning his other writings.[22] Only in the twelfth century would these comments be put aside, and Origen's significance as an exegete be fully realized.

Ambrose frequently mentioned Origen's phrase *Ecclesia vel anima*, but interpreted the soul as virginal, as a way of emphasizing its purity. Augustine never repeats Origen's phrase, preferring to interpret the bride simply as the Church.[23]

[18] For the phrase *Ecclesia uel anima*, see Origen, *Commentarium in Canticum Canticorum*, 2, 3, ed. by Baehrens, pp. 167, 185, 190, 202. On Origen's reading of the Song, see Matter, *The Voice of my Beloved*, pp. 25–31.

[19] Origen, *Commentarium in Canticum Canticorum*, Prol., ed. by Baehrens, pp. 78–79; see also *Commentarium in Canticum Canticorum*, 1, 2, 4, ed. by Baehrens, pp. 100, 119–20, 141, 148, 240.

[20] Origen, *Commentarium in Canticum Canticorum*, 2, ed. by Baehrens, p. 166: 'Quid ergo interest, utrum in Cantico canticorum sponsa "perunguat unguento" sponsum an in Evangelio discipula magistrum et Maria Christum sperans, ut diximus, redire ad se ex hoc "unguento odorem" Verbi et fraglantiam Christi, ut et ipsa dicat: "bonus odor sumus Deo"?'.

[21] See for example Augustine, *De civitate Dei*, 11.23, ed. by Dombart and Kalb, p. 342. In seeking to promote the importance of Origen in the Latin West, de Lubac passes over Augustine's reserve about Origen, emphasizing those authors who spoke more highly of his influence, *Exégèse médiévale*, I, 213–14.

[22] *Decretum Gelasianum*, widely reprinted, including in the *Sic et Non* of Peter Abelard, ed. by Boyer and McKeon, p. 107: 'Item Origenis nonnulla opuscula, quae vir beatissimus Ieronimus non repudiat, legenda suscipimus. Reliqua autem omnia cum auctore suo dicimus esse renuenda'.

[23] Asiedu, 'The Song of Songs and the Ascent of the Soul'.

He never quotes its opening verse about kissing on the mouth or its injunction (Canticles 5. 1) to eat, drink, and get drunk ('Comedite amici, bibite et inebriamini'). One of its few phrases of which he was fond, 'ordinate me in caritatem' (Canticles 2. 4), Augustine interprets as reflecting the ideal love offered by the City of God, in contrast to human selfishness: 'For love itself is to be loved in an ordered way (*ordinate*), by which what is to be loved is loved well, so that in us is the virtue by which we live well. Thus it seems to me that a brief and true definition of virtue is the order of love, because of which the bride of Christ, the city of God, sings in the holy Song of Songs: "Order in me love" (*ordinate in me caritatem*). Thus with love (*caritas*), namely intimacy and passion (*dilectionis et amoris*), disturbed, the sons of God [cf. Genesis 6. 2] neglected God and loved the daughters of men'.[24] Augustine reads the bride not as an individual soul, but allegorically as the heavenly city. His relatively limited references to the Song consistently emphasize the gulf between physical and spiritual love, and the corruption of the human will. Augustine frequently invokes Psalm 35. 9, 'inebriabuntur ab ubertate domus tuae' ('They shall be inebriated with the plenty of thy house'), but interprets it as about the collective ecstasy of paradise rather than as about individual enjoyment.[25] For Augustine, inebriation referred to the condition of the saints in heaven, not a possibility for souls here and now. His exegesis is overwhelmingly allegorical, not tropological. His ecclesiological reading of the Song, of profound influence in the early medieval period, reflects his own increasing caution about what he perceived as the excessively personal exegesis promoted by Origen, still present in the writing of Ambrose. As a bishop, charged with watching over the Christian community, Augustine feared the social consequences of reading the Song as about individual longing, in the manner of Julian of Eclanum. He preferred to emphasize the greatness of God's love and fallen human nature, rather than the parity of two lovers, implied by the Song.

While Gregory does not doubt that the bride can be understood as *Ecclesia* he was not so troubled by Origen's understanding of it as also the soul. He recognizes that the bride's primary role is to inspire us to a higher love, in the same

[24] Augustine, *De civitate Dei*, 15.25, ed. by Dombart and Kalb, p. 488: 'Nam et amor ipse ordinate amandus est, quo bene amatur quod amandum est, ut sit in nobis uirtus qua uiuitur bene. Vnde mihi uidetur, quod definitio breuis et uera uirtutis ordo est amoris; propter quod in sancto cantico canticorum cantat sponsa Christi, ciuitas dei: *Ordinate in me caritatem*. Huius igitur caritatis, hoc est dilectionis et amoris, ordine perturbato deum filii dei neglexerunt et filias hominum dilexerunt'.

[25] Augustine, *Enarrationes in Psalmos*, 35.14, ed. by Dekkers and Fraipont, p. 333.

way as Job was a virtuous gentile and an exemplar of Christ. 'For the soul who longs to be purged through love, who seeks to gaze on the vision of her beloved, says, "Let him kiss me with the kiss of his mouth"'.[26] Augustine, always conscious of the corruption of the will, never made such a claim. Gregory frequently picks up the notion of Origen that there is close link with the desire of the Church and that of the soul: 'We speak to this church, to this soul, to this lover, to this one burning in love for her beloved, so that she may grasp great desire, from which she may grasp awareness of his divinity'.[27] Yet while Gregory is more open to the Song's imagery than Augustine, he is still cautious about inebriation. Like Augustine, he never mentions the verse 'Eat, drink, and get drunk', presumably because it runs too far against his view of the passions as to be transcended rather than celebrated. For him, the inebriation recalled in the Song is that of 'knowledge, which intoxicates, the memory of breasts that which inebriates, which recalls knowledge of gifts'.[28]

Gregory connected the bride in the Song of Songs, not just to the Church, but to the figure of Mary Magdalene in his homily (25) on Christ's Resurrection: 'She first sought, therefore, and did not find, she persevered so that she sought, and sought so that it happened that she found, and it happened that her spread out desires grew, and seized the growing things that they had found'.[29] Gregory may well have been familiar with early Christian interpretation of the Song as articulating the voice of Mary Magdalene, attested by the presence of a rubric to Canticles 3. 1, 'on my bed at night I sought him whom my soul loves' ('in cubilo meo in noctibus quaesivi quem diligit anima mea') in two surviving manuscripts of the Vetus Latina version: *Vox Marie Magdalene ad Ecclesiam* ('The

[26] Gregory the Great, *Expositio in Canticum Canticorum*, 18, ed. by Verbraken, p. 21: 'Anima ergo, quae iam per amorem conpungi desiderat, quae iam contemplari uisionem sponsi sui appetit, dicat: *Osculetur me osculo oris sui*'.

[27] Gregory the Great, *Expositio in Canticum Canticorum*, 21, ed. by Verbraken, p. 22: 'Dicamus huic ecclesiae, dicamus huic animae, sic amanti, sic aestuanti in amorem sponsi sui, unde tantum desiderium perceperit, unde notitiam diuinitatis eius apprehenderit'.

[28] Gregory the Great, *Expositio in Canticum Canticorum*, 30, ed. by Verbraken, p. 22: 'Vinum enim est scientia, quae inebriat; memoria uberum, quae debriat, quae ad cognitionem donorum reuocat'.

[29] Gregory the Great, *Homiliae in evangelia*, 25.2, ed. by Etaix, p. 205: 'Quaesivit igitur prius et minime invenit, perseveravit ut quaereret, unde et contingit ut inveniret, actumque est ut desideria dilate crescerent, et crescentia caperent quod invenissent'. See also *Homiliae in evangelia*, 33 on Luke 7. 36–50, ed. by Etaix, pp. 288–98.

Voice of Mary Magdalen to the Church').[30] This linking of Mary Magdalene to the Song may well be influenced by recognition of its imagery in the account of how she searched out the body of Christ in John 20. 1–19.[31] In another homily (33), Gregory dwells at length on Mary as the *peccatrix* described by Luke as kissing and anointing the feet of Jesus (without ever explicitly identify her as the Magdalene), initiating the pattern of emphasizing her interior penitence.[32] Gregory's focus on Mary Magdalene as emblematic of the bride in the Song of Songs derives from his reading of Origen's interpretation of that text as about the soul as much as the Church.

While Bede's influential commentary on the Song of Songs often repeats Origen's phrase, with a slight caution, that the bride is *Ecclesia vel anima fidelis* (or *electa*), the rubrics he applies to the Song introduce the bride first as *Synagoge* and then as *Ecclesia*.[33] In the introduction to his commentary Bede sharply criticizes the otherwise unknown exposition offered by Julian of Eclanum, whom he considers has given unhealthy approval to human sexuality.[34] Against Julian, Bede repeats what Ambrose had said about the virginal quality of the bride. For Bede, inebriation was a purely heavenly state that referred to the future ecstasy of the Church, rather than any form of personal experience.[35] The injunction of Canticles 3. 1 to rejoice and get drunk he sees as about a collective future state: 'For when he said that he had eaten the honeycomb with its honey and drunk wine with its milk, namely that he had collected the saints to increase his heav-

[30] De Bruyne, 'Les Anciennes Versions latines du Cantique des Cantiques'. He edits the Vetus Latina version, found in Salzburg, Stiftsbibliothek Sankt Peter, MS a.IX.16 (s. viii–ix) and Graz, Universitätsbibliothek, Fol. 167 (s. xii), at p. 100, noting that *Magdalene* has been deleted in the Salzburg copy. See the introduction to *Canticum canticorum*, ed. by Schulz-Flügel, pp. 20–24.

[31] Winsor, *A King Is Bound in the Tresses* and Carr, *Erotic Word*, pp. 155–70.

[32] Jansen, *The Making of the Magdalen*, pp. 32–35; Mews, 'Singing the Song of Songs at the Paraclete'.

[33] Bede, *In Canticum canticorum*, 1.2, ed. by Hurst, pp. 217, 220; 3.4 (p. 254); 3.5 (p. 280); 4.6 (pp. 301, 305); 4.7 (p. 318).

[34] Bede, *In Canticum canticorum*, 1.2, ed. by Hurst, p. 190. These excerpts from Julian's *In Canticum canticorum* are edited by De Coninck; cf. p. 398: 'Dicit eundem quamdiu nihil de genitalitatis uoluptate desiderat, quasi ad solius animi moueri arbitrium, et in actibus suis habere iucunditatem, ut perturbationis immunem, ita etiam libertate gaudentem'.

[35] Bede, *In Cantica canticorum*, 3.4, ed. by Hurst, pp. 258–59: 'Vbi intimatum est typice quod litteralis obseruatio legis finem esset acceptura et ea quae in littera uelabatur euangelii gratia reuelanda atque amore spiritali domum esset nuptiarum inebriatura caelestium, hoc est sanctam ecclesiam quam sibi Christus sponsam consecrare dignatus est'.

enly body, soon he turns his face and words to the inhabitants of heaven saying: "Eat, my friends, drink and get drunk, dearest", which is a way of saying in other words: "Congratulate me because I have found the sheep of mine that had been lost"'.[36] Bede's perspective, shaped by that of Augustine, shapes the fundamentally ecclesiological foundation for other exegetes of the Carolingian period and later.[37]

Anselm of Laon and the Song of Songs

The eleventh century witnessed an upsurge in the writing of commentaries on the Song of Songs, very often by monks connected to a reform movement that looked back to the example of Pope Gregory the Great for its inspiration. As Matter has argued, the commentary by Robert of Tombelaine (1010–1080), a monk of Mont St-Michel, picks up on the ecclesiological interpretation of earlier writers, but also picks up on the ideal of monastic perfectionism to promote the vision of the bride as purified Church that had emancipated itself from the impurity of the world.[38] Yet, although this reforming vision initially started within a monastic milieu, by the early twelfth century it would be taken up in a fresh but influential way by a secular master, equally committed to ideals of reform. Relatively little attention has been given to the contribution of Anselm of Laon (d. 1117), celebrated by his students in the twelfth century as a great authority on scripture.[39] In part, this neglect has been provoked by scholarly uncertainty about his literary output. Yet the fact that so many copies survive of his marginal and interlinear glosses on the Song, as well as three continuous commentaries on the Song either attributed to Anselm or linked to his school, highlights his interest in this book of the Bible.[40]

[36] Bede, *In Cantica canticorum*, 3.5, ed. by Hurst, p. 273: 'Cum enim se dixisset fauum cum melle suo comedisse et uinum bibisse cum lacte suo, id est sanctos in caelestis sui corporis augmenta collegisse, mox ad ipsos caeli incolas uultum et uerba conuertit dicens: Comedite amici mei et bibite et inebriamini carissimi, quod est aliis uerbis dicere: Congratulamini mihi quia inueni ouem meam quae perierat'.

[37] Haimo, *Commentarium in Cantica Canticorum*, ed. by Migne.

[38] Robert of Tombelaine, *Commentariorum in Cantica Canticorum*, of which the first part (I.1–11) is printed in *PL*, CL, cols 1361–70, with the remainder attributed to Gregory the Great in *PL*, LXXIX, cols 493–548; see Matter, *The Voice of my Beloved*, pp. 106–11.

[39] On their reputation, see Giraud, *Per verba magistri*, pp. 150–61, and Herman of Tournai, *Les Miracles de sainte Maie de Laon*, ed. by Saint-Denis, pp. 132–34.

[40] Giraud, 'Lectiones magistri Anselmi' (with edition of the A and B prefaces on pp. 195–200), referring to *Enarrationes in Cantica Canticorum*, edited in *PL*, CLXXXII, cols 1187C–1228B (Incipit: *In initiis*), attributed to certain manuscripts to Anselm.

While these glosses have often been dismissed as largely dependent on the Fathers, the critical edition by Mary Dove shows that they combine many extracts from Origen's homilies (not Origen's commentary) on the Song of Songs, Gregory the Great, and Bede with some two hundred glosses not derived from patristic tradition.[41] Suzanne LaVere has persuasively argued that they demonstrate an unusual interest in the role of preaching. In its interpretation of the bride as a purified *Ecclesia*, it combines traditional patristic exegesis with the reforming vision of exegetes like Robert of Tombelaine.[42] Anselm emphasizes education and preaching, as in his own comments on Canticles 2. 12: 'You must not cease preaching for the sake of quietness, because Christ, who was in great quietness with the Father, to an extent interrupted quietness for the sake of preaching'.[43] Although preaching is a theme that Bede mentions within his commentary, Anselm gives it particular emphasis. While maintaining the perspective that the final end of the Song is contemplative, the *Glossa* cites Bede to call the faithful soul to engage in preaching.[44] Anselm's reading of the two cheeks of the bride as preachers (picked up by Gratian in his *Decretum*) has no precedent in patristic tradition.[45] He expands on a comment of Bede on 'ubera tua botris' ('your breasts are likened to clusters of grapes'; Canticles 7. 7), '*breasts*, that is masters temper their teaching according to the capacity of their hearers', by adding: '*grapes* gladdening hearts and making each person sublimely drunk with the richness of the house of God'.[46] This emphasis draws on

[41] *Glossa ordinaria. In Canticum canticorum*, ed. by Dove, p. 47; their number and importance is identified by LaVere, 'From Contemplation to Action'. See also *The Glossa Ordinaria on the Song of Songs*, trans. by Dove, pp. xxi–xxii.

[42] Robert's influence on the *Glossa ordinaria* is noted by Matter, *The Voice of my Beloved*, p. 121 and by Dove, *The Glossa Ordinaria on the Song of Songs*, pp. xx–xxi (noting that Anselm omits many of Robert's comments on corruption in the Church).

[43] *In Cant.* 2.12, *Glossa ordinaria*, 111, ed. by Dove, p. 175 (trans. by Dove, p. 54): 'Pro quiete tua non debes dimittere predicationem, quia Christus qui in magna quiete erat cum patre quietem quodammodo pro predicatione intermisit'. Besides this reference, the opening quotation in LaVere's study, see *In Cant.* 2.1, *Glossa ordinaria*, 1, ed. by Dove, p. 139, a quotation from Bede: 'Quod non potest impleri nisi intermissa quiete qua delectaris ad officium predicationis accingaris'. Also *In Cant.* 2.2, *Glossa ordinaria*, 6, ed. by Dove, p. 175 (from Alcuin): 'et maior est fructus predicationis quam quietis'.

[44] *In Cant.* 3.7, *Glossa ordinaria*, 6, ed. by Dove, p. 211 (from Bede): 'Utrumque lectulum ambiunt fortissimi quia et presentem quietem et pacem ecclesiae predicatores contra incursus tuentur et in eternam patriae celestis requiem quique perfectiores fixa intentione speculantur'.

[45] *In Cant.* 1.9, *Glossa ordinaria*, 136–37, ed. by Dove, p. 121; trans. by Dove, p. 25.

[46] *In Cant.* 7.7, *Glossa ordinaria*, 57, ed. by Dove, p. 364: 'id est magistri qui pro capacitate

an exegetical tradition, mentioned by Bede and going back to Apponius, which compared 'your breasts' to doctors of the Church, because they give 'the milk of instruction to the little ones of Christ'.[47] The comparison prompted Anselm to think of inebriation not simply as the ecstasy of the heavenly Jerusalem, but as a process by which a teacher could intoxicate students with their learning. Anselm draws on elements of patristic tradition to promote the importance of preaching alongside that of contemplation.

There also survive three continuous commentaries on the Song of Songs attributed to Anselm or closely linked to his school.[48] The commentary *In initiis* (A) communicates similar ideas to the briefer comments found in the *Glossa ordinaria*. It proposes that *oculi tui* (Canticles 1. 14) are 'your preachers', educating the faithful by word and example.[49] The term *Surge* (Canticles 3. 2) is taken as another way of saying 'preach'.[50] As in the *Glossa ordinaria*, the inebriation of false teaching (of philosophy) is contrasted with the true inebriation of spiritual teaching.[51] The verse 'Thy navel is like a round bowl never wanting cups' ('umbilicus tuus crater tornatilis numquam indigens poculis'; Canticles 7. 2), an image that Ambrose had interpreted as about completeness of knowledge, is interpreted with a new twist, as about the seedbed of reproduction, in

audientium suam temperant doctrinam et unumquemque ad sublimia ab ubertate domus Dei inebriant et corda exhilarant'.

[47] Bede, *In Cantica canticorum*, 5.7, ed. by Hurst, p. 331: 'Vbera ut saepe dictum est ecclesiae sunt doctores cum lac primae eruditionis paruulis Christi ministrant'.

[48] Stirnemann, 'Où ont été fabriqués les livres de la glose ordinaire dans la première moitié du XIIe siècle', p. 262.

[49] Anselm of Laon, *In initiis*, ed. by Migne, col. 1195CD: '*Oculi tui,* id est praedicatores tui, qui tibi provident ut oculi corpori, erunt *columbarum.* Intransitive dictum est, id est, erunt revera columbae, id est septem virtutes habentes, quae denotantur per septem naturas columbae. Columba enim secus fluenta habitat, ut, viso accipitre, se mergat et evadat; meliora grana eligit, alienos pullos nutrit, rostro non lacerat, felle caret, in cavernis petrae nidificat, gemitum pro cantu habet. Ita praedicatores sancti secus divinae Scripturae fluenta, quibus eorum irrigantur corda, inhabitant, ut eorum munimento ab incursu diabolico evadant. Meliora grana, id est, meliores sententias, scilicet non haereticorum eligunt. Alienos pullos, id est homines, primum a Christo alienatos, qui pulli, id est, filii diaboli fuerant, doctrina sua nutriunt et exemplo'.

[50] Anselm of Laon, *In initiis* [Ct. 3.2], ed. by Migne, col. 1200A: 'Dico, surge, praedica, et praedicatio tua non erit infructuosa'.

[51] Anselm of Laon, *In initiis* [Ct. 5.1], ed. by Migne, col. 1211AB: 'etiam fide et veritate ferventes et alios inebriantes doctrina *cum lacte,* id est cum simplicibus meis qui sunt nutriti lacte, id est doctrina fidei, non alta sentientes, et hos bibi, id est cum delectatione et sine labore mihi incorporavi, vel bibi, quia maturos tales ad beatitudinem assumpsi'.

that married women generate sons for God, and that they are like a drinking vessel, 'inebriating others with the love of God'. The commentary's explanation of 'ubera tua botris' (Canticles 7. 7) as like wine that intoxicates 'just like your teachings' is very similar to that of the *Glossa ordinaria*.[52] Without abandoning the ideal of contemplation, Anselm was urging readers of the Song of Songs to defend the Church and engage in effective preaching. Even though a secular cleric rather than a monk, he imitated their interpretation of the Song of Songs as about ecclesial renewal rather than about the desire of the individual soul.

Bernard of Clairvaux and Monastic Reading of the Song of Songs

The bride was often understood as a purified *Ecclesia*, embodied by the Virgin Mary, in monastic commentaries of the early twelfth century. This is the case with Rupert of Deutz (*c.* 1075 – *c.* 1129) and Honorius Augustodunensis (1080–1154), two monks who both read the Song of Songs as applying to the Virgin Mary as the icon par excellence of a reformed Church.[53] Yet both Rupert and Honorius, like Anselm of Laon, focus on the bride as the ideal Church, rather than in terms of the soul. Even though Anselm of Laon had access to the homilies of Origen on the Song, his use of this text was relatively limited. The next revolution in exegetical approach would only come with Bernard's appreciation of Origen's commentary on the Song.

The importance of Origen to the monks of Clairvaux is evident from the surviving first leaf of a library catalogue compiled in the first half of the twelfth century. After listing manuscripts of the Bible and works of Augustine, it then cites under *Libri Origenis* eight different manuscripts of his writings, followed by its holdings of Hilary, Ambrose, and Jerome.[54] Precisely when Bernard

[52] Anselm of Laon, *In initiis* [Ct. 7.7], ed. by Migne, col. 1221C: 'Sicut enim palma in altum semper fertur, ita fideles isti semper tendunt ad altitudinem virtutum, *et ubera tua*, id est, doctrinae tuae similes sunt *botris*, id est vino, sicut enim vinum, ita doctrinae tuae inebriant'.

[53] Rupert of Deutz, *Commentaria in Canticum Canticorum*, ed. by Haacke; Honorius Augustodunensis, *Expositio in Cantica Canticorum*, ed. by Migne. On Rupert's commentary, see Matter, *The Voice of my Beloved*, pp. 159–63, and on that of Honorius, pp. 58–76.

[54] Edited by Vernet, *La Bibliothèque de l'abbaye de Clairvaux du* XII*^e^ au* XVIII*^e^ siècle*, pp. 34–56, with introduction on pp. 3–16. Only the first folio survives of the catalogue, in large format, copied probably before 1147. The copy of Origen's commentary on the Song (now Troyes, Médiathèque, MS 1412) was copied in the first half of the twelfth century. Leclercq discusses the prominence of Origen in this catalogue in 'Origène au XIIe siècle', p. 428, and the coincidence that Bernard's sermons on the Song of Songs did not go further than the incomplete commentary of Origen on the Song in this copy.

came across the text is not certain. The Clairvaux copy of Origen's commentary on the Song of Songs, from the early twelfth century, does not go beyond Canticles 2. 15, close to where Bernard's own homilies on the Song conclude.[55] It could have been from relatively early in his time at Clairvaux, a community he founded in 1115, after requesting ordination as abbot from William of Champeaux (d. 1121), perhaps the most important disciple of Anselm of Laon. According to William of Saint-Thierry, Bernard became a close intimate of William over the next five years, frequently spending time with him at Châlons, while also inviting William to Clairvaux: 'What more? From that day and from that hour, they became one heart and one soul in the Lord, so much that often one would consider the other as henceforward his guest, and the house of the bishop of Châlons was his own, while Clairvaux became not only the house of the bishop, but through him [Bernard], the whole city of Châlons'.[56] Through his contact with William of Champeaux, it would be surprising if Bernard had not come across the writings of Origen, as also with the commentaries of Anselm of Laon. For Bernard, close reading of the original commentary of Origen provided a liberating experience. Rather than focus on the bride as *Ecclesia*, Bernard examined the Song of Songs for what it had to say about the longing of the soul.

William of Saint-Thierry speaks about how, during a period of convalescence at Clairvaux, he first started to share Bernard's understanding of the Song of Songs in a passage in which he speaks about his exposition of that text *moraliter*, and delivering the voice of experience:

> Itaque tunc disseruit mihi de Cantico canticorum, quantum tempus illud infirmitatis meae permisit, moraliter tantum, intermissis mysteriis Scripturae illius, quia sic volebam, et sic petieram ab eo. Singulisque diebus quaecunque super hoc audiebam, ne mihi effugerent, scripto alligabam, in quantum mihi Deus donabat, et memoria me juvabat. In quo cum benigne et sine invidia exponeret mihi, et communicaret sententias intelligentiae et sensus experientiae suae, et multa docere niteretur inexpertum, quae nonnisi experiendo discuntur, etsi intelligere non poteram adhuc quae apponebantur mihi, plus tamen solito intelligere me faciebat quid ad ea intelligenda deesset mihi.

[55] On Bernard's defence of Origen, see *Sermones de diversis*, Sermo 34, *SBO*, VI.1, 228–33.

[56] William of Saint-Thierry, *Vita prima* I.7, ed. by Migne, cols 245C–246A: 'Quid multa? Ex illa die et ex illa hora facti sunt cor unum et anima una in Domino, in tantum ut saepe alter alterum hospitem deinceps haberet, et propria esset domus Episcopi Clara-Vallis; Clarae-Vallensium vero efficeretur non sola domus Episcopi, sed et per ipsum tota civitas Catalaunensis'.

[Therefore he then expounded to me *morally* about the Song of Songs, in as far as that period of my illness allowed, putting aside the mysteries of that Scripture, because I wanted thus, and thus I requested of him. For whatever I heard on individual days, I put into writing lest they escape from me, as far as God allowed me and memory helped. In which since he expounded to me kindly and without jealousy, and communicated the judgements of intelligence and the meanings of his experience, he strove to teach someone inexpert many things which are only learned by experience; although I could not understand what was being put to me, yet more than normal he made me understand what I lacked to understand those things.][57]

De Lubac rightly observes that Bernard's reading of the Song of Songs was mediated by his particularly personal response to the commentaries of both Gregory the Great and Origen.[58] Verdeyen has suggested that this was the occasion (perhaps in the course of 1128) that Bernard and William of Saint-Thierry jointly made their discovery of the Song of Songs, through the commentary of Origen.[59] In fact, Bernard had already started to write about the law of love in a letter to the early Carthusian community (*c.* 1124/25), in which he is already familiar with the Song of Songs, ideas much expanded by the early 1130s in his *De diligendo Deo*.[60] Yet the project of writing a series of homilies about the Song of Songs only had started to germinate in the mid-1130s. William, who had written a treatise *De natura et dignitate amoris* around 1120, had been influenced by his own conversations with Bernard when he produced his own commentary on the Song of Songs.[61] Both William and Bernard focus their attention on what it has to say about the soul and the nature of love. William's analysis, however, consistently turns around on the notion of a contrast between carnal and spiritual love. Bernard, a more eloquent preacher, uses the Song to speak more about the evolution of love, from self-concern to selfless love, for the sake of God. The Song provides him with a template for reflecting on these themes.

Bernard's more personal interpretation of the Song is evident from his interpretation of the verse Canticles 5. 1, to drink and get drunk: 'He calls those who

[57] William of Saint-Thierry, *Vita prima* 1.12.59, ed. by Migne, col. 259BC.

[58] De Lubac, *Exégèse médiévale*, I.2, 586–99.

[59] Verdeyen, 'Un théologien de l'expérience', p. 570.

[60] Bernard of Clairvaux, Ep. 11, ed. by Leclercq, Talbot, and Rochais, *SBO*, VII, 52–60; Bernard of Clairvaux, *De diligendo Deo*, ed. by Leclercq, Talbot, and Rochais, *SBO*, III, 119–54.

[61] William of Saint-Thierry, *De natura et dignitate amoris*, in *Deux traités de l'amour de Dieu*, ed. by Davy, pp. 71–137; William of Saint-Thierry, *Expositio super Cantica Canticorum*, ed. by Déchanet.

work in the body to food; those who rest, laying down their body he calls to drink; resuming their bodies he impels those whom he calls dearest, he calls be filled to excess with love'.[62] He then invokes Psalm 22. 5, 'my inebriating cup', to describe how one who loves God may become drunk in the house of God, without any concern for himself, 'drinking it with Christ in the house of his Father'.[63] While Augustine had written eloquently in the *Confessions* about the disturbed state of his soul in loving God, no one before Bernard had written a systematic reflection on how the individual soul might grow in loving God. By introducing imagery of inebriation from the Song of Songs and the Psalms, Bernard was giving a personal cast to a notion traditionally interpreted in terms of corporate eschatology. 'When the good and faithful servant is introduced into the joy of the Lord and be made drunk by the overflowing of the house of God, forgetful of himself in a marvellous kind of way and completely weak in himself, he will advance totally to God, and adhering to him, shall be one spirit with him'.[64]

Bernard is not here speaking about the mystical state of the Church in paradise. Rather he is using the Song of Songs to urge his listeners to identify with the bride in their journey to spiritual illumination. A recurring theme of his *sententiae* is the contrast between carnal and spiritual inebriation: 'There is a twofold inebriation, one from the wine of carnal desire, as in "He made me drunk with absinth", the other from the wine of pure prayer: "and be drunk from the overflowing of the house of God"'.[65] Inebriation is the fruit of personal prayer, not simply the state of the heavenly Jerusalem.

[62] Bernard of Clairvaux, *De diligendo Deo* 31, ed. by Leclercq, Talbot, and Rochais, *SBO*, III, 145: 'Audi et sponsum in Canticis ad profectum hunc trimodum invitantem: *comedite*, inquit, amici, *et bibite, et inebriamini carissimi*. Laborantes in corpore vocat ad cibum; iam posito corpore quiescentes ad potum invitat; resumentes corpora, etiam ut inebrientur impellit, quos et vocat carissimos, nimirum caritate plenissimos'.

[63] Bernard of Clairvaux, *De diligendo Deo* 32. ed. by Leclercq, Talbot, and Rochais, *SBO*, III, 146: 'Tum demum ad crateram admissa sapientiae, illam de qua legitur: *et calix meus inebrians quam praeclarus est*! quid mirum iam si inebriatur ab ubertate domus Dei, cum, nulla mordente cura de proprio, secura bibit purum et novum illud cum Christo in domo Patris eius?'

[64] Bernard of Clairvaux, *De diligendo Deo* 39, ed. by Leclercq, Talbot, and Rochais, *SBO*, III, 153: 'Erit autem procul dubio, cum introductus fuerit servus bonus et fidelis in gaudium Domini sui, et inebriatus ab ubertate domus Dei: quasi enim miro quodam modo oblitus sui, et a se penitus velut deficiens, totus perget in Deum, et deinceps adhaerens ei, unus cum eo spiritus erit'.

[65] Bernard of Clairvaux, *Series 3. Sententia* 97, ed. by Leclercq, Talbot, and Rochais, *SBO*, VI.2, 159: 'Est igitur duplex ebrietas, altera ex vino concupiscentiae carnalis; unde legitur: *inebriavit me absinthio*, et altera ex vino purae orationis, unde: *et inebriamini ab ubertate domus Dei*'.

Bernard's intensely personal reading of the Song can be illustrated by a sermon that he preached on 'the three kinds of kiss', inspired by its opening line, 'Let him kiss me with the kisses of his mouth'.[66] Whereas Origen uses the verse to contrast carnal and spiritual love, Bernard uses it to reflect on stages of spiritual growth. He posits three kinds of kiss, the first involving remission of sins, the second the acquisition of virtue, the third contemplation of heavenly intimacy. While one kind of contemplation was that of self-inflated wisdom, the other was genuinely the work of grace. He relates these three stages to the verse 'Eat, friends, drink and get drunk' (Canticles 5. 1).[67] This verse, completely avoided by Augustine and Gregory the Great, excites Bernard as a way of thinking about spiritual life. Bernard avoids schematic labels of whether he is pursuing allegorical, moral, or analogical exegesis. With a free-ranging style, close to that of Origen as translated by Rufinus, he reflects on love in a psychological way that goes beyond Gregory's simple contrast between the lower love of the bride in the Song with the 'higher love' to which we are called. Bernard may retain the traditional allegorical reading of the bridegroom as the Word of God, but reads the Song as about his recurring visits to the individual soul. To use the image of the Song, the bride — namely the soul — is brought into the wine cellar of her beloved and ordered in love. Whereas Augustine had used that verse (2. 4) to lament on the disturbance to ordered love among humanity without grace, Bernard uses the Song to show how the individual soul moves through the experience of eating and drinking to reach final inebriation. His psychological reading of the Song was very different from the Augustinian ecclesial focus that had prevailed among exegetes since the time of Bede.

Conclusion

Bernard's interpretation of the Song of Songs personalized traditional monastic thinking about the bride as *Ecclesia* by reading its account of anticipated pleasure as first of all about the desire of the soul to escape suffering in the world through union with the Word of God. His emphasis on arguing from experience would have a great impact in subsequent interpretations of the Song of Songs, opening the way to those who believed that ecstasy and spiritual inebriation were available to women as much as men, even outside the confines of the monastic life, in ways he could scarcely have imagined. The conventional reading of the Song, as expounded by a reforming generation of monks in the late elev-

[66] Bernard of Clairvaux, *Sermones de diversis*, no. 87, *SBO*, VI.1, 329–33.

[67] Bernard of Clairvaux, *Sermones de diversis*, no. 87, *SBO*, VI.1, 331.

enth and early twelfth centuries, had been shaped by comments of Augustine, picked up by Bede in his exposition of the bride as allegorically the Church and anagogically as foreshadowing the heavenly Jerusalem. Augustine's argument with Julian of Eclanum, a married bishop, pushed him to de-emphasize the overtly erotic aspect of its imagery. In the early twelfth century, the neglected glosses of Anselm of Laon on the Song of Songs extend this ecclesiological reading of the bride, attaching particular importance to the task of preaching. To describe the thought of Bernard of Clairvaux as characteristic of 'monastic theology' fails to recognize the radical innovation of his psychological reading of the Song of Songs, and thus of intoxication as personal experience.

Bernard was here expanding upon Origen's reading of the bride in the Song of Songs as either *Ecclesia* or the soul, deepened by his reading of Gregory the Great, who had similarly been provoked by Origen to produce a commentary on the Song of Songs. While Augustine was fascinated by the experience of love, his controversy with Pelagius and the claims of asceticism to pursue the path of perfection made him much more cautious than his mentor, Ambrose, about reading the Song of Songs. Bede's influential commentary on the Song of Songs, critical of the more naturalistic reading of the Song offered by Julian of Eclanum, reflected the influence of Augustine's ecclesiological focus, which dwelt on God's saving grace bestowed on the Church rather than on the mutuality of two lovers. Drawing on both Origen and Gregory, Bernard subtly departed from Augustine, in giving a moral reading of the Song of Songs as about not external behaviour, but the psychology of the soul in its desire for her beloved, and her dependence on the visits made by her beloved. Augustine may have been fascinated by the experience of love, but he always struggled with perception of his own inadequacy compared to divine love. Although still shaped by Augustine, Bernard had a greater sense of the Song as making possible a theory of love that evolves through grace, namely the visit of the beloved, to a state of spiritual inebriation. The Song called the friends of the bride to eat, drink, and get drunk. Bernard may have been fascinated by both Origen and Gregory in their expositions of the Song, but neither had taken these words of the Song so much to heart. In his way, Bernard was as original as both Abelard and Heloise in thinking about love.

I leave aside here the question of whether in choosing to focus on the Song of Songs Bernard might have been responding to wider interest in the theme of love outside the monastery. We know that in the early 1130s, Bernard visited Heloise at the Paraclete.[68] The Abbot of Clairvaux would certainly have been

[68] Abelard to Bernard, *Letters IX–XIV*, Letter 10, ed. by Smits, pp. 239–47.

aware of the idealism surrounding love, as well as of the potential for reading what the Song of Songs says about longing for the pleasure of intimate contact between a man and a woman in a more human way. In the *Epistolae duorum amantium*, certainly written in the early twelfth century, we find an educated young woman alluding to the metaphor of Canticles 5. 1 when she proclaims that 'if a droplet of knowability (*guttula scibilitatis*) trickled down to me from the honeycomb of wisdom, I would try to portray in the jottings of my letter various things with a fragrant nectar for your nourishing love'.[69] This imagery alludes to the injunction of Canticles 5. 1 about eating honey from the honeycomb. The Song of Songs did not just provoke spiritual intoxication. Its imagery provided a powerful resource to express the emotions of love, and the intoxication of a relationship that went beyond reason. While Bernard was fascinated by the psychology of love described in the Song, he never interpreted its dialogue in its most obvious naturalistic way, as about the delight of two lovers in the realm of the senses. Bernard's reading follows that of Origen in being concerned for the journey of the soul rather than of the body. His understanding of pleasure is that of spiritual intoxication rather than of delight in the senses. In the eyes of his admirers, however, Bernard did open up new ways of thinking, in seeming to be intoxicated with the delight of divine love.

[69] Letter 53 of the *Epistolae duorum amantium*, trans. by Mews and Chiavaroli, p. 259.

Works Cited

Manuscripts

Graz, Universitätsbibliothek, Fol. 167
Salzburg, Stiftsbibliothek Sankt Peter, MS a.IX.16
Troyes, Médiathèque, MS 1412

Primary Sources

Abelard, Peter, *Letters IX–XIV*, ed. by E. R. Smits (Groningen: Bouma's Boekhuis, 1983)

——, *Sic et Non*, ed. by B. Boyer and R. McKeon (Chicago: Chicago University Press, 1976–77)

Ambrose, *Expositio evangelii secundum Lucam*, ed. by Marc Adriaen, CCSL, 14 (Turnhout: Brepols, 1957)

Anselm of Laon, *In initiis* (*Enarrationes in Cantica canticorum*, in *PL*, CLXXXII, cols 1187A–1227B

Augustine, *Contra duas epistolas Pelagianorum*, ed. by C. F. Urba and J. Zycha, CSEL, 60 (Wien: Tempsky, 1913)

Augustine, *De civitate Dei*, ed. by Bernhard Dombart and Alfons Kalb, CCSL, 47–48 (Turnhout: Brepols, 1955)

——, *Enarrationes in Psalmos*, ed. by E. Dekkers and J. Fraipont, CCSL, 38 (Turnhout: Brepols, 1956)

Bede, *In Cantica canticorum*, ed. by D. Hurst, CCSL, 119B (Turnhout: Brepols, 1983)

Bernard of Clairvaux, *Sancti Bernardi Opera*, ed. by Jean Leclercq, Charles Talbot, and Henri Rochais, 8 vols (Roma: Editiones Cistercienses, 1957–77)

Biblia sacra, ed. by Bonifatius Fischer and others (Stuttgart: Deutsche Bibelgesellschaft, 1983)

Canticum canticorum, ed. by Eva Schulz-Flügel, Vetus Latina 10.3 (Freiburg: Herder, 1992)

Cassian, John, *Conlationes*, ed. by M. Petschenig, CSEL, 13 (Wien: Tempsky, 1886)

Epistolae duorum amantium, trans. by Constant J. Mews and Neville Chiavaroli, in Constant J. Mews, *The Lost Love Letters of Heloise and Abelard: Perception of Dialogue in Twelfth-Century France*, 2nd edn (New York: Palgrave, 2008). pp. 214–313

Eucherius of Lyons, *Formulae spiritualis intelligentiae. Epist. Ad Veranum*, ed. by C. Mandolfo, CCSL, 66 (Turnhout: Brepols, 2004)

Gilbert of Hoyland, *Sermones in cantica*, in *PL*, CLXXXIV, cols 11–298

Glossa ordinaria. In Canticum canticorum, ed. by Mary Dove, CCCM, 170.22 (Turnhout: Brepols, 1997); *The Glossa Ordinaria on the Song of Songs*, trans. by Mary Dove (Kalamazoo: Medieval Institute Publications, 2004)

Gregory the Great, *Expositio in Canticum Canticorum*, ed. by P. Verbraken, CCSL, 144 (Turnhout: Brepols, 1963), pp. 3–46

——, *Homiliae in evangelia*, ed. by R. Etaix, CCSL, 141 (Turnhout: Brepols, 1999)

——, *The Letters of Gregory the Great*, trans. by John R. C. Martyn (Toronto: Pontifical Institute of Mediaeval Studies, 2004)
——, *Moralia in Job*, ed. by M. Adriaen, CCSL, 143 (Turnhout: Brepols, 1979)
Haimo, *Commentarium in Cantica Canticorum*, in *PL*, CXVII, cols 295–308
Herman of Tournai, *Les Miracles de sainte Marie de Laon: Miracula sancte Marie Laudunensis*, ed. by Alain Saint-Denis (Paris: CNRS, 2008)
Honorius Augustodunensis, *Expositio in Cantica Canticorum*, in *PL*, CLXXII, cols 347–496
Jerome, *Commentiaria in Ezekielem*, ed. by F. Glorie, CCSL, 75 (Turnhout: Brepols, 1964)
Julian of Eclanum, *Expositio in Job*, ed. by L. De Coninck, CCSL, 88 (Turnhout: Brepols, 1977), pp. 3–109
——, *In Canticum canticorum*, ed. by L. De Coninck, CCSL, 88 (Turnhout: Brepols, 1977), pp. 398–401
Pseudo-Jerome [Aponius], *Expositio sancti Hieronimi presbiteri in libro Cantici canticorum*, ed. by B. de Vregille and L. Neyrand, CCSL, 19 (Turnhout: Brepols, 1986), pp. 315–90
John of Ford, *Sermones super extremam partem Cantici Canticorum*, ed. by Edmund Mikkers and Hilary Costello, CCCM, 17–18 (Turnhout: Brepols, 1970)
The Song of Songs: Interpreted by Early Christian and Medieval Commentators, ed. by Richard A. Norris, Jr (Grand Rapids, MI: Eerdmans, 2003)
Origen, *Commentarium in Canticum Canticorum*, ed. by W.A. Baehrens, GCS, 33 (Leipzig: J. C. Hinrichs, 1925), pp. 61–241
——, *Homélies sur le Cantique des Cantiques*, ed. by Olivier Rousseau, Sources chrétiennes, 37bis (Paris: Cerf, 1966)
——, *In Genesim homiliae, In Leviticum homiliae*, trans. by Rufinus, ed. by W. A. Baehrens, GCS, 29 (Leipzig: J. C. Hinrich, 1920)
Robert of Tombelaine, *Commentariorum in Cantica Canticorum*, in *PL*, CL, cols 1361–70, and *PL*, LXXIX, cols 493–548
Rupert of Deutz, *Commentaria in Canticum Canticorum*, ed. by H. Haacke, CCCM, 26 (Turnhout: Brepols, 1974)
William of Saint-Thierry, *Deux traités de l'amour de Dieu*, ed. M.-M. Davy (Paris: Vrin, 1953), pp. 71–137
——, *Expositio super Cantica Canticorum*, ed. by J. M. Déchanet, Sources chrétiennes, 82 (Paris: Cerf, 1962)
——, *Sancti Bernardi Vita prima*, in *PL*, CLXXXV, cols 225A–268A

Secondary Works

Asiedu, F. B. A., 'The Song of Songs and the Ascent of the Soul: Ambrose, Augustine, and the Language of Mysticism', *Vigiliae Christianae*, 55.3 (2001), 299–317
Astell, Ann W., *The Song of Songs in the Middle Ages* (Ithaca, NY: Cornell University Press, 1990)
Carr, David M., *Erotic Word: Sexuality, Spirituality and the Bible* (Oxford: Oxford University Press, 2003)

Clooney, Francis X., *His Hiding Place Is Darkness: A Hindu-Catholic Theopoetics of Divine Absence* (Stanford: Stanford University Press, 2014)

De Bruyne, D., 'Les Anciennes Versions latines du Cantique des Cantiques', *Revue Bénédictine*, 38 (1926), 97–122

Giraud, Cédric, 'Lectiones magistri Anselmi: Les Commentaires d'Anselme de Laon sur le Cantique des Cantiques', in *The Multiple Meaning of Scripture: The Role of Exegesis in Early-Christian and Medieval Culture*, ed. by Ineke van't Spijker (Leiden: Brill, 2009), pp. 177–201

——, *Per verba magistri: Anselme de Laon et son école au XIIe siècle* (Turnhout: Brepols, 2010), pp. 150–61

Jansen, Katherine L., *The Making of the Magdalen: Preaching and Popular Devotion in the Later Middle Ages* (Princeton, NJ: Princeton University Press, 2000)

LaVere, Suzanne, 'From Contemplation to Action: The Role of the Active Life in the *Glossa ordinaria* on the Song of Songs', *Speculum*, 82 (2007), 54–69

Leclercq, Jean, *L'Amour des lettres et le désir de Dieu: Initiation aux auteurs monastiques du moyen age* (Paris: Cerf, 1957); *The Love of Learning and the Desire for God: A Study of Monastic Culture*, trans. by Catherine Misrahi (New York: Fordham University Press, 1961)

——, 'Origène au XIIe siècle', *Irénikon*, 21 (1951), 425–39

Lubac, Henri de, *Exégèse médiévale: Les Quatre sens de l'Écriture*, 4 vols (Paris: Aubier, 1959–64); *Medieval Exegesis: The Four Senses of Scripture*, trans. by Mark Sebanc (vol. I) and by E. M. Macierowski (vols II–III) (Grand Rapids, MI: Eerdmans, 1998–2009)

Matter, E. Ann, *The Voice of my Beloved: The Song of Songs in Western Medieval Christianity* (Philadelphia: University of Pennsylvania Press, 1990)

Mews, Constant J., 'Singing the Song of Songs at the Paraclete: Abelard, Heloise, and Gregory the Great on Mary Magdalen as Lover and Bride', *Cîteaux*, 59 (2008), 299–313

Mews, Constant J., and Claire Renkin, 'The Legacy of Gregory the Great in the Latin West', in *A Companion to Gregory the Great*, ed. by Bronwen Neil and Matthew Dal Santo (Leiden: Brill, 2013), pp. 315–42

Ohly, Friedrich, *Hohelied-Studien: Grundzüge einer Geschichte der Hoheliedauslegung des Abendlandes bis um 1200* (Wiesbaden: Franz Steiner, 1958)

Stirnemann, Patricia, 'Où ont été fabriqués les livres de la glose ordinaire dans la première moitié du XIIe siècle', in *Le XIIe siècle: Mutations et renouveau en France dans la première moitié du XIIe siècle*, ed. by Françoise Gasparri, Cahiers du Léopard d'Or (Paris: Léopard d'Or, 1994), pp. 257–85

Straw, Carole E., *Gregory the Great: Perfection in Imperfection* (Berkeley: University of California Press, 1988)

Turner, Denys, *Eros and Allegory: Medieval Exegesis of the Song of Songs*, Cistercian Studies Series, 156 (Kalamazoo: Cistercian Publications, 1995)

Verdeyen, P. 'Un théologien de l'expérience', in *Bernard de Clairvaux: Histoire, mentalités, spiritualité*, ed. by Dominique Bertrand and Guy Lobrichon, Sources chrétiennes, 380 (Paris: Cerf, 1992), pp. 557–77

Vernet, André, *La Bibliothèque de l'abbaye de Clairvaux du* XIIe *au* XVIIIe *siècle* (Paris: CNRS, 1979)

Winsor, Ann Roberts, *A King Is Bound in the Tresses: Allusions to the Song of Songs in the Fourth Gospel* (New York: Lang, 1999)

Pleasure in Medieval Christian Mystical Literature: The Analysis of John of Ruusbroec (1281–1381) and Hadewijch (Thirteenth Century)

Rob Faesen
Translated by John Arblaster

Following Jacques Lacan and others, several recent studies have focused on the presence of the topic of 'pleasure' in mystical texts, and many have done so in reference to the thirteenth-century Middle Dutch mystic Hadewijch. Indeed, Middle Dutch mystical literature makes abundant use of the term *ghebruken* ('to enjoy', cf. the Latin *frui*).[1] One might wonder, however, *what*, according to the texts, the mystic is enjoying, why precisely this is an experience of *enjoyment*, and whether this enjoyment relates to *physical or spiritual* pleasure or an interrelation of both. This contribution investigates a number of crucial passages concerning mystical pleasure or enjoyment in the works of John of Ruusbroec (1283–1381) and his forerunner Hadewijch (thirteenth century) in order to address the above questions. Both these authors are of central importance in the Middle Dutch mystical tradition. John of Ruusbroec (in part through the translation of his works into Latin by Laurentius Surius)

[1] Naturally, the strict distinction between *uti* and *frui*, one of the central themes in the work of Augustine (*De doctrina christiana* I; *De Trinitate* X, XI and XIII; *De civitate Dei* XI, XIX; cf. Cayré, '*Frui* et *uti*'), forms part of the background of Middle Dutch mystical thought. One must bear in mind, however, that Middle Dutch does not make the distinction lexicologically, and consequently it does not occur as such in the texts. We shall thus not consider it in this contribution.

Rob Faesen (rob.faesen@theo.kuleuven.be) is in the Faculty of Theology and Religious Studies, KU Leuven, at the Faculty of Theology, Tilburg University, and Ruusbroecgenootschap, University of Antwerp.

Pleasure in the Middle Ages, ed. by Naama Cohen-Hanegbi and Piroska Nagy, IMR 24 (Turnhout: Brepols, 2018), pp. 353–378 BREPOLS PUBLISHERS 10.1484/M.IMR-EB.5.113474

profoundly influenced the later mystical tradition in the West.[2] Hadewijch was one of his most important sources. Along with Beatrice of Nazareth and the *Limburg Sermons*, her work marks the very beginning of vernacular mystical literature in Western Europe.[3] Despite the fact that her work also occupies a prominent position in European literature, it was not as famous or as widely circulated as that of John of Ruusbroec.

John of Ruusbroec

Let us first examine the meaning and significance of 'enjoyment' in the work of John of Ruusbroec. He was born in 1293 in a town between Brussels and Halle, called Ruisbroek, and received his initial intellectual formation at the chapter school of Saint Gudule in Brussels. He was ordained a priest in 1317 and was chaplain of Saint Gudule until 1343 when he, together with two other priests, withdrew into the solitude of the forest, in Groenendaal. In 1350, the community adopted the Rule of Saint Augustine. John of Ruusbroec died in 1381.[4] The tremendous importance of his oeuvre in the history of Western mystical literature is often emphasized.[5] It is here — in a male author's works — that we find the most perceptive analysis of *ghebruken* (enjoyment) in Middle Dutch mystical literature.[6] We shall examine this on the basis of his *Little Book of Enlightenment*, a text he wrote in approximately 1362, following a request from the Carthusians of Herne for a clear and concise summary of his mystical doctrine.[7]

[2] Cf. Andriessen, 'Ruusbroec's Influence until *c.* 1800'.

[3] Cf. Arblaster and Faesen, 'Mysticism in the Low Countries before Ruusbroec'.

[4] For further information, see Arblaster and Faesen, 'John of Ruusbroec's Life and Works'.

[5] Cf. McGinn, 'The Significance of Ruusbroec's Mystical Theology'.

[6] In line with Jacques Lacan (who discusses Hadewijch, among others), *jouissance* is often associated with femininity; cf. Depoortere, '*Fruitio Dei* and/or *jouissance féminine*?'. The term occurs more frequently in Ruusbroec's work than in Hadewijch's. On the other hand, Hadewijch's oeuvre is considerably shorter than Ruusbroec's. As the editor of the critical edition of Hadewijch, Jozef van Mierlo, notes, however: 'the word [*ghebruken*] does not yet have a distinct, technical meaning, and especially not an erotic meaning; in fact it rarely means anything more than to possess, possession: enjoyable, restful, untroubled, secure possession' (Hadewijch, *Strofische gedichten*, ed. by Van Mierlo, p. 301). And in his commentary on the *Letters*: 'An ordinary word that does not always express (the highest) enjoyment, but often simply means: to enjoy, to possess enjoyably, or to associate with or have free disposal of: the meanings are often difficult to distinguish' (p. 301).

[7] Cf. Ruusbroec, *Boecsken der verclaeringhe*, ed. by de Baere, p. 109, lines 24–29; see also

The first time Ruusbroec uses the term *ghebruken* is precisely in the middle of his exposition. In the preceding paragraphs, Ruusbroec describes how the human person is united with God through the mediation of God's grace and the person's virtuous life. To Ruusbroec, the latter implies that the human person dedicates himself entirely to God.[8] He describes this as follows:

> Wanneer dat hem al selc levende mensche, met gheheelheiden sijns selves ende met allen sinen crachten, op recht ende te gode voeghet met levender werkeleker minnen, soe ghevoelt hi dat sine minne in haren gronde, daer si beghent ende indet, *ghebrukeleec* es ende sonder gront. Wilt hi dan voert in dringhen met sijnre werkeleker minnen in die *ghebrukeleke* minne, al daer moeten wiken alle die crachte siere zielen, ende moeten liden ende ghedoghen die doregaende waerheit ende goetheit die god selve es.[9]

> [When he who lives in this manner raises himself with the totality of his self and with all his powers and turns to God with lively active love, then he feels that his love, in its ground, there where it begins and ends, is *enjoyable* and fathomless. If he then wishes further to penetrate this *enjoyable* love with his active love, there all the powers of his soul must give way, and suffer and endure the piercing truth and goodness which is God himself.]

In other words, Ruusbroec refers here to a certain aspect of the human experience of love. In the actual, active experience of love, it is possible for the human person to experience that the ground of that (human) love is enjoyable and fathomless ('ghebrukeleec ende sonder gront'). The metaphor 'ground' is often used to denote the foundation of something.[10] For example, certain human actions or behaviours may have a certain reason or ground. Here, Ruusbroec says that the 'depth' of human love is 'fathomless', that is, it has no 'ground', no definable cause or foundation. In other words, the foundation of love is an infinite abyss. Ruusbroec connects this to the notion of 'enjoyment'. Moreover, it is impossible for the human person to access this ground independently, that is, through his or her own efforts and activities. The only way this might be achieved is if the human person becomes receptive to the activity of God.

the introduction by Paul Mommaers (pp. 24–26); Faesen, 'Ruusbroec at the Charterhouse of Herne'; and Faesen, 'We Were Perplexed by What He Wrote'.

[8] Which evidently implies love for one's neighbour; cf. Ruusbroec, *Boecsken der verclaeringhe*, ed. by de Baere, p. 111, lines 48–51.

[9] Ruusbroec, *Boecsken der verclaeringhe*, ed. by de Baere, p. 129, lines 246–49.

[10] Cf. Verwijs and Verdam, *Middelnederlandsch Woordenboek*, *s.v.*

In this passage, Ruusbroec locates enjoyment (*ghebruken*) on the level of the 'ground' of love, or more accurately perhaps, he locates enjoyment *in* the 'ground'. He specifies that the ground is where love 'begins and ends'. This implies that by 'ground' Ruusbroec does not mean an isolated foundation, but the source from which (human) love flows. Indeed, in another work he clarifies this meaning using the metaphor of a rising source and the hidden stream from which the source is constantly fed. He even adds that the ground is also the location to which love flows back. In other words, he refers to both the foundation and the consummation principle of love. Furthermore, he articulates this idea in the present tense, which is itself telling: the 'ground' is not so much that from which human love once flowed forth (past tense) or will at some point return (future tense), but rather it is a principle that is constantly both origin and consummation in the present.

Furthermore, it is notable that Ruusbroec combines 'enjoyable' and 'fathomless'. That which is the foundation and consummation principle of love does not itself have a 'ground' — in other words, it is not rooted in anything. This suggests to the reader that Ruusbroec is referring to a *divine* reality. This suggestion is later developed explicitly, as we shall discuss below. We may first briefly mention that Ruusbroec is explicitly responding to a thirteenth-century theological dispute concerning the extent to which human love for God and the Holy Spirit might be identified. In the twelfth century, Peter Lombard had adopted a radical position in this regard, entirely consonant with his contemporaries William of Saint-Thierry and Hugh of Saint-Victor. He writes that the Holy Spirit is the mutual love between the Father and the Son as well as the human person's love for God, when it is completely united with God's love.[11] Later

[11] Cf. book I, distinction 17 (Lombard, *Sententiae*, pp. 141–52). Peter Lombard suggests that this refers to human love in so far as it is completely united to God in *Sent*. I, d. 17, c. 6, a. 4. William of Saint-Thierry describes this point very clearly in his *Golden Epistle*: 'Super hanc autem et alia adhuc est Dei similitudo; haec de qua iam aliquanta dicta sunt, in tantum proprie propria, ut non iam similitudo, sed unitas spiritus nominetur; cum fit homo cum Deo unus spiritus, non tantum unitate idem volendi, sed expressiore quadam veritate virtutis, sicut iam dictum est, aliud velle non valendi. Dicitur autem haec unitas spiritus, non tantum quia efficit, vel afficit eis spiritum hominis Spiritus sanctus, sed quia ipsa ipse est Spritus sanctus' ('In addition to this there is yet another likeness, of which something has been said already. It is so close in its resemblance that it is styled not merely a likeness but unity of spirit. It makes man one with God, one spirit, not only with the unity which comes of willing the same thing but with a greater fullness of virtue, as has been said: the inability to will anything else. It is called unity of spirit not only because the Holy Spirit brings it about or inclines a man's spirit to it, but because it is the Holy Spirit himself'). Guillemus a Sancto Theoderico, *Epistola ad Fratres de Monte Dei*, ed. by Verdeyen, p. 282 (William of Saint-Thierry, *The Golden Epistle*, trans. by Berkeley, pp. 95–96).

commentators on his *Sentences* such as Thomas Aquinas and Bonaventure, however, insisted that the master needed to be corrected on this point. According to these authors, the relationship between human love and the Holy Spirit as the intra-Trinitarian love cannot be direct, but must necessarily be mediated. Ruusbroec, on the other hand, aligns himself completely with the basic conviction of the twelfth-century authors mentioned, but reformulates the position in light of the objections raised in the thirteenth century. He states that human love for God is not identical as such with the Holy Spirit (for the human would therefore cease to be human), but that divine love is present in human love as its constant source and destination. In other words, God is personally present in human love. Incidentally, this is completely consonant with his view of the way in which God is present in the 'being' (*wesen*) of the human person.[12]

Ruusbroec later explicitly indicates that enjoyment (*ghebruken*) is characteristic of the Trinitarian life of God himself. Love is enjoyable (*ghebrukelijc*): this is true in a certain sense for human love and it is true in an absolute sense for absolute love, namely that of the Trinitarian loving unity. It is precisely because the human person shares in the absolute, divine love — and the extent to which it does so — that human love is *enjoyable*:

> Dat ghevoelen dat es onse overweseleke salecheit, die een *ghebruken gods* es ende alle sinre gheminde. Dese salecheit dat es die duustere stille die altoes ledech steet. Si es gode weseleec, ende allen creaturen overweseleec. Ende daer eest te nemene dat die persone wiken ende verwielen in die weseleke minne, dat es, in ghebrukeleker enecheit, ende nochtan altoes staende bliven na persoenleker aert in werken der drieheit. Ende aldus moghedi proeven dat die godleke nature ewech werkende es na wise der persoene, ende ewech ledech steet ende wiseloes na eenvoldecheit haers wesens. Ende hieromme, aldat god vercoren hevet ende begrepen met ewegher persoenleker minnen, dat hevet hi al weseleke beseten, *ghebrukeleke in enecheiden*, met weseleker minnen. Want die godleke persone behelsen hen onderlinghe in.i. ewech behaghen met grondeloeser werkeleker minnen in enecheit. Ende dit werc vernuwet altoes in dat levende leven der drivoldecheit. Want daer es altoes nuwe ghebaren in nuwe bekinnen, nuwe behaeghen ende nuwe ute gheesten in een nuwe behelsen met nuwer vloet van eweger minnen. In desen behaghene sijn behelset alle die utevercorne, ingle ende menschen, vanden lesten tote den iersten. Ane dit behaeghen hanghet hemel ende erde, wesen, leven, werc ende onthout alre creaturen, sonder allene die avekeer van gode in sonden.[13]

[12] Cf. Faesen, '"Poor in Ourselves and Rich in God"'.

[13] Ruusbroec, *Boecsken der verclaeringhe*, ed. by de Baere, pp. 137–39, lines 329–47. The English translation of the Middle Dutch mitigates the dimension of 'enjoyment' somewhat.

[This experience is our superessential beatitude which is an *enjoyment of God* and of all his beloved. This beatitude is the dark silence that is always inactive. It is essential to God and superessential to all creatures. And there we assume that the Persons yield and lose themselves whirling away in essential love, that is, *in enjoyable unity*; nevertheless, they always remain according to their personal properties in the working of the Trinity. You may thus understand that the divine nature is eternally active according to the mode of the Persons and eternally at rest and without mode according to the simplicity of its essence. It is why all that God has chosen and enfolded with eternal personal love, he has possessed eternally, *enjoyably in unity*, with essential love. For the divine Persons embrace mutually in eternal complacency with an infinite and active love in unity. This activity is constantly renewed in the living life of the Trinity. There is continuously new birthgiving in new knowledge, new complacency and new breathing forth of the Spirit in a new embrace with a new torrent of eternal love. All the elect, angels and men, from the last to the first, are embraced in this complacency. It is in this complacency that heaven and earth are suspended, existence, life, activity, and maintenance of all creatures, save only the aversion from God through sin.]

The quotation above describes the enjoyment (*ghebruken*) of God, which for the human person is 'superessential'.[14] In Ruusbroec's thought, the term 'superessential' means that which is higher (*super-*) than the 'being' (*-essence*) of the human person as a creature, and thus that which is part of the life of the Creator.[15] Before we discuss Ruusbroec's description of this divine enjoyment, we must address a preliminary epistemological question of a more general nature: Is it actually possible to say anything about 'divine enjoyment'? In view of the fact that God is radically transcendent, one might object that it is impossible to express anything about what God 'experiences'. The highest knowledge human beings might ever acquire about God consists in acknowledging that we do not know who or what he is — since he is radically transcendent. Twelfth- and thirteenth-century theology increasingly emphasized this point.[16] Ruusbroec, however, has a different, though unfashionable, fundamental conviction. He by no means denies that God is absolutely transcendent, and that he is com-

In Middle Dutch, the words *salecheit* and *behaeghen* have strong connotations of 'enjoyment', which is far less the case with 'beatitude' and 'complacency'.

[14] In the expression 'which is God's enjoyment', 'God's' is not an objective genitive, but a subjective genitive.

[15] 'Our *overwesen* is the divine *wesen*': de Baere, 'Explanation of Technical Terms', p. 275.

[16] Cf. Deblaere, 'La Littérature mystique au Moyen Âge'.

pletely unknowable to human reason.[17] But according to Ruusbroec, on a more profound level than human rationality, the human person is adopted into the life of God. This by no means terminates the activity of the human intellect, since this life is the very foundation of that intellect. It is not on the level of the higher faculties, but rather on the level of 'being' that the human person is adopted into the life of God. Consequently, it is possible for the human person to experience something of the divine enjoyment (*ghebruken*), considering that the human person is actually implicated in the life of the Transcendent. The statement 'this experience is our superessential beatitude, which is an enjoyment of God and of all his beloved' is a concise expression of this conviction.[18]

This raises then the question of what divine enjoyment (*ghebruken*) actually is. Ruusbroec again provides a concise, programmatic formulation: 'and there we assume that the Persons yield and lose themselves whirling away in essential love, that is, in enjoyable unity; nevertheless, they always remain according to their personal properties in the working of the Trinity'. Ruusbroec thus refers to the love of the three divine Persons, which is *weselijc* — that is, on the level of their 'being'. The mutual loving self-gift of the Father and the Son in the Holy Spirit is total. There is not a single aspect of each of their Persons that is not implicated in the total and free gift to the other ('the Persons yield and lose themselves whirling away in essential love'). This implies complete mutual belonging, and more even, a loving unity — 'my beloved is mine and I am his' (Canticles 2. 16) — and it is precisely *this* that Ruusbroec describes as enjoyment ('in enjoyable unity'). This would obviously make little sense if the total gift of the self were to result in the disappearance of the Persons, the fusion of one into the other or into an impersonal substance. Enjoyment (*ghebruken*) here refers on the one hand to the complexity of love, which consists in the Persons giving themselves to each other entirely and without reservation, and on the other hand in the fact that they remain entirely 'persons' nonetheless. The latter is a prerequisite for the Persons to continue to gift themselves to each

[17] As Ruusbroec states in the *Espousals*, for example: 'Dit est dat hoochste kinnisse gods dat de mensche hebben mach in werkende levene: dat hi bekinne in lichte dies gheloofs, dat god ombegripelijc ende ombekinlijc is' (This is the highest knowledge of God that a person may have in active life: that he recognize, in the light of faith, that God is incomprehensible and unknowable). Ruusbroec, *Die geestelike brulocht*, ed. by Alaerts, p. 277, line 998.

[18] The title of this section in Surius's Latin translation emphasizes this point: 'De complacentia divinarum personarum: itemque de complacentia mutua inter Deum et homines bonos' (Ruusbroec, *Die geestelike brulocht*, ed. by Alaerts, p. 136). This is, of course, an interpretive addition on the part of Surius himself, since Ruusbroec's texts contain no titles.

other. As Ruusbroec says: 'that the Persons yield and lose themselves whirling away in essential love, that is, in enjoyable unity; nevertheless, they always remain according to their personal properties in the working of the Trinity'. If any of these components were to be lacking or were to cease, the enjoyment too would cease. Indeed, the 'enjoyable unity' (*ghebrukeleke enecheit*) is only possible because the Persons actually gift themselves to each other, which presumes their enduring alterity and free activity. If, by contrast, this mutual gift were not to be total and definitive, but only partial or temporary, it would not constitute genuine unity, and ipso facto not an enjoyable unity.[19]

Ruusbroec describes this divine life (or rather: 'the living life of the Trinity') poetically in the following sentence, with an allusion to the novelty motif that often recurs in Hadewijch's work: 'There is continuously new birthgiving in new knowledge, new complacency and new breathing forth of the Spirit in a new embrace with a new torrent of eternal love'. Created reality, and thus human life, is consequently not detached from this 'living life'; on the contrary, it is adopted into this embrace: 'All the elect, angels and men, from the last to the first, are embraced in this complacency. It is in this complacency that heaven and earth are suspended, existence, life, activity, and maintenance of all creatures'.

Ruusbroec's conception of the different forms of human enjoyment is based on this consciousness of the absolute, divine love and the enjoyment that characterizes it. This implies that according to him, love (and the enjoyment of it) belongs to the most fundamental level of human reality, namely the origin of 'being' itself. It is not limited to the physical or emotive dimensions. In fact, Ruusbroec specifies that on these levels, enjoyment (*ghebruken*) is merely accidental.[20] On the most fundamental level, however — that of 'being' (*wesen*) — the human person is adopted into 'our superessential beatitude'. This is related to Ruusbroec's fundamental conviction that relationality is not accidental, as

[19] *Minne* (love) has three components: (1) It 'flows out' meaning that it constitutes the alterity; it does not fuse but is, on the contrary, the foundation of the otherness (*anderheit*). (2) It 'draws in', meaning that the other is a beloved (*geliefde*) other; the persons do not turn away from one another, but love one another and give their unqualified assent to this love. Furthermore, they do not keep to a safe distance from one another, but the one gives himself entirely to the other and lives in the other. (3) It is 'above distinction in enjoyment', meaning that the delight and the enjoyment of the love of one partner (the love with which he loves, is loved, and gifts himself to the other) is not qualitatively inferior to the love of the other; in no respect whatsoever is there 'one-way traffic' in love. It is total and mutual and there is thus no difference between the mutual happiness enjoyed by both partners. Cf. Faesen, 'We Were Perplexed by What He Wrote', p. 227.

[20] Cf. lines 268–69 (Middle Dutch text).

is the case in nominalist thought,[21] but rather that it is proper to the 'being' of the human person. In other words, enjoyment (*ghebruken*) on the other levels of human reality is a consequence of the most fundamental human reality. Physical or emotive enjoyment is a logical consequence of humanity's fundamental existential structure. It is precisely because the human person is relational on the level of *wesen* that all the other levels — including the physical — experience joy in love. Ruusbroec articulates this as follows:

> Siet, dese eweghe minne die in den gheeste levet, daer hi mede gheenecht es sonder middel, si ghevet hare licht ende hare ghenade in alle die crachte der zielen. Ende dit es die orsake alre doeghede. Want die ghenade gods gherijnt die overste crachte, ende daer ute ontspringhet karitate ende kinnesse der waerheit, minne tote alre gherechtecheit, oefeninghe der rade gods na beschedenheit, onghebeelde vriheit ende alle dinc verwennen sonder aerbeit, ende overmidts minne ontgheesten in enecheit. Alsoe langhe alse de mensche in deser oefeninghen blivet, soe es hi hebbelec te scouwene ende eninghe te ghevoelne sonder middel. Ende hi ghevoelt dat gherinen gods in hem, dat ene vernuwinghe es sijnre gratien ende alle sijnre doghede. Want ghi selt weten dat die gratie gods dorvloeit tote in die nederste crachte ende gherijnt des menschen herte. Ende daer af comt herteleke liefde ende ghevoellec lost te gode. Ende liefde ende lost doregaen herte ende sen, vleesch ende bloet ende alle die lijfleke nature, ende maken in den mensche perse ende ongheduer in sine lede, alsoe dat hi hem dicwile hoe hebben en weet. Want hem es te moede alse enen dronckenen mensche, die sijns selves niet en es. Ende hier af comt meneghe selsene wise die selke morwherteghe menschen niet wel bedwinghen en connen, dat es dat si dicwile hare hoet op heffen met openen ogen in den hemel overmids onghedurech verlanghen; alse nu bliscap, alse nu wenen; alse nu singhen, alse nu criten; nu wel, nu wee, ende dicwile beide te gadere in een; springhen, lopen, hande

[21] The basic axiom of nominalism is the fundamental individuality of beings, which coincide entirely with themselves. Indeed, Ockham sought to avoid the paradox that the relationship as such constitutes an independent, existing reality that might be attributed to beings ad hoc, so that for example 'being a father' (as a relational category) might theoretically be attributed to somebody who has never had a child: 'Omnem rem quam Deus conservat sine alia re potest Deus de novo producere etiam si illa res alia non sit vel nunquam fuisset; si ergo paternitas qua refertur pater ad filium sit alia res a patre et filio, et Deus eam conservat sine generatione, quia illa praeterita est, ergo potest vel potuit Deus eam paternitatem de novo producere etsi numquam fuisset illa generatio, et per consequens poterit aliquid esse pater illius quem non genuit' (William of Ockham, *Summa logicae*, ed. by Boehner, Gál, and Brown, p. 161). From the above it is clear that Ruusbroec evidently avoids this paradox, since there is no relationship without the persons. On the other hand, he also avoids the ill-fated conclusion of the fundamental individuality and existential isolation of beings (as in nominalism). According to Ruusbroec, persons are never without relationship.

te gadere slaen, knielen, neder bughen, ende aldustanech baraet in menegher wijs. Alsoe langhe alse de mensche hier bi blivet ende met openre herten op gherecht steet toe der rijcheit gods die in sinen gheeste levet, so ghevoelt hi nuwe gerinen van gode ende nuwe ongheduer van minnen. Ende soe vernuwen alle dese dinghe. Ende hier omme moet de mensche overmidts dit lijfleke ghevoelen biwilen doreliden in een geestelec ghevoelen, dat redelec es; ende overmids dat geesteleke gevoelen doreliden in een godlec ghevoelen, dat boven redene es; ende overmidts dat godleke ghevoelen hem selven ontsinken in een onbewechlec salech gevoelen. Dat ghevoelen dat es onse overweseleke salicheit, die een ghebruken gods es ende alre sine gheminde.[22]

[See, this eternal love, which lives in the spirit and to which it is united without intermediary, gives its light and its grace in all the powers of the soul, and this is the source of all virtue. For the grace of God touches the higher powers and from this spring charity and knowledge of truth, love of all justice, practice of the councils of God with discretion, imageless freedom and the overcoming of all things without effort, and a transport into unity through love. As long as man continues this exercise, then he is able to contemplate and to experience union without intermediary. And he feels the touch of God in him that is a renewal of his grace and all his virtues. For you must know that the grace of God flows down to the lower faculties, and touches the heart of man, and from that comes heartfelt affection and sensitive desire for God. And affection and desire penetrate the heart and senses, flesh and blood, and all the corporeal nature and cause in him strain and restlessness in his body, so that often he does not know what to do with himself. He is in the state of a man who is so drunk that he is no longer in possession of himself. And from this comes much eccentric behaviour, which these soft-hearted men cannot well control, that is, they often lift their heads to heaven with eyes wide open because of the restless desire; sometimes joy, sometimes weeping, now singing and now shouting, now weal and now woe, and often both together at once; leaping, running, clapping their hands together, kneeling, bowing down, and making similar fuss in many ways. As long as man remains in this state and stands with open heart raised up to the richness of God who lives in his spirit, he experiences new touching from God and new impatience of love. And so all these things are renewed. And for this reason man must at times pass through this bodily feeling to a spiritual feeling which is rational, and through the spiritual feeling pass to a divine feeling which is above reason, and through this divine feeling sink away from himself into an experience of motionless beatitude. This experience is our superessential beatitude which is an enjoyment of God and of all his beloved.]

Ruusbroec provides a strikingly physical description of enjoyment in this passage.[23]

[22] Ruusbroec, *Boecsken der verclaeringhe*, ed. by de Baere, pp. 133–37, lines 297–330.

[23] Incidentally, we may note in passing that this physical description finds a surprising echo in Erasmus's *In Praise of Folly*: 'Hoc nimirum est quod pollicetur propheta: "Oculus non

That which is proper to the 'being' of the human person, namely participation in the enjoyment of the divine, intra-Trinitarian love, also affects the 'lower faculties', the heart (conceived as the emotive power) and the physical aspects of the human person. From Ruusbroec's perspective, this should not be considered surprising. Indeed, the human person's 'being' — and the relationality that characterizes it — includes naturally the physical dimension, the human person's 'flesh and blood'. Since the human person's body really exists, it shares in the relationality of the human person's 'being'. The body enjoys precisely because it loves, or in other words because it participates in the human person's love, which is more fundamental than the physical dimension and which is rooted in absolute love. The fact that the contemplative experiences this as a kind of drunkenness is indicative of the measurelessness of divine love, which exceeds the human capacity to bear it.

vidit nec auris audivit nec in cor hominis ascenderunt quae praeparavit deus diligentibus se". Atque haec est moriae pars, quae non aufertur commutatione vitae, sed perficitur. Hoc igitur quibus sentire licuit (contigit autem perpaucis), ii patiuntur quiddam dementiae simillimum, loquuntur quaedam non satis cohaerentia nec humano more, sed dant sine mente sonum, deinde subinde totam oris speciem vertunt. Nunc alacres, nunc deiecti, nunc lachrymant, nunc rident, nunc suspirant, in summa, vere toti extra se sunt. Mox ubi ad sese redierint, negant se scire ubi fuerint, utrum in corpore an extra corpus, vigilantes an dormientes: quid audierint quid viderint, quid dixerint, quid fecerint, non meminerunt nisi tanquam per nebulam ac somnium, tantum hoc sciunt, se felicissimos fuisse dum ita desiperent. Itaque plorant sese resipuisse nihilque omnium malint, quam hoc insaniae genus perpetuo insanire. Atque haec est futurae felicitatis tenuis quaedam degustatiuncula' ('This is surely what the prophet promises: "Eye has not seen, nor ear heard, nor have there entered into the heart of man the things which God has prepared for them that love Him" (1 Cor. 2:9). And this is the good part of folly which is not taken away by the transformation of life but is perfected. So those who are granted to have a foretaste of this — and very few have the good fortune — experience something which is very like madness. They speak incoherently and unnaturally, utter sounds without sense, and their faces suddenly change expression. One moment they are excited, the next depressed, they weep and laugh and sigh by turns; in fact, they are truly quite beside themselves. Then when they return to themselves, they say they do not know where they have been, in the body or outside it (2 Cor. 12:2), awake or asleep. They cannot remember what they have heard or seen or said or done, except in a mist, like a dream. All they know is that they were happiest when they were out of themselves in this way, and they lament their return to themselves, for all they want is to be mad for ever with this kind of madness. And this is only the merest taste of the happiness to come'). Erasmus, *Opera omnia*, ed. by Miller, pp. 193–94 (Erasmus, *Praise of Folly*, trans. by Radice, pp. 207–08). The great humanist visited the Priory of Groenendaal in approximately 1493/94 and spent some time working in the library. It is also possible that he was introduced to Ruusbroec's work by Thomas More, who was well acquainted with the Carthusians in London (Alaerts, 'De prins van de humanisten', p. 12).

Let us now reconsider our three initial questions. First, *what* is enjoyed? In response, Ruusbroec describes a specific kind of love. He refers to the 'enjoyment of God' (*ghebruken gods*), which of course must not be interpreted in the sense that God is the object of enjoyment, but rather as 'an enjoyment that is proper to God'. It is even incorrect to say that love is the object of enjoyment; it would be more accurate to conceive of enjoyment as an intrinsic experiential aspect of love. Love is the Trinity's complete, unreserved, and mutual gift of the self to the other (while retaining personhood). For the human person, this is experienced in the 'ground' of human love. In this sense, according to Ruusbroec, absolute love is not an abstract (Platonic) idea, but a very real and personal reality. Secondly, how is this an *enjoyment* for the human person? The enjoyment is simply rooted in the fact that the human experience of love corresponds to the structure of human existence, namely the 'ground' of the self.[24] And, thirdly, since this enjoyment is an integral part of being, it ipso facto involves the *physical* dimension of life.

[24] It may be useful to repeat Erasmus's words here: 'Primum igitur existimate Platonem tale quiddam iam tum somniasse, cum amantium furorem omnium felicissimum esse scriberet. Etenim qui vehementer amat, iam non in se vivit, sed in eo quod amat quoque longius a seipso digreditur et in illud dimigrat, hoc magis ac magis gaudet. [...] Porro quo amor est absolutior, hoc furor est maior ac felicior. Ergo quaenam futura est illa coelitum vita, ad quam piae mentes tanto studio suspirant? [...] Deinde spiritus a mente illa summa mire absorbebitur, quippe infinitis partibus potentiore. Ita ut iam totus homo extra se futurus sit, nec alia ratione felix futures nisi quod extra sese positus, patietur quiddam ineffabile a summo illo bono omnia in se rapiente. [...] Fit ut praemii quoque illius aliquando gustum aut odorem aliquem sentiant. Id tametsi minutissima quaedam stillula est ad fontem illum aeternae felicitates, tamen longe superat universas corporis voluptates, etiam si omnes omnium mortalium deliciae in unum conferantu' ('First consider how Plato imagined something of this sort when he wrote that "the madness of lovers is the highest form of happiness" (*Phaedrus* 245B). For anyone who loves intensely lives not in himself but in the object of his love, and the further he can move out of himself into his love, the happier he is. [...] The more perfect the love, the greater the madness — and the happier. What, then, will life in heaven be like, to which all pious minds so eagerly aspire? [...] The spirit will be in a marvellous manner taken by the supreme Mind, which is more powerful than its infinite parts. And so when the whole man will be outside of himself, and be happy for no reason except that he is out of himself, he will enjoy some ineffable share in the supreme good which draws everything into itself. [...] The pious occasionally have a foretaste of the reward to come. It is only the tiniest drop in comparison with the fount of eternal bliss, yet it far exceeds all pleasures of the body, even if all mortal delights were rolled into one'). Erasmus, *Opera omnia*, ed. by Miller, pp. 192–93 (Erasmus, *Praise of Folly*, trans. by Radice, pp. 206–07, slightly modified). It is striking that this prince among humanists conceives of the glory of heaven as the joy of love. The central issue of the passage quoted above is the conviction that the spiritual joy of love hinges on the fact that the human person does not live 'in

Hadewijch

Let us now go a little further back in time to explore the oeuvre of the thirteenth-century mystic Hadewijch, to whom Ruusbroec often refers, though without ever mentioning her name. In other words, Hadewijch precedes Ruusbroec chronologically, but Ruusbroec's analysis is more detailed than Hadewijch's. Furthermore, Ruusbroec is helpful to bring the theological significance that is implicit in Hadewijch's work to the fore, and thus to inquire whether the emphases she places are different from his.

No biographical information about Hadewijch has been transmitted. Generally, one may assume that she lived in the Duchy of Brabant during the first half of the thirteenth century. It is clear from her work that she was familiar with courtly culture and with Cistercian spirituality.[25] Her oeuvre consists of thirty-five poems (probably all originally songs), fourteen visions, and thirty-one letters, as well as sixteen rhymed letters — all written in Middle Dutch. A number of these texts were translated into Latin,[26] but these translations are no longer extant. The Carthusians of Herne — the addressees of Ruusbroec's *Little Book of Enlightenment* — owned two of the four known manuscripts of Hadewijch's work.

Her conception of enjoyment (*ghebruken*) is most clearly formulated in her first letter, which almost programmatically introduces all the central themes in her thought.[27] The letter we shall examine here is the very first in the collection, but this does not necessarily imply that it was written first chronologically.

himself' but 'in the one he loves'. Joy is proportional to the extent to which the one loves the other. Although Erasmus does not state it explicitly, he seems to suggest that this corresponds precisely to the vocation of human beings. The more human beings live in the other, the more human they become; joy and happiness are the clearest indications that this is the case. The fulfilment of a human life, according to Erasmus, lies in the complete *esse ad Alium*, namely when the human lives entirely in the other, and does not live in himself in any way. Humans are able to foretaste this immense joy — which is correlated to the complete gift of self to the other — in this life. Erasmus calls this a 'folly', which, in this context, must be considered an honorific title.

[25] Cf. Faesen, 'Was Hadewijch a Beguine or a Cistercian?'.

[26] The Carthusians of Zelem owned a copy of the Latin translations of Hadewijch's visions and letters; cf. Axters, 'Nederlandse mystieken in het buitenland', pp. 209–10.

[27] The letter was presumably circulated in broader circles, since part of it was copied in the treatise 'The Book of the Orchard' (*Dbuec vanden bogarde*), which is in the thirteenth-century collection — probably made in a Cistercian milieu — known as the 'Limburg Sermons'; cf. *Limburgsche Sermoenen*, ed. by Kern, pp. 538–46.

Indeed, as we have no historical information whatsoever about Hadewijch, we do not know to whom these letters were addressed or when they were written. In fact, some of the 'letters' are more like treatises. Nevertheless, as mentioned above, this first letter contains a number of central insights that are developed further in other letters. This is the case, for example, with the theme of *enjoyment*.

The letter consists of three main sections:[28] a descriptive section (lines 1–17); an exhortation (lines 18–55); and a personal-exemplarist section (lines 56–82). The first section is a profound reflection on the clarity (one might also translate: the glory, cf. John 17. 1–5) of the noble love that is God,[29] and especially on the total abandonment to this love, as a result of which God can become active in this human striving. Hadewijch does not yet use the term enjoyment (*ghebruken*) in this passage. For our purposes, it is especially important that Hadewijch emphasizes active human striving and effort from the very beginning and combines this with her reflections on human abandonment to God:

> God, die de clare minne, die onbekint was verclaerde bi siere doghet daer hi alle doghet bi verlichte in siere claerheit der minnen, hi moet u verliechten ende verclaren metter claerre claerheit daer hi hem selven claer met es ende al sinen vrienden ende sinen naesten gheminden. Die alre meeste claerheit die men hebben mach in ertrike, dat es ghewaricheit in ieghenwordeghen werken van gherechticheden, ende van allen wesenen waerheit te pleghene omme claerheit der edelre minnen, die god es. Ay, hoe groete claerheit es dat datmen gode ghewerden late met siere claerheit. Daer in werct minne hem selven ende allen creaturen elken na sijn recht, dat hem sine goetheit gheorconden mach te ghevene met gherechticheden in claerheyden.[30]

> [God, who clarified clear love — that was unknown — by his life, by which He clarified all life with the clarity of love, He may enlighten and clarify you with the clear clarity by which He is clear to himself and to all his friends and his nearest beloved. The greatest possible clarity one may have on earth, is to be true in real

[28] The editor of Hadewijch's work, Jozef Van Mierlo, distinguishes between only two sections (Hadewijch, *Brieven*, p. 11).

[29] We may also note the following: 'love' is not capitalized here. Hadewijch thus plays with the ambiguity of whether the word refers to human love or divine love. There has been much discussion about how this word is to be understood (concise bibliographical overview in Hadewijch, *Liederen*, ed. by Fraeters and Willaert, p. 426). On my reading, this discussion has failed to appreciate the full importance of the interrelationship of divine and human (indwelling) love discussed above, for example as it was articulated by Peter Lombard, and later misunderstood and rejected as problematic. Hence the continuing discussion of whether Hadewijch refers to human or divine love, while the issue is precisely that the one is within the other.

[30] Hadewijch, *Brieven*, ed. by Van Mierlo, p. 16.

works of righteousness, and to practice truth in everything for the sake of the clarity of the noble love who is God. Ah, what great clarity it is to let God have his way with his clarity! Therein love, for himself and all creatures according to their right, brings about that which his goodness notifies him to give rightfully in clarity.][31]

Hereafter, the second, central section of the letter explicitly discusses enjoyment (*ghebruken*). We will first cite the following, longer text, before analysing the theme of enjoyment in Hadewijch's thought.

Hier omme bidic u alsoe vrient sinen lieven vrient ende mane u alse suster haere liever suster ende hete u alse moeder haren lieven kinde ende ghebiede u van uwen gheminden alse brudegom ghebiedet siere liever bruyt dat ghi ontpluuct die oghen uwer herten claerlike ende besiet u in gode heilichleke. Leert te besiene wat god es: hoe hi es waerheit alre dinghen ieghenwerdichilike ende goetheit alre rijcheit vloyeleke ende gheheelheit alre doghet gheheeleke omme de welke men singhet.iij. sanctus inden hemel omme dattie.iij. namen in haren enighen wesene alle doechde versamenen van welken ambachte si sijn ute desen.iij. wesenen. Siet hoe vaderlike u god ghehuet hevet ende wat hi u gheghevet hevet ende wat hi u gheloeft hevet. Besiet hoe hoghe minne es deen vor dander, ende danckes hem met minnen, wildi dit besien hoe god dit es ende werken in hem in siere claerheit *ghebrukeleke*, in glorilecheiden ende toenleke in claerheiden alle dinc te verlichtene ende te demsterne na hare wesen. Om dies dit god es, daer omme salmenne *sijns selves laten ghebruken* in al sinen werken van siere claerheit sicut in celo et in terra altoes met woerden ende met werken te segghene fiat voluntas tua. Ay, lieue kint, soe sine gheweldeghe ghewout meer verclaert wert in u, soe sijn heileghe wille bat in u ghesciet ende soe sijn claere waerheit naere in u schijnt, soe en spaert dan niet sueter rasten te darven omme die grote gheheelheit gods. Verclaert u wesen ende chiert u met doechden ende met gherechten werken. Widet uwe sinne met hogher begherten der gheheelheit gods ende ordineert u ziele *ten groten ghebrukene der al gheweldegher minnen* ons alte suets gods.[32]

[This is why I pray you as a friend would his dear friend, and I admonish you as a sister her dear sister, and I demand of you as a mother her dear child, and I order you from your Beloved, as the bridegroom orders his dear bride, that you open up the eyes of your heart in clarity and regard yourself as holy in God. Learn to see what God is. How He is the truth that lends presence to all things, and the goodness that makes all richness flow, and the wholeness that makes all life into a whole, for which they sing *sanctus* three times in heaven, because those three names in their one being gather all powers, whatever their working, from these three beings. See how as a father God has guarded you and what He has given you and what He

[31] Hadewijch, *The Complete Letters*, trans. by Mommaers and Daróczi, slightly modified.

[32] Hadewijch, *Brieven*, ed. by Van Mierlo, pp. 16–17.

> has promised you. See how high love is: the one for the other, and thank Him for it with love — namely see how God is that, and work in Him in His clarity, *enjoying*, in glory, and also revealing in clarity all things, so as to lighten and to darken them according to their being. Because this is what God is, therefore one shall *let Him enjoy Himself* in all the works of His clarity, *sicut in caelo et in terra*, always with words and with works saying: *fiat voluntas tua*. Ah, dear child, the more His tremendous power becomes clearer in you, the more His holy will is done better in you, and the more closely His clear truth shines in you, for the sake of God's wholeness, do not, then, avoid deprivation of sweet rest, clarify your being and adorn yourself with virtues and righteous works. Broaden your mind through high desiring for God's wholeness. And prepare your soul *for the great enjoyment of the sovereign Love* of our all too sweet God.][33]

The exhortative but also loving tone of this passage is entirely consonant with Saint Bernard's prologue to his *De consideratione*,[34] in which he also tells his readers that he does not wish to instruct them as a master, but rather as a mother, and especially as a lover.[35]

In the first instance, this passage uses the term enjoyment (*ghebruken*) to describe the life of God. Indeed, the reader is encouraged to see what love actually is — namely, 'the one for the other', or in other words, total mutual belonging. Hadewijch emphasizes that this is precisely what constitutes God's life. God is mutual relationship, love, absolute mutual belonging. The reader is exhorted to contemplate this, and at the same time to work in God. This life is constituted by enjoyment (*ghebruken*) and glory. Clearly Hadewijch does not conceive of this life as a chronological sequence of action and contemplation, in the way one might conceive of the Benedictine *ora et labora*. On the contrary, this life consists of virtues and righteous works, but works which are practised in such a way that their enduring source is in the absolute love that is God.

Hadewijch then specifies that from this perspective, it is essential for the human person to let God enjoy God's self — on earth (human reality) as in heaven (divine reality) — by saying, in word and in deed, your will be done. From these two brief references to enjoyment (*ghebruken*), it is apparent that it is an enjoyment of God's love, that is, of the total mutual belonging of the Father and the Son in the Spirit. This is the case in heaven (*in celo*), and it is only thus that God can enjoy God's self on earth (*in terra*).

[33] Hadewijch, *The Complete Letters*, trans. by Mommaers and Daróczi, slightly modified.

[34] As Columba Hart notes, Hadewijch, *The Complete Works*, trans. by Hart, p. 364.

[35] 'Monebo te proinde, non ut magister, sed ut mater: plane ut amans': Bernard of Clairvaux, *Sancti Bernardi Opera*, ed. by Leclercq and Rochais, III, 394.

Hadewijch treats human enjoyment at the very end of this section of her letter. She exhorts her addressee 'to widen the mind with a desire for God's totality'. In the context of the above, it is clear that she does not mean a desire for God as an object that can be possessed enjoyably. Rather, she refers to a desire for the same quality of relationship with God as God is in God's self (*sicut in celo et in terra*).

The fact that Hadewijch uses the word *gheweldech* as an adjective to qualify love is entirely understandable if (unlike many others) we do not translate it as 'powerful' but as 'sovereign'. Indeed, the primary meaning of *ghewelt* is 'sovereignty'. *Al gheweldech* thus means 'absolutely sovereign, having completely free disposal'. This is precisely what the phrase *fiat voluntas tua* seeks to express: persons who belong to each other entirely and mutually, who give themselves completely and reciprocally at the disposal of one another. As is often the case, the background to this insight is again the verse from the Song of Songs: 'my beloved is mine, and I am his'.[36] Hadewijch evokes a complete abandonment in love without any reservation, in which the beloved belongs more to the other than to herself. The reader is exhorted to desire this love, and in this way to become 'wide' by desiring it.

In the third section of the letter, which (at least at a cursory glance) appears much more personal and attesting, the tone abruptly appears to change, and the opposite of enjoyment comes to the foreground:

> Ay, lieve kint, al seggic alte suete, dat es mi over oncont, sonder inden wensch van miere herten dat mi doghen suete hevet gheweest om sine minne. Mer mi hevet hi wredere gheweest dan mi nye duvel was, want si en consten mi nie benemen hem te minnene noch nieman dien hi mi beval te vorderne. Mer hi hevet mi selve benomen. *Dat hi es, dat verteert hi selve in siere sueter ghebrukenissen ende laet mi dus dolen buten dien ghebrukene ende laet mi emmer sere verladen met minnen onghebruken*, ende laet mi demster van ghebruken alre yoyen die mi te guede souden werden. Ay arme, dat selve dat hi mi boet ende ghegheuen hadde te werder van ghebrukene van gherechter minnen, dat hevet hi dus nu laten varen, alse ghi een deel wel wet. Ay, wet god, ic hieltene herde sere over here ende eyschede hem luttel vordere dan hi selve woude. Mer dat hi mi boet, dat haddic gherne ghenomen in ghebrukene, had hijs mi willen hulpen. Biden eersten waest mi leet ghenoech ende

[36] Cf. *Thirteenth Letter*: 'Ende dat es hare [= minnende herte] begherte attoes ende hare bede, in enicheiden van minnen te sine, alsoe men leset in die canteken "Dilectus meus mihi et ego illi"' (And this is always their [= loving hearts'] desire and their prayer: to be in the unity of love, as one reads in the Song of Songs: *Dilectus meus mihi et ego illi*) Hadewijch, *Brieven*, ed. by Van Mierlo, pp. 113–14, lines 11–14.

> liet mi vele bieden, eer icker na vinc. Mer nu benic ghevoert alse een dien met yet te spele biedet ende alse hi daer na veet soe sleetmenne op de hant ende seghet godsat hebbe die waers waende ende houdet dat op datmen hem boet.[37]
>
> [Ah, dear child, although I say all too sweet, that is to me more than unknown, unless — in my heart's wish — suffering has been sweet to me for the sake of his love. Yet, to me He has been more cruel than ever a devil was, for they could never keep me from loving Him or someone He ordered me to advance. Yet He has kept me from it himself. *What He is, that He digests himself in His sweet enjoyment, and thus lets me wander about out of that enjoyment, and lets me always be bowed down with the non-enjoyment of love*, and leaves for me in the dark the enjoyment of all the joys which should be my share. Ah, poor me, precisely that which He offered me and had given me in pledge of the enjoyment of righteous love, that He thus has now abandoned, as you partly know. Ah, God knows, I recognized Him very much as the Lord and I demanded of Him hardly more than He himself wanted to give. Yet, what He offered me, I would gladly have accepted it to enjoy it, if He had granted me. At first it gave me sorrow enough and I let love offer me much before I reached for it. But now I am slapped down like someone offered something in jest, and as he reaches for it, one smacks his hand saying: 'the wrath of God on the one who thought this true', and what was offered is withdrawn.][38]

The letter ends with these rather sombre observations. In other words, Hadewijch describes her own situation as in darkness — John of the Cross would later describe this as the 'night of the soul' — and without enjoyment.[39] She says that God enjoys God's self, but that she is excluded from the enjoyment. God has even taken the pledge of the enjoyment from her.

These closing paragraphs of this programmatic first letter — which are echoed on numerous occasions in the *Poems in Stanzas* — drastically nuance, and perhaps even contradict, contemporary reflections on the *jouissance féminine* in Hadewijch.[40] Hadewijch does not present herself as someone who experiences enjoyment. Rather, she describes herself as someone whose very pledge of enjoyment has been taken away by God himself.

Nevertheless, we must not lose sight of the letter's inherent thematic coherence. Indeed, in the second part of the letter, Hadewijch exhorts her reader

[37] Hadewijch, *Brieven*, ed. by Van Mierlo, p. 18.

[38] Hadewijch, *The Complete Letters*, trans. by Mommaers and Daróczi, slightly modified.

[39] The expression 'as you partly know' ('alse ghi een deel wel wet') indicates that the addressee was familiar with Hadewijch's spiritual situation. The identity of this addressee is unknown.

[40] Cf. Depoortere, '*Fruitio dei* and/or *jouissance féminine*?'.

to complete abandonment to the divine will — *sicut in celo et in terra* — and thus 'to widen the mind with a desire for God's totality'. From this perspective, the third part of the letter provides an exemplary description of what such abandonment might entail. Every form of enjoyment that resides in less than the totality of God, and thus reduces enjoyment to a certain experience ('sweet rest', i.e. physical, emotional, affective, or religious pleasure), finds satisfaction in something inferior to God and consequently maintains a certain 'measure' in the abandonment in love. Hadewijch encourages her readers to engage in a loving abandonment that is far more profound and which implies no measure or limitation. She describes her own spiritual situation as an example of such a far-reaching loving abandonment. The crucial point in this regard is that in the context of her foregoing reflections, this constitutes precisely what enjoyment is. In other words: enjoyment does not cease but is stripped of an unduly narrow definition. She formulates this succinctly in the sixteenth letter: 'the lack of this enjoyment is the sweetest enjoyment' (lines 17–19). In the first part of the first letter, Hadewijch elevates the concept of enjoyment (*ghebruken*) from the obvious meaning of delightful pleasure to a very different and exceptionally demanding level: the divine.[41]

The use of the term enjoyment (*ghebruken*) in Hadewijch's oeuvre is thus complex. This refers, on the one hand, to the enjoyment that belongs to God's own Trinitarian life — namely the total, mutual possession of the Father and the Son in the unity of the Holy Spirit — and, on the other hand, to the human person's complete participation in this love. The latter is only fully the case when the human person belongs to God in an equally radical manner and abandons him/herself to God in the same way as the Persons of the Trinity do to one another. This implies that the human person is prepared ultimately to relinquish enjoyment. One might say that Hadewijch refers to an enjoyment (*ghebruken*) that has no pleasure, that is, an enjoyment on the level of 'being' rather than the level of 'experiencing'.

To clarify this further, we may turn to another example, from her *Fortieth Poem in Stanzas*. The fifth stanza (lines 33–40) reads as follows:

[41] Cf. *Seventeenth Poem in Stanzas*: 'Ay wat ic meine ende hebben ghemeent | Heeft god den edelen wel versceent | Dien hi quale van minnen heeft verleent | Omme ghebruken van minnen natuere | Eert al met al wert vereent | Smaect men bitteren suere' ('Ah! What I mean and always have meant | God has indeed caused to dawn upon gentle persons | To whom he has granted torment of love to hold in fee | For the sake of fruition of love's nature. | Before all is united to all | One savours acridity and acid'). Hadewijch, *Strofische gedichten*, ed. by Van Mierlo, pp. 110–11, line 73–78 (Hadewijch, *Poetry*, trans. by Van Baest, p. 137).

Dien minne verwint dat hise verwinne,
Hem wert hare suete natuere noch cont.
Als hi ghevoelt die soete minne,
Wort hi met haren wonden ghewont.
Als hi met wondere hare wondere kinnet,
Sughet hi met niede der aderen gront,
Altoes met dorste van nuwen beghinne,
Eer hi ghebruct der zueter minnen.

[To whoever love overthrows so that he may overpower her.
Her sweet nature will yet become manifest.
When he feels this sweet love,
He is wounded with her wounds.
When in wonder he perceives her wonders,
He ardently sucks the ground of love's veins,
Always thirsting after beginning afresh,
Until he has fruition of sweet love.][42]

The first line refers to complete loving abandonment, but also contains a paradoxical expression stating that this abandonment is the way in which one overpowers love — an idea Hadewijch develops in the twelfth letter, in her interpretation of Jacob wrestling with the angel (lines 177–203), and even more explicitly in the expression that Mary's humility drew God 'into herself' (lines 4–5).[43] Those who abandon themselves completely in this love come to know the 'sweet nature' of love. This obviously refers to a pleasurable experience. The second sentence takes up this theme again, but immediately adds that those who feel sweet love are wounded by the wounds of love. Hadewijch does not specify what exactly these wounds of love are, but they presumably refer to the wounds of Christ. In his humanity, the abandonment of his love only became absolute when he spoke the words *consummatum est*, that is, on the cross.[44] The external, physical wounds in his humanity are externalizations of his complete personal, interior abandonment.[45]

[42] Hadewijch, *Strofische gedichten*, ed. by Van Mierlo, p. 257; Hadewijch, *Poetry*, trans. by Van Baest, p. 269.

[43] An unusual expression that was later also used by Eckhart. Cf. also Hadewijch's *Poem in Stanzas* 29 (Hadewijch, *Strofische Gedichten*, ed. by Van Mierlo, pp. 186–91).

[44] Cf. the sixteenth letter (Hadewijch, *Brieven*, ed. by Van Mierlo, pp. 132–33, lines 32–40).

[45] The theme of the wounds of love is explicitly developed by Richard of Saint-Victor in his *De quattuor gradibus violentae caritatis*. He clarifies that for the human person, these wounds signify complete submission to the will of the divine other (cf. nos 41–42; Richard of Saint

Hadewijch follows these reflections with a play on words: from 'wound' to 'wonder' and 'wonderment'. Those who become conscious of the absolute gift of the self in love are astounded by it.[46] Hadewijch then refers to the insatiable desire: the lover 'sucks the deepest from the veins of love'. According to the *Middle Dutch Dictionary*, 'vein' may refer here to 'bloodstream in the body' (which seems unlikely in this context) or 'vein or jet of water' (which is more probable). The 'ground' of the water vein is its source, a reservoir of water beneath the earth. Applied to love, this means 'the deepest, divine origin of all forms of love'. It is precisely there that the lover enjoys the 'sweet love'.

This stanza thus combines two aspects, each consisting of four lines: (1) total abandonment (being overpowered by love) — tasting the sweet nature of love — being wounded by the wounds of love = *enjoyment*; (2) coming to know the wonder of love with amazement — insatiable thirst for the deepest ground of love. Logically, one might be inclined to reverse this order (first desire, then enjoyment), but in a very refined way, Hadewijch cuts across this logic by noting the two aspects in reverse order. Logically, the enjoyment precedes desire.

It is evident from these texts that Hadewijch also treats divine enjoyment. Her reflection begins from divine enjoyment, which consists in the complete mutual possession of the divine Persons in *minne*. Human participation in this enjoyment is based in the radical gratuitousness of love — *minne sonder waeromme*[47] — that is proper to God's own life. Hadewijch underscores this gratuitousness and illustrates her concern with reference to the lack of experience in her own life. This results in the paradoxical situation that according to her, the most fundamental participation in the divine enjoyment consists of being stripped of all 'experience'.

Victor, *Les quatre degrés*, ed. by Dumeige, pp. 169–71). This is also Hadewijch's presupposition. Considering that the divine Persons *are* complete loving submission to one another ('hoghe minne es deen vor dander'; 'high love is: the one for the other'), divine love is not a wound for them. For humanity, however, it is a wound, but is beneficial and curative — to the extent that the human person has become estranged from complete loving submission of God. Cf. also Bernard's *De diligendo Deo* (Bernard, *Sancti Bernardi Opera*, ed. by Leclercq and Rochais, III, 124).

[46] In the twenty-second letter, Hadewijch describes that the human person's insatiable desire is caused by amazement at the measureless and uncalculated love of God (Hadewijch, *Brieven*, ed. by Van Mierlo, pp. 195–96, lines 183–212).

[47] This expression is used by Hadewijch's contemporary Beatrijs van Nazareth (1200–1268), *Seven maniren van minne*, ed. by Reypens and Van Mierlo, p. 7, and by John of Ruusbroec (Tabernacle 4:1366: 'minne sonder waeromme die ons salech maect', *Van den geesteliken tabernakel*, ed. by Mertens, V, 475). Although the content of Hadewijch's work indicates precisely the same point, we do not find this literal expression in her work.

Conclusion

What may we conclude from this investigation into a number of key passages in the works of John of Ruusbroec and Hadewijch?

First, enjoyment (*ghebruken*) features prominently in their works. These mystical authors assign a central place to the dimension of enjoyment in the union with God. Both Hadewijch and Ruusbroec base their reflections on the conviction that enjoyment is proper to God's life, namely the absolute and mutual personal belonging in the intra-Trinitarian love. Consequently, an interpretation of enjoyment (*ghebruken*) in Hadewijch and Ruusbroec requires an inquiry into their fundamental Trinitarian theology: God is not a supra-personal, unmoved divine substance but is the essentially relational, loving, mutual, complete, and definitive gift of the self between the Persons.

Furthermore, both authors situate the fullest human enjoyment on the level of 'being'. Given that God is the origin of human existence, and God's inner life is the absolute enjoyment of love, human enjoyment involves the level of 'being' as such, which bears the characteristics of its source. Hadewijch and Ruusbroec refer to a joy that is proper to existence, and which is experienced as such on that level. Considering that from their perspectives, there is no interruption, discontinuity, or distance between the creating God and the created human person, the most intimate contact with God can also be experienced as measureless, overwhelming joy.

Third, with respect to the concrete description of this experience, there appears to be a difference between the male author Ruusbroec, who unproblematically describes the various levels of enjoyment, including its physical dimensions, and the female author Hadewijch, who is far more radical in her focus on enjoyment (*ghebruken*) without any form of pleasure.[48] Historically, this may be the result of the different spiritual contexts in which Ruusbroec and Hadewijch lived. In Hadewijch's time, pleasure may have become a goal in itself, while Ruusbroec's period was characterized more by the imageless, emotionless, loveless contemplation of the Free Spirit. However, the difference may be smaller than first appears. Indeed, Ruusbroec also refers to the passing (*doreliden*) from the physical and spiritual to the divine feeling (*ghevoelen*).

[48] Much of the secondary literature refers to an opposition between male and female mystical authors; for Hadewijch and Ruusbroec, see for example Warnar, '"Ex levitate mulierum"'. This opposition is often ungrounded, however. As far as our subject is concerned, Jacques Lacan's association between *jouissance* and *féminine* (based on his reading of Hadewijch) is not entirely justified.

And both situate genuine enjoyment (*ghebruken*) in the participation in the love of the Trinity, about which both Hadewijch and Ruusbroec exclaim with equal passion: 'love Love!' ('mint de Minne!').[49]

[49] Ruusbroec, *Van seven trappen*, ed. by Faesen, p. 213, line 1100; Hadewijch, *Poem in Stanza* 25 (*Strofische Gedichten*, ed. by Van Mierlo, p. 162, line 51).

Works Cited

Primary Sources

Beatrijs van Nazareth, *Seven manieren van minne*, ed. by L. Reypens and J. Van Mierlo, Leuvense studiën en tekstuitgaven, 11 (Leuven: De Vlaamsche Boekenhalle, 1926)

Bernard of Clairvaux, *Sancti Bernardi Opera*, vol. III, *Tractatus et opuscula*, ed. by Jean Leclercq and Henri M. Rochais (Roma: Editiones Cistercienses, 1963)

Erasmus, Desiderius, *Opera omnia*, IV.3, ed. by Clarence H. Miller (Amsterdam: North-Holland, 1979)

Erasmus of Rotterdam, *Praise of Folly and Letter to Martin Dorp 1515*, trans. by Betty Radice, Penguin Classics (Harmondsworth: Penguin Books, 1976)

Guillemus a Sancto Theoderico, *Epistola ad Fratres de Monte Dei*, ed. by Paul Verdeyen, CCCM, 88 (Turnhout: Brepols, 2003)

Hadewijch, *Brieven*, ed. by Jozef Van Mierlo, vol. I, *Tekst en commentaar*; vol. II, *Inleiding*, Leuvense studiën en tekstuitgaven, 14 (Antwerpen: Standaard, 1947)

——, *The Complete Letters*, ed. by Paul Mommaers and Aniko Daróczi (Leuven: Peeters, forthcoming)

——, *The Complete Works*, trans. and introd. by Columba Hart (New York: Paulist Press, 1980)

——, *Liederen*, ed., introd., trans., and commented by Veerle Fraeters and Frank Willaert, with a reconstruction of the melodies by Louis Peter Grijp (Groningen: Historische Uitgeverij, 2009)

——, *Poetry of Hadewijch*, introd., trans., and notes by Marieke Van Baest, Studies in Spirituality Supplement, 3 (Leuven: Peeters, 1998)

——, *Strofische Gedichten*, ed. by Jozef Van Mierlo, vol. I, *Tekst en commentaar*; vol. II, *Inleiding*, Leuvense studiën en tekstuitgaven, 13 (Antwerpen: Standaard, 1942)

Limburgsche Sermoenen, ed. by Johan Hendrik Kern, Bibliotheek van Middelnederlandsche letterkunde (Groningen: Wolters, 1895)

Lombard, Peter, *Magistri Petri Lombardi Sententiae in IV libri distinctae*, vol. I, Spicilegium Bonaventarium, 4 (Grottaferrata: Collegii S. Bonaventurae Ad Claras Aquas, 1971)

[Richard of Saint-Victor], *Ives, Épitre à Séverin sur la charité; Richard de Saint-Victor, Les quatre degrés de la violente charité*, ed. by Gervais Dumeige, Textes philosophiques du Moyen Âge, 3 (Paris: Vrin, 1955)

Ruusbroec, Jan van, *Boecsken der verclaeringhe*, ed. by Guido de Baere, vol. I of *Opera omnia*, CCCM, 101 (Turnhout: Brepols, 1989)

——, *Die geestelike brulocht*, ed. by Joseph Alaerts, vol. III of *Opera omnia*, CCCM, 103 (Turnhout: Brepols, 1988)

——, *Van den geesteliken tabernakel*, ed. by Thom Mertens, vols V–VI of *Opera omnia*, CCCM, 105–06 (Turnhout: Brepols, 2006)

——, *Van seven trappen*, ed. by Rob Faesen, vol. IX or *Opera omnia*, CCCM, 109 (Turnhout: Brepols, 2003)

William of Ockham, *Guillelmi de Ockham Summae logicae*, ed. by Philoteus Boehner, Gedeon Gál, and Stephanus Brown (New York: St. Bonaventure, 1974)
William of Saint-Thierry, *The Golden Epistle: A Letter to the Brethren at Mont Dieu*, trans. by Theodore Berkeley, introd. by Jean-Marie Déchanet, Cistercian Fathers Series, 12 (Collegeville: Liturgical Press, 1971)

Secondary Works

Alaerts, Jos, 'De prins van de humanisten: Desiderius Erasmus (1467/69–1536)', *Acta Medica Catholica*, 1 (1992), 7–12
Andriessen, Jos, 'Ruusbroec's Influence until *c.* 1800', in *A Companion to John of Ruusbroec*, ed. by John Arblaster and Rob Faesen, Brill's Companions to the Christian Tradition, 51 (Leiden: Brill, 2014), pp. 286–302
Arblaster, John, and Rob Faesen, 'John of Ruusbroec's Life and Works', in *A Companion to John of Ruusbroec*, ed. by John Arblaster and Rob Faesen, Brill's Companions to the Christian Tradition, 51 (Leiden: Brill, 2014), pp. 47–80
——, 'Mysticism in the Low Countries before Ruusbroec', in *A Companion to John of Ruusbroec*, ed. by John Arblaster and Rob Faesen, Brill's Companions to the Chrstian Tradition, 51 (Leiden: Brill, 2014), pp. 5–46
Axters, Stephanus, 'Nederlandse mystieken in het buitenland: Van Rupert van Deutz tot Ruusbroec', *Verslagen en mededelingen van de Koninklijke Vlaamse Academie voor Taal- en Letterkunde*, nieuwe reeks, 1965, 163–328
Baere, Guido de, 'Explanation of Technical Terms', in Jan van Ruusbroec, *Opera omnia*, II, ed. by Guido De Baere, CCCM, 102 (Turnhout: Brepols, 1989), pp. 263–78
Cayré, F., '*Frui* et *uti*', in *Oeuvres de Saint Augustin*, 1e série: *Opuscules*, XI: *Le Magistère chrétien*, ed. and trans. by G. Combès and J. Farges (Paris: Desclée, 1949), pp. 558–61
Deblaere, Albert, 'La Littérature mystique au Moyen Âge', in *Albert Deblaere (1916–1994): Essays on Mystical Literature*, ed. by Rob Faesen, Bibliotheca Ephemeridum Theologicarum Lovaniensium, 177 (Leuven: University Press & Peeters, 2004), pp. 291–315
Depoortere, Frederiek, '*Fruitio dei* and/or *jouissance féminine*? An Exploration', in *Mystical Anthropology: Cross-Religious Perspectives*, ed. by Ineke Cornet, Rob Faesen, and Martin Sebastian Kallungal, Annua Nuntia Lovaniensia, 66 (Leuven: Peeters, 2012), pp. 61–78
Faesen, Rob, '"Poor in Ourselves and Rich in God": Indwelling and Non-identity of Being (*wesen*) and Suprabeing (*overwesen*)', *Medieval Mystical Theology*, 21 (2012), 147–69
——, 'Ruusbroec at the Charterhouse of Herne: How Did the Carthusians React to the Eckhart-Shock?', in *A Fish Out of Water? From Contemplative Solitude to Carthusian Involvement in Pastoral Care and Reform Activity*, ed. by Tom Gaens and Stephen J. Molvarec, Studia Cartusiana, 2 (Leuven: Peeters, 2013), pp. 107–25
——, 'Was Hadewijch a Beguine or a Cistercian? An Annotated Hypothesis', *Cîteaux*, 55 (2004), 47–64
——, 'We Were Perplexed by What He Wrote: The Cartusians and a Crucial Moment in the Development of Mystical Literature in the Low Countries', in *The Cartusians*

in the Low Countries: Studies in Monastic History and Heritage, ed. by Krijn Pansters, Studia Cartusiana, 4 (Leuven: Peeters, 2014), pp. 217–32

McGinn, Bernard, 'The Significance of Ruusbroec's Mystical Theology', *Louvain Studies*, 31 (2006), 19–41

Verwijs, E., and J. Verdam, eds, *Middelnederlandsch Woordenboek*, 10 vols (Den Haag: Nijhoff, 1885–1941)

Warnar, Geert, '"Ex levitate mulierum": Masculine Mysticism and Jan van Ruusbroec's Perception of Religious Women', in *The Voice of Silence: Women's Literacy in a Men's Church*, ed. by Thérèse de Hemptinne and Maria Eugenia Góngora (Turnhout: Brepols, 2004), pp. 193–206

Index

Abelard: xiv, 11, 13, 173, 335 n. 22, 338 n. 32, 347
abstinentia: 240 n. 58, 312
accidentia anime: 61, 64
Adam of Dryburgh: 3, 5, 7, 14
Aelred of Rievaulx, St: 12, 14, 16, 147
Aesop: 51
affectiones, *affectus*: 5–7, 16–17, 173, 175, 230, 235, 240–41
affectivity: 225, 227 n. 4, 236 n. 36, 241
  affect: xv, xviii, xix–xx, 4–6, 12, 61, 136, 144–47, 227–28, 233–34
  anthropology of: 226, 229, 238
  definition of medieval emotion: 227
  medieval understanding of: 225
  see also affectiones, *affectus*
Agnes Blannbekin: 8–9
'Aisha bint Talha: 120, 123
Albert of Bologna: 43, 44 n. 21, 45 n. 25
Albert the Great, St: 184, 230, 232, 235, 316 n. 19
Alcuin: xx, 167–71, 173–77, 287 n. 23, 289 n. 33, 340 n. 43
Alice Vaughan: 28
Al-Mutawakkil, caliph: 116 n. 8, 126
Ambrose, St: 146, 289, 333 n. 11, 334–36, 338, 341–42, 347
amor: 12 n. 26, 64, 71–72, 182, 189, 217 n. 45, 231 n. 19, 235 n. 34, 285, 302, 323, 333, 336, 337 n. 26, 337 n. 27, 338 n. 35, 364
Andrew Borde: 28, 30–31
anima: 12 n. 25, 33, 46, 51 n. 47, 61, 64, 167, 169, 173–74, 176, 189, 190 n. 25, 204, 211 n. 25, 225, 230–31, 284, 302, 320, 333, 335, 337–38, 343 n. 56
Anselm of Canterbury, St: xiv, 11–12, 151
Anselm of Laon: 339–43, 347
Anthony of Parma: 45, 47 n. 31, 48 n. 34
Aristotle: xi, 12–13, 171, 172 n. 23, 196, 204–11, 212 n. 30, 213–16, 217 n. 44, 220–21, 230, 240, 242, 252
Arnaldus de Villanova: 43, 44 n. 16, 48 n. 35, 50–53
Arnaut Guilhem de Marsan: 148–49
Arnoul Gréban: 261–62, 263 n. 37, 264
Augustine, St: xii, 6–7, 146–47, 172–73, 174 n. 37, 175, 190, 204–05, 226, 229, 240, 243, 273, 289, 294, 297, 303 n. 86, 330, 334–37, 339, 342, 345–47, 353 n. 1, 354
Avicenna: 29, 46 n. 28, 48–49, 230

Bartolomeo of Varignana: 43
Bartholomeus Anglicus: 22–23, 30, 33, 211
Bartholomeus Montagnana: 69–70
Bartholomeus of Salerno: 66
Baudri de Bourgueil: 11
Beatrice of Nazareth: 354, 373 n. 47
Beatrix Smyth: 28
Bede the Venerable: xxi, 281, 285, 288–304, 333, 338–41, 346–47

Benedetto Reguardati da Norcia: 61
Bernard of Clairvaux, St: xxii, 11, 13, 77–78, 150, 152, 173, 190–91, 233, 234 n. 28, 235–36, 329–32, 342–48, 368, 373 n. 45
Bernard de Gordon: 43, 72, 210 n. 22
Bonaventure, St: 357
Borso d'Este, Duke of Ferrara: 65
Brunetto Latini: 188

Caesarius of Heisterbach: 15
caritas: 189, 234, 237–38, 331, 336, 345 n. 62
carnality: xiii, 7–8, 15, 77–78, 88–89, 114, 189–90, 226, 228–33, 235, 238, 242, 287, 303 n. 86, 311, 314–18, 321–23, 344–46
Catherine of Genoa, St: 10
Chaucer, Geoffrey: 188, 314
Charles V, King of France: 204 n. 8
chastity: 131 n. 4, 153, 217, 255, 321, 325
Christ: xii, xiv, 5, 9–10, 12, 22, 33–34, 77 n. 1, 80, 92, 96, 98–100, 105–06, 150 n. 56, 228, 237, 251, 259–60, 263 n. 37, 264, 266, 291 n. 38, 292, 294–99, 302–03, 311, 329, 333–34, 337–38, 340–41, 345, 372
  Passion of: xiii, 80, 96, 260–61, 265, 272
Cicero: 12, 173, 175–76, 206
coitus: 67–68, 72
compassion: 9, 173, 250, 252–53, 257, 258 n. 28, 259, 264, 270–73
consolation, solace: 168–69, 171, 176, 229, 251
  see also solatium
Constantine the African: 63, 71
Cyprian, St: 251, 256, 273
Dananir al-Barmakiyya: 126

Dante Alighieri: xi, 188
David Aubert: 256, 257 n. 23
Defensor of Ligugé: 171
delectatio: xv, 3–4, 7, 8 n. 10, 42–43, 45 n. 22, 45 n. 23, 64, 70, 176, 184, 191–92, 194–96, 207 n. 15, 208, 216, 226, 228–30, 233, 324, 341 n. 51
delicia: xv, xx, 40, 42–44, 45 n. 24, 45 n. 25, 46, 47 n. 31, 195, 283, 285 n. 15, 364 n. 24
delight: xiii, xvi, xx–xxii, 3–4, 7–8, 10, 13, 17, 64, 67, 69, 84, 103, 114, 176, 185, 197, 229–30, 250, 254, 256–57, 284, 303, 324, 348, 360 n. 19, 364 n. 24
  see also suavitas
demons: 15, 17, 172 258–59, 269, 283, 291 n. 38
desire: xvi, xx–xxi, 5, 42, 66, 68–69, 71–72, 78, 84–85, 90, 92, 98, 100–02, 104–05, 107, 114, 118, 122, 124, 128, 133, 141, 143, 146, 153, 155–06, 158, 172, 175–76, 182, 190–91, 195, 209, 214, 218, 227, 230, 235–36, 239, 282–85, 287, 290–91, 296, 300–01, 303, 311, 313, 315, 322–25, 331, 335, 337, 345, 362, 369, 371, 373
  sexual: 42, 71, 114, 122, 124, 128, 131, 133, 141, 153, 156–58, 282
Devil: 33, 234, 258, 268, 271, 289 n. 32, 316
devils: 15, 253 n. 12, 254, 258–60, 262, 264–73, 370
Dino del Garbo: 43
displicentia: 182
dolor: 12 n. 26, 44, 45 n. 23, 46 n. 26, 48 n. 33, 194, 240, 273 n. 62
Domnin, St: 258
Dunstan, St: 259

Eckhart, Meister: 372 n. 43
Edmund de Stonor: 26
Edward V, King of England: 29
Elizabeth Clere: 25
emotion. *See* affectivity
enjoyment: xiii, xvi, xxi–xxii, 4–7, 10–11, 14, 17, 33, 45 n. 21, 52, 65, 69, 78, 87, 118, 147–48, 150–52, 168, 207 n. 15, 208, 215 n. 38, 218 n. 48, 230, 233–34, 236, 238–39, 250–51, 258–59, 269, 272–74, 285, 303, 313, 316, 331, 336, 353–71, 373–75
  see also frui, fruitio; *ghebruken*
Erasmus: 362 n. 23, 364 n. 24
Ethelwold of Winchester, St: 259
Evagrius of Pontus: 4 n. 2, 172, 283, 284 n. 11, 333–34

felicitas: 4, 204, 207 n. 15, 209, 363 n. 23, 364 n. 24

fitna: 114, 121, 123
frui, fruitio: xv, 7, 229, 353

Galen: 43–45, 46 n. 28, 47 n. 32, 48–49, 66, 206, 282 n. 2
Ganymedes: 151, 185
Gaucher de Châtillon d'Autresche: 82, 84, 91, 98
gaudium: xv, 4, 22, 33, 40, 46, 51 n. 47, 64, 65, 92, 169, 175, 190 n. 25, 207 n. 15, 210 n. 20, 229–31, 233–34, 238, 240, 315, 323 n. 37, 324, 338 n. 34, 345 n. 64, 364 n. 24
Gentile da Foligno: 43, 45 n. 22, 46 n. 29, 47 n. 32, 48 n. 33, 48 n. 35, 49
Geoffrey, count of Anjou: 150
Geoffrey of Vigeois: 153, 156 n. 73
George Cely: 26, 28
ghebruken: 353–62, 364–69, 371–72, 374–75
Gilbert of Hoyland: 330
Giles of Rome: xxi, 203–06, 207 n. 15, 208–21
Gilles Deschamps: 204 n. 8
Giovanni Matteo Ferrari da Grado: 66–68, 69 n. 26. 69 n. 27, 70–71
gluttony: xxi, 17, 90, 170, 189–90, 220, 231, 281, 283, 285–88, 291 n. 38, 304, 315
see also gula
God: xiii, xix, xxi, 11, 14, 22 n. 2, 25–26, 32–33, 63, 65, 92, 96–97, 146–47, 150, 157, 172–76, 191–93, 225, 228–39, 241–43, 251, 255, 271–72, 281, 289–90, 293, 296, 302, 312–13, 319, 323–25, 332, 334, 336, 340, 342, 344–47, 355–59, 362, 363 n. 23, 364, 366–74
Gregory I, St: xxii, 170–72, 175–76, 184, 190, 197, 256 n. 20, 287 n. 25, 289, 290 n. 35, 291 n. 41, 302, 314–18, 322, 331–40, 344, 346–47
Gregory VII, St: xxi, 309–11, 313–14, 317–25
Guibert of Gembloux, St: 13
Guibert of Nogent: 9
gula: 8 n. 10, 231 n. 19, 281, 287, 312 n. 5

Hadewijch: xxii, 353–54, 360, 365–75
Hajar: 122
happiness: xiii, 4, 6–7, 10, 24, 28, 36, 53, 65, 118–19, 124, 145, 168–70, 175–76, 185, 206–09, 217, 229, 231, 235, 238–39, 284 n. 11, 360, 363, 364 n. 24
see also felicitas; *laetitia*
Heinrich of Nördlingen: 14
Heinrich von Langenstein: 188
Heloïse: 11
see also Abelard
Henri de Gauchi: 204
Henry II, King of England: 149–50, 152
Henry IV, King of England: 320–21
Henry VI, King of England: 27, 33
Henry the Young King: 149
Hildebrand, bishop of Tours: 134, 153
Hildegard of Bingen, St: 8–9, 10 n. 15, 13, 15, 63
Holy Spirit: 96, 98, 174, 323, 332, 356–57, 359, 371
Honorius Augustodunensis: 342
Hugh of Saint-Victor: 5, 356
Humbert of Romans: 188, 196, 197 n. 45

iocundus: 3, 24, 26–27, 33, 176, 190 n. 25, 230, 231, 236, 338 n. 34
Isidore of Seville, St: 171
Ivo of Chartres, St: 151

Jacob: 372
jāriya (concubine): 113
Jaume II, King of Aragon: 49, 51, 53
Jean de Saint-Amand: 42–44
Jean de Vignay: 256–57
Jean Gerson: 189
Jean Wauquelin: 204 n. 8
Jeremiah: 322, 332
Jerome, St: 146, 191, 281 n. 1, 285 n. 15, 289, 291 n. 40, 294 n. 53, 330, 333–35, 342
Joan Bukley: 25
Joanna, Queen of Sicily: 148–49
Job: 314, 333–34, 337
John Cassian, St: 171, 172, 283–87, 291–92, 300–01, 333, 334 n. 13
John Crote: 28
John Doddington: 26
John Lydgate: 29–30, 32 n. 36
John Mirk: 34
John of Ford: 330

John of Ruusbroec: xxii, 353–65, 374–75
John of Salisbury: 14, 149–50, 151 n. 57
John Veron: 24
joy: xiii, xv–xvi, xx–xxii, 3–4, 7–8, 10, 17, 24, 27–29, 32–34, 35 n. 46, 40–41, 49–52, 54, 61–62, 64–65, 72, 78, 145, 169–70, 173, 175–76, 182, 226, 228–30, 234, 236, 240–41, 249–50, 257, 273–74, 281, 298, 300, 323–24, 345, 361–62, 364 n. 24, 370, 374
see also gaudium; Virgin Mary
Julian of Eclanum: 334, 336, 338, 347
Julian the Hospitaler, St: 258
Justin Martyr, St: 250–51

Katherine Ryche: 26–27

Lactantius: 185
laetitia: xv, 4, 170 n. 17, 175–76, 229–31, 238, 296, 331
Lapo da Castiglionchio the Younger: 185
Laurentius Surius: 353
Lorenzo Valla: 7
love: xi, xiii, xx–xxii, 6, 11–12, 15, 22, 64, 71–72, 89, 117, 119, 121, 126, 136, 141, 145–47, 150 n. 56, 152, 154, 156–58, 168, 174, 181–82, 189, 191, 198, 209, 215, 226, 229, 234–35, 237, 241, 251 n. 8, 266, 285, 289 n. 30, 291, 302, 304, 314–15, 320, 324, 329–33, 335–37, 342, 344–48, 355–75
see also amor; *minne*

Maino de Maineri: 65
Malik bin Anas: 122–23
Margaretha Ebner, St: 10, 14
Margaret Paston: 25
Margery Kempe: 5 n. 5, 32–33
Mary Magdalene: 337–38
merriment, merry: xx, 3, 24–35, 62
Michel Beheim: 188
Michele Savonarola: 65, 67, 70
minne: 355, 357, 360 n. 19, 361–62, 366–67, 369, 371 n. 41, 372–73, 375
Muhammad: 120, 122, 317
Mu'awiya: 123

Niccolò III d'Este, Marquis of Ferrara: 65

Odilo of Cluny, St: 15
Orderic Vitalis: 151
Origen: xxii, 227, 233, 289 n. 31, 292 n. 45, 330–38, 340, 342–44, 346–48
Ovid: 153, 194 n. 37, 196

pain: xii–xiii, 5, 9–10, 12–14, 40, 42–45, 48, 61, 65, 92, 136, 139–42, 145, 182, 184–85, 195, 207 n. 15, 210, 215, 220, 228, 254–55, 258–59, 263, 267, 272–73, 297
see also dolor
passio, *passiones*: 44, 45 n. 24, 46 n. 26, 167, 172, 208, 240
passion, passions: 5, 7, 11, 22–23, 60–61, 68–69, 71–72, 116, 127, 146, 181, 184–85, 208, 210, 214–15, 220, 229–32, 240, 265, 336–37, 375
see also Christ; *passio*, *passiones*
Paul, St: 146, 250 n. 4, 332
Peter Damian, St: 132, 150, 311–13, 315, 317, 321
Peter Lombard: 132, 356, 366 n. 29
Peter of Abano: 6
Peter of Limoges: 182, 183 n. 4, 184
Peter of Spain: 44 n. 20, 72
Philip I, King of France: 151
Philip IV, King of France: 82, 203–04
Pierre the Chanter: 151
Plato: xi, 146, 210, 364 n. 24
Pseudo-Augustine: 4, 66, 171
Pseudo-Dionysius the Areopagite: 290 n. 33

qayna: 113–14, 115 n. 6, 117, 125–27

Ralph of Coggeshall: 257, 258 n. 26
Reginald Pecock: 22
Richard Cely: 26, 28
Richard I, King of England: 148
Richard Hill: 34
Richard of Saint-Victor: 372 n. 45
Richard Rolle: xxi, 225–26, 232–38, 241–43
Robert Estienne: 24, 35
Robert of Arbrissel: 158
Robert of Tombelaine: 339–40
Roger Bacon: 196
Rufinus of Aquileia: 330, 333 n. 11, 346
Rupert of Deutz: 342

Schadenfreude: 250, 256, 269, 273
sensation: xiii, xv–xvi, xxi–xxii, 4–6, 45–48, 53–54, 64–65, 103, 144, 228, 233–36, 238, 242, 257
senses: xv, 4–5, 7, 10, 28, 41–42, 46, 90, 103–05, 107, 114, 145, 186, 192, 210–11, 235, 293 n. 45, 301, 303 n. 86, 348, 362
Simone Fidati: xxi, 225–26, 232, 236–43
sin: xxi, 16, 31, 33, 62, 65–67, 69, 82, 87–91, 101, 107, 132, 146, 151, 158, 173, 175–76, 181–95, 197–98, 217–18, 220, 228–33, 237, 239–40, 253–55, 258–60, 268, 270–71, 281, 283, 285, 287, 291 n. 38, 318–19, 322–23, 331, 346, 358
solatium: 169, 234
sonder gront (fathomless): 355
soul: xii–xiii, xv–xvi, xxii, 10, 17, 29, 31–32, 36, 46, 50–51, 60–65, 68–69, 146–47, 150, 169, 173–74, 176, 182, 190, 210–12, 214, 218, 227–35, 238–42, 282, 283 n. 7, 291, 302–03, 330–33, 335–38, 342–48, 355, 362, 368, 370
  and body: xiii–xvi, 36, 46, 62, 64, 84, 97, 146, 173, 182, 190, 210–11, 218, 227, 229, 238, 241, 273 n. 60, 282, 291, 332, 348
  spirit: xii, 29, 33, 51–53, 68, 70, 97, 153, 169, 173–74, 191, 231, 273 n. 60, 283 n. 7, 284, 345, 356 n. 11, 362, 364 n. 24
  see also accidentia anime; *anima*
Sozzinus Benzi: 68
Stephen of Blois, King of England: 150
suavitas: 3–4, 8 n. 10, 235–36
surriya: 122

temperance: 190, 232
Tertullian: 185, 250–51, 256, 273
Thomas Aquinas, St: 10, 13, 204 n. 5, 206, 216, 230–31, 240, 260, 357
Thomas Becket, St: 148 n. 47, 149, 152
Thomas Betson: 26
Thomas More, St: 363 n. 23
Thurkill: 258–60, 272
Tnugdal: 253, 256, 272
  see also Tondalus
Tondalus: 253
  see also Tnugdal
tristitia: 33, 46 n. 26, 48 n. 33, 48 n. 34, 51 n. 47, 170 n. 17, 172, 176, 207 n. 15, 208, 210 n. 20, 216 n. 41, 239 n. 49

Ugo Benzi: 66, 68

Venus: 185
vice: xiii, xx–xxi, 13, 22, 32, 69, 167, 170–73, 175–76, 181–82, 184–85, 187–91, 193–94, 196–98, 215, 225, 229, 231–32, 239, 242, 283, 286–87, 290, 294, 304
Vincent de Beauvais: 206, 219, 253, 257–58
Virgin Mary: 27, 34, 80–81, 88, 91–93, 96–103, 105–07, 342, 372
  Joys of the: 80–81, 91–92, 96–103, 105–07
virtues: xx–xxi, 3, 7, 12–13, 22, 32–33, 98, 167, 170–73, 175, 184, 187–89, 195, 197, 206–07, 209, 211, 213–14, 215 n. 37, 220–21, 225, 229, 232, 234, 237–38, 240, 259 n. 30, 284–87, 294–95, 302 n. 82, 303 n. 86, 304, 334, 336, 346, 356 n. 11, 362, 368
voluptas: xv, 7–8, 16–17, 226, 228–30, 233–34, 273 n. 62, 285, 296, 303, 321, 364

Walter Map: 149
Wido, count: xx, 167, 169–71, 177
William, Giles of Rome's translator: 204 n. 8, 205, 214, 215 n. 36, 217–19, 220 n. 52, 221
William II, King of Sicily: 149
William IX, Duke of Aquitaine: 131, 133–35, 150, 152–58
William of Auxerre: 182
William of Champeaux: 343
William of Ockham: 361 n. 21
William of Saint-Thierry: 191 n. 26, 343–44, 356
William Paston: 25
William Peraldus: xxi, 181, 182 n. 2, 184–85, 187–98
William Plumpton: 26
William II, King of England: 151

International Medieval Research

All volumes in this series are evaluated by an Editorial Board, strictly on academic grounds, based on reports prepared by referees who have been commissioned by virtue of their specialism in the appropriate field. The Board ensures that the screening is done independently and without conflicts of interest. The definitive texts supplied by authors are also subject to review by the Board before being approved for publication. Further, the volumes are copyedited to conform to the publisher's stylebook and to the best international academic standards in the field.

Titles in Series

Across the Mediterranean Frontiers: Trade, Politics, and Religion, 650–1450, ed. by Dionisius A. Agius and Ian Richard Netton (1997)

Dictionaries of Medieval Germanic Languages: A Survey of Current Lexicographical Projects, ed. by K. Van Dalen-Oskam, K. Depuydt, W. J. J. Pijnenburg, and T. H. Schoonheim (1997)

From Clermont to Jerusalem: The Crusades and Crusader Societies 1095–1500, ed. by Alan V. Murray (1998)

The Community, the Family and the Saint: Patterns of Power in Early Medieval Europe, ed. by Joyce Hill and Mary Swan (1998)

The Vocation of Service to God and Neighbour: Essays on the Interests, Involvements and Problems of Religious Communities and their Members in Medieval Society, ed. by Joan Greatrex (1998)

Negotiating Secular and Ecclesiastical Power: Western Europe in the Central Middle Ages, ed. by Arnoud-Jan A. Bijsterveld, Henk Teunis, and Andrew Wareham (1999)

Christianizing Peoples and Converting Individuals, ed. by Guyda Armstrong and Ian N. Wood (2000)

Decorations for the Holy Dead: Visual Embellishments on Tombs and Shrines of Saints, ed. by Stephen Lamia and Elizabeth Valdez del Álamo (2002)

Time and Eternity: The Medieval Discourse, ed. by Gerhard Jaritz and Gerson Moreno-Riaño (2003)

The White Mantle of Churches: Architecture, Liturgy, and Art around the Millennium, ed. by Nigel Hiscock (2003)

Love, Marriage, and Family Ties in the Later Middle Ages, ed. by Isabel Davis, Miriam Müller, and Sarah Rees Jones (2003)

The Medieval Household in Christian Europe, c. 850–c. 1550: Managing Power, Wealth, and the Body, ed. by Cordelia Beattie, Anna Maslakovic, and Sarah Rees Jones (2003)

Exile in the Middle Ages: Selected Proceedings from the International Medieval Congress, University of Leeds, 8–11 July 2002, ed. by Laura Napran and Elisabeth van Houts (2004)

Representations of Power in Medieval Germany, 800–1500, ed. by Björn Weiler and Simon MacLean (2006)

Aspects of Power and Authority in the Middle Ages, ed. by Brenda Bolton and Christine Meek (2008)

Behaving like Fools: Voice, Gesture, and Laughter in Texts, Manuscripts, and Early Books, ed. by Lucy Perry and Alexander Schwarz (2011)

Languages of Love and Hate: Conflict, Communication, and Identity in the Medieval Mediterranean, ed. by Sarah Lambert and Helen Nicholson (2012)

Medieval Life Cycles: Continuity and Change, ed. by Isabelle Cochelin and Karen Smyth (2013)

Problems and Possibilities of Early Medieval Charters, ed. by Jonathan A. Jarrett and Alan Scott McKinley (2013)

The Tree: Symbol, Allegory, and Mnemonic Device in Medieval Art and Thought, ed. by Pippa Salonius and Andrea Worm (2014)

Travels and Mobilities in the Middle Ages: From the Atlantic to the Black Sea, ed. by Marianne O'Doherty and Felicitas Schmieder (2015)

Approaches to Poverty in Medieval Europe: Complexities, Contradictions, Transformations, c. 1100–1500, ed. by Sharon Farmer (2016)

In Preparation

Miracles in Medieval Canonization Processes: Structures, Functions, and Methodologies, ed. by Christian Krötzl and Sari Katajala-Peltomaa